W9-CKJ-961

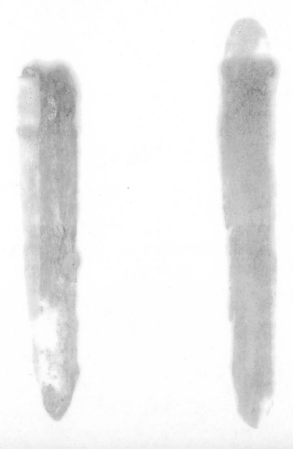

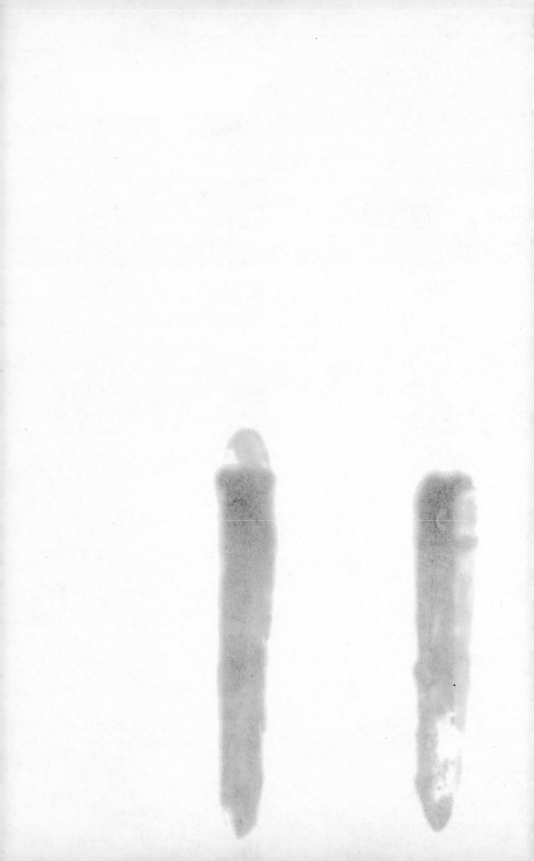

BEHAVIORAL TREATMENTS OF OBESITY

Edited by

JOHN PAUL FOREYT

Baylor College of Medicine, Houston, Texas

PERGAMON PRESS

OXFORD · NEW YORK · TORONTO
SYDNEY · PARIS · FRANKFURT

U. K.	Pergamon Press Ltd., Headington Hill Hall, Oxford OX3 0BW, England
U. S. A.	Pergamon Press Inc., Maxwell House, Fairview Park, Elmsford, New York 10523, U.S.A.
CANADA	Pergamon of Canada Ltd., 75 The East Mall, Toronto, Ontario, Canada
AUSTRALIA	Pergamon Press (Aust.) Pty. Ltd., 19a Boundary Street, Rushcutters Bay, N.S.W. 2011, Australia
FRANCE	Pergamon Press SARL, 24 rue des Ecoles, 75240 Paris, Cedex 05, France
WEST GERMANY	Pergamon Press GmbH, 6242 Kronberg-Taunus, Pferdstrasse 1, West Germany

Copyright © 1977 Pergamon Press Ltd

All Rights Reserved. No part of this publication may be reproduced, stored in a retrieval system or transmitted in any form or by any means: electronic, electrostatic, magnetic tape, mechanical, photocopying, recording or otherwise, without permission in writing from the publishers

First edition 1977

Library of Congress Cataloging in Publication Data
Main entry under title:
Behavioral treatments of obesity.
(Pergamon general psychology series; 61)
Includes bibliographies and indexes.
1. Corpulence — Psychological aspects. 2. Behavior therapy. I. (Foreyt,) John Paul. [DNLM: 1. Obesity— Therapy. 2. Behavior therapy. WD210 F718b]
RC628.B354 1975   616.3'98'065   75-23272
ISBN 0-08-019902-X (Hardcover)

Printed in Great Britain by Page Bros (Norwich) Ltd

RC
628
.B354
1977z

Contents

PART III. COVERT SENSITIZATION

PART IV. COVERANT CONDITIONING

PART V. THERAPIST REINFORCEMENT TECHNIQUES

PART VI. SELF-CONTROL TECHNIQUES

Introduction. D. Balfour Jeffrey   299

Preface

If you are overweight and have tried any of the hundreds of popular diets or treatment programs, chances are you stuck with it for awhile, perhaps even lost a few pounds, then discarded it, regained the lost weight, and began looking for another, easier way.

Don't feel alone. There are perhaps 80 million overweight individuals in the United States alone, most of them apparently doing the same thing. Weight reduction is one of the most difficult, most frustrating problems we face in our urbanized, mechanized society. Whether the treatment is a specific regimen of diet, medication, and exercise prescribed by a doctor, psychotherapy from a psychiatrist, or this month's fad diet from a favorite periodical, most people simply find themselves unable to reduce their weight or maintain any significant amount of loss.

In the last decade, behavior therapists have begun focusing their attention on treating obesity. By viewing the development of eating behaviors as similar to the development of other learned patterns of behavior, they have investigated a number of psychological techniques, broadly based on learning principles, aimed at helping obese persons achieve control over their eating by manipulating the antecedent and consequent conditions of their behavior. This research has brought some remarkable advances in our knowledge of obesity and its treatment. These techniques hold promise for many who have previously been unable to control their weight.

Five trends have developed in the behavioral research for treating obesity. These trends are: overt aversive techniques, covert sensitization, coverant conditioning, therapist reinforcement techniques, and self-control techniques.

The purpose of this book is to bring together in one source a collection of articles, including both case studies and experimental reports, describing and evaluating each of these five trends. The articles selected include the "classic" oft-quoted ones, along with studies describing creative, promising techniques as yet unevaluated. Each chapter is preceded by an introduction reviewing the specific trend.

These studies represent the most impressive attack on the problem to date. It is hoped that these reports will provide the impetus for future advances in the treatment of obesity.

I am indebted to the authors and publishers of the selections reprinted for their very kind cooperation in making their work available. I especially want to thank Drs. Richard A. Frohwirth, Richard L. Hagen, and D. Balfour Jeffrey for their outstanding contributions and Drs. Antonio M. Gotto, Jr., Wallace A. Kennedy, Jim T. Parks, and Ben J. Williams for their encouragement and support. Special appreciation is extended to Ms. Susi LeBaron for her skillful typing and assistance in the preparation of the manuscript.

Thanks also to Mr. William Kortas and Ms. Barbara White for their help with the final page proofs. The support of the Diet Modification Clinic of the National Heart and Blood Vessel Research and Demonstration Center, Baylor College of Medicine, a grant-supported research program of the National Heart, Lung, and Blood Institute, National Institutes of Health, Grant No. 17269, is also deeply appreciated.

Contributors

1. Dr. Edward E. Abramson
   Department of Psychology
   California State University at Chico
   Chico, California 95926

2. Dr. Stanley B. Baker
   318 Social Science Building
   Pennsylvania State University
   University Park, Pennsylvania 16802

3. Dr. John L. Bernard
   Department of Psychology
   Memphis State University
   Memphis, Tennessee 38111

4. Dr. Betty L. Borden
   206 St. Joseph Avenue
   Long Beach, California 90803

5. Dr. P. T. Brown
   35/37 Fitzroy Street
   London, WIP 5AF, England

6. Dr. David Castell
   The Laurels, Doctor's Row
   Blofield, Norwich NR13LLF, England

7. Dr. Joseph R. Cautela
   10 Phillips Road
   Sudbury, Massachusetts 01776

8. Dr. Edwin R. Christensen
   Murray–Jordan–Tooele Mental Hygiene
   Center
   5130 South State Street, Suite B
   Murray, Utah 84107

9. Mr. John Colwick
   Department of Psychology
   Partlow State Hospital
   Tuscaloosa, Alabama 35401

10. Dr. A. H. Crisp
    Department of Psychiatry
    St. George's Hospital Medical School
    Clare House
    Blackshaw Road, London, SW 17, England

11. Dr. Blaine C. Crum
    Department of Psychology
    University of South Alabama
    Mobile, Alabama 36608

12. Mr. Charles Diament
    Psychology Clinic
    Professional School of Psychology
    Rutgers University
    New Brunswick, New Jersey 08854

13. Dr. Michael Dinoff
    Psychology Department
    University of Alabama
    Tuscaloosa, Alabama 35401

14. Dr. Charles B. Ferster
    4708 Linnean Avenue N.W.
    Washington, D.C. 20008

15. Dr. Ross D. Filion
    756 South Darien Street, R–7
    Philadelphia, Pennsylvania 19147

16. Dr. John Paul Foreyt
    Director, Diet Modification Clinic
    6608 Fannin, Suite 1009
    Houston, Texas 77030

17. Dr. Sonja Fox
    854 North 29th Street
    Philadelphia, Pennsylvania

18. Dr. Richard M. Foxx
    Psychology Department
    University of Maryland and Baltimore
    County
    5401 Wilkens Avenue
    Baltimore, Maryland 21228

19. Dr. Richard A. Frohwirth
    Psychometric Associates, Inc.
    Greenwich, Connecticut 06803

20. Dr. Richard L. Hagen
Department of Psychology
Florida State University
Tallahassee, Florida 32306

21. Dr. Robert G. Hall
850 Lurline
Foster City, California 94404

22. Dr. Sharon M. Hall
850 Lurline
Foster City, California 94404

23. Dr. Erin S. Hallbauer
6721 Barnhart N.E.
Albuquerque, New Mexico 87109

24. Dr. Richard W. Hanson
206 St. Joseph Avenue
Long Beach, California 90803

25. Dr. Morton G. Harmatz
Department of Psychology
University of Massachusetts
Amherst, Massachusetts 01002

26. Dr. L. Garth Harrington
Veterans Administration Mental Hygiene
Clinic
803 South Salina Street
Syracuse, New York 13202

27. Dr. Mary B. Harris
Educational Foundations Department
University of New Mexico
Albuquerque, New Mexico 87131

28. Dr. Alan M. Hoffman
306 Education Building
Wayne State University
Detroit, Michigan 48202

29. Dr. John J. Horan
315 Social Science
Pennsylvania State University
University Park, Pennsylvania 16802

30. Dr. Gilbert L. Ingram
8181 West Quincy
Littleton, Colorado 80123

31. Dr. Louis H. Janda
Department of Psychology
Old Dominion University
Norfolk, Virginia 23508

32. Dr. D Balfour Jeffrey
Department of Psychology
University of Montana
Missoula, Montana 59801

33. Dr. R. Gilmore Johnson
433 Erickson Hall
Michigan State University
East Lansing, Michigan 48823

34. Dr. Wallace A. Kennedy
Department of Psychology
Florida State University
Tallahassee, Florida 32306

35. Dr. Bernard Klein
3206 Clubhouse Road
Merrick, New York 11566

36. Dr. Paul S. Lapuc
173 Columbia Drive
Amherst, Massachusetts 01002

37. Dr. Eugene Levitt
Director, Section of Psychology
Department of Psychiatry
Indiana University Medical Center
Indianapolis, Indiana 46202

38. Dr. Leonard S. Levitz
Department of Psychiatry
University of Pennsylvania
Philadelphia, Pennsylvania 19174

39. Dr Michael J. Mahoney
Department of Psychology
Pennsylvania State University
University Park, Pennsylvania 16802

40. Dr. Barry M. Maletzky
1345 S.E. Harney Street
Portland, Oregon 97202

41. Dr. Ronald A. Mann
Division of Child Psychiatry
University of Texas Medical Branch
Galveston, Texas 77550

42. Dr. Beatrice I. Manno
1 University Place, Apartment 8E
New York, New York 10003

43. Dr. Albert R. Marston
    Psychology Research Service Center
    University of Southern California
    734 West Adams Boulevard
    Los Angeles, California 90007

44. Ms. Mavis McLaren-Hume
    Nutrition Department
    The New York Hospital
    525 East 68th Street
    New York, New York 10021

45. Dr. Victor Meyer
    Department of Psychiatry
    Medical School
    Middlesex Hospital
    London W1, England

46. Dr. Charles H. Moore
    Psychology Department
    East Carolina University
    Greenville, North Carolina 27834

47. Dr. Kenneth Morganstern
    Department of Psychology
    University of Oregon
    Eugene, Oregon 97403

48. Dr. Nanci G. M. Moura
    Rua Almirante
    Guillobel 110 Apto 308
    Lago, Rio de Janeiro
    Guanabara, Brasil

49. Dr. David C. Murray
    V. A. Mental Hygiene Clinic
    803 South Salina Street
    Syracuse, New York 13202

50. Ms. Judith G. Newton
    Head Nurse
    Brockton Veterans Administration Hospital
    Brockton, Massachusetts 02401

51. Dr. John I. Nurnberger
    Institute of Psychiatric Research
    1100 West Michigan Street
    Indianapolis, Indiana 46202

52. Dr. James P. Pappas
    100 Oldin Union
    University of Utah
    Salt Lake City, Utah 84112

53. Dr. Jim T. Parks
    Psychology.Service
    Veterans Administration Center
    Temple, Texas 76501

54. Dr. Sydnor B. Penick
    Department of Psychiatry
    Princeton Hospital
    Princeton, New Jersey 08540

55. Dr. Louis H. Primavera
    1799 Collins Street
    Seaford, New York 11783

56. Dr. Henry C. Rickard
    Psychology Department
    University of Alabama
    University, Alabama 35401

57. Dr. David C. Rimm
    Department of Psychology
    Southern Illinois University at Carbondale
    Carbondale, Illinois 62901

58. Dr. Raymond G. Romanczyk
    Department of Psychology
    S.U.N.Y. at Binghamton
    Binghamton, New York 13901

59. Dr. Lewis B. Sachs
    Psychology Service
    Veterans Administration Hospital
    4150 Clement Street
    San Francisco, California 94121

60. Dr. E. Schmidt
    Shovecroft
    Leafy Lane
    Pudloe, Corsham
    Wilts, England

61. Dr. Robert E. Shute
    1001 University Drive
    Pennsylvania State University
    State College, Pennsylvania 16801

62. Dr. William E. Simon
    678 Allwyn Street
    Baldwin, New York 11510

63. Dr. Richard L. Steele
    HPCCMHC
    201 East 7th Street
    Hays, Kansas 67601

64. Dr. Gary E. Stollak
Department of Psychology
Michigan State University
East Lansing, Michigan 48823

65. Dr. James H. Straughan
Psychology Service, Res. 14A
Veterans Administration Hospital
Sheridan, Wyoming 82801

66. Dr. Richard B. Stuart
Department of Psychiatry
University of British Columbia
Vancouver, B.C. V6T 1W5, Canada

67. Dr. Albert Stunkard
Department of Psychiatry
Stanford University Medical Center
Stanford, California 94305

68. Dr. G. L. Thorpe
Bangor Mental Health Institute
Box 926
Bangor, Maine 04401

69. Dr. J. G. Thorpe
Department of Psychiatry
Manor Hospital
Epsom, Surrey, England

70. Dr. Dorothy A. Tracey
4702 Langdrum Lane
Chevy Chase, Maryland 20015

71. Dr. Vernon O. Tyler, Jr.
Department of Psychology
Western Washington State College
Bellingham, Washington 98225

72. Dr. Dennis Upper
Department of Psychology
Veterans Administration Hospital
Brockton, Massachusetts 02401

73. Dr. Terry C. Wade
Department of Psychology
Hawaii State Hospital
Kaheohe, Hawaii 96744

74. Dr. B. Wijesinghe
Psychology Department
Claybury Hospital
Woodford Bridge, Essex, England

75. Dr. G. Terence Wilson
Graduate School of Applied and
Professional Psychology
Rutgers University
New Brunswick, New Jersey 08903

76. Dr. Janet P. Wollersheim
Department of Psychology
University of Montana
Missoula, Montana 59801

The Editor

John Paul Foreyt (Ph.D., Florida State University) is an assistant professor in the Departments of Medicine and Psychiatry at Baylor College of Medicine, Houston, Texas. In addition to teaching and consulting, Dr. Foreyt serves as project director of the Baylor College of Medicine National Heart and Blood Vessel Research and Demonstration Center's Diet Modification Program.

Dr. Foreyt has published widely in the area of behavioral treatments of obesity, behavior modification techniques in institutions and psychological assessment. Before coming to Baylor College of Medicine, Dr. Foreyt was Director of the Behavior Modification Token Economy Program at Florida State Hospital, Chattahoochee, and a faculty member in the Department of Psychology, Florida State University.

Introduction

JOHN PAUL FOREYT
Baylor College of Medicine

and

RICHARD A. FROHWIRTH
Psychometric Associates, Inc., Greenwich, Connecticut

Over the past decade interest in the behavioral treatments of obesity has increased at a rapid rate. This rise in interest may be attributed to two factors. First, traditional medical and psychotherapeutic treatments of obesity have had little success in dealing with this extremely difficult and common problem (Penick and Stunkard, 1972; Stuart and Davis, 1972; Stunkard, 1972; Stunkard and McLaren-Hume, 1959). Most investigations of weight reduction are methodologically inadequate, particularly in terms of subject sampling procedures and in length of follow-up (U.S. Public Health Service, 1966) and it is difficult to interpret findings. However, investigators generally still agree with Stunkard's (1958, p. 79) summary of the results of traditional approaches to obesity: "Most obese persons will not stay in treatment for obesity. Of those who stay in treatment, most will not lose weight, and of those who do lose weight, most will regain it." Behavioral approaches, on the other hand, have been viewed as very promising (Stuart, 1971; Stuart and Davis, 1972; Stunkard, 1972; Kiell, 1973; Mann, 1974), although more recent findings (Hall, 1973; Hall *et al.*, 1974) are also beginning to cast doubt on the efficacy of some of these newer techniques in the maintenance of long-term weight loss.

The second reason for the current popularity of these techniques is that weight reduction offers an excellent arena in which to test theoretical and conceptual problems in behavior therapy, while at the same time, preserving clinical relevance. Criterion measures are readily specified and quantified, the population of potential experimental subjects is large, volunteers are easily obtained, and manipulation of independent variables (i.e. treatment conditions) is fairly easily achieved. Thus, basic research issues such as therapist contact (Hagen, 1974), temporal sequences in conditioning (Sachs and Ingram, 1972), and locus of control of reinforcement (Hall, 1972) can be investigated without resort to analog studies of trivial problems (e.g. snake phobia) which are so common in the literature on systematic desensitization and implosive therapy.

Two major procedural lines may be discerned in the application of behavioral techniques to obesity. The first evolved from the classical conditioning paradigm, and involves attempts to create conditioned aversion responses to certain classes of foods or to overeating in general. Aversive conditioning, or aversion therapy as it is generally known, has not been especially popular in weight reduction, although it has seen wide application in the elimination of other addictive, compulsive, and persistent behavior disorders, primarily alcoholism and sexual deviations. Aversion therapy refers a wide variety of techniques in which a noxious, aversive unconditioned stimulus is repeatedly paired with a target stimulus (conditioned stimulus) or with the stimulus components of the behavior to be eliminated in order to reduce the attractiveness of the conditioned stimulus. Electric shock, chemical nauseants, foul odors, and imagery of unpleasant scenes have served as unconditioned stimuli, while actual stimulus objects (e.g. food), photographs of such objects or of the individual engaging in the problematic behaviour, and imaginal representation of both objects and behaviors have been used as conditioned stimuli (Rachman and Teasdale, 1969). The rationale for the use of such procedures in the treatment of obesity is that the learned avoidance of particular foods will result in reduction of caloric intake, and hence in weight loss. Similarly, aversive conditioning of actual eating behavior (e.g. Meyer and Crisp, 1964), food obsessionality (e.g. Thorpe, *et al.*, 1964; Wolpe, 1954), of merely thinking about problematic foods (e.g. Tyler and Straughan, 1970) has been considered to be at least potentially useful in lessening the appeal of eating. Aversion therapy in the treatment of obesity has been considered to have advantages over other behavioral methods in that while other procedures may teach an individual how to control his food intake, they do nothing to reduce craving for problematic foods (Foreyt, 1969). To date, this advantage has not been borne out empirically. It is generally conceded that the results of aversion therapy with obesity have been poor, and at best, it might be used adjuctively with other specific techniques (Abramson, 1973; Hall and Hall, 1974; Stuart, 1973; Stuart and Davis, 1972) although a few investigators have seen more promise for aversive methods (Foreyt and Kennedy, 1971; Kennedy and Foreyt, 1968). Even the more optimistic writers view aversion therapy as possibly helpful only when used in combination with other methods. Nonetheless, scattered reports of success with individual cases (e.g. Ashem, Poser, and Trudell, 1972; Morganstern, 1974; Wijesinghe, 1973; Wolpe, 1969) and with experimental groups (Foreyt and Kennedy, 1971) as well as the general methodological inadequacy of previous research in the area suggest a need for further investigation of a more rigorously experimental nature.

The second and more prominent approach has come from the Skinnerian or operant conditioning learning paradigm. Such procedures typically involve control over stimulus conditions surrounding eating, self-monitoring of weight and food intake, and contingency management (e.g. Hagen, 1974; Harris, 1969;

Harris and Hallbauer, 1973; Penick, *et al.*, 1971; Stuart, 1967, 1971; Stuart and Davis, 1972; Wollersheim, 1970). The therapeutic outcome of these procedures has been claimed to be generally encouraging. Mean weight losses in the range of 8 to 10 lb for groups of individuals treated with procedures based upon operant principles are not uncommon, and some investigators (e.g. Penick *et al.*, 1971; Stuart, 1971) have reported more substantial weight losses (over 20 lb) in a fair percentage of treatment subjects. In reviewing this line of research, Stuart (1971, p. 179) concluded that "It is probably true that behaviour therapy has offered greater promise of positive results than any other type of treatment." Relatively short follow-up intervals, confounding by non-specific factors, and subject sampling difficulties, however, all of which are characteristic of much of the behavioral weight loss research, make interpretation of results difficult. At the present time it appears more accurate to conclude that operant approaches to weight loss have been relatively successful in comparison to other treatments in short-term weight reduction. More definitive conclusions must await 5- and 10-year follow-up results.

All of the behavioral techniques apparently work with some individuals, at least in producing initial weight losses. The most helpful techniques for the clinician to use when treating overweight clients seems to involve some *combination* of the following:

1. Self-control techniques for habit change (Ferster, Nurnberger and Levitt, 1962; Jeffrey, 1974; Mahoney, 1974; Romanczyk *et al.*, 1973; Stuart, 1971; Stuart and Davis, 1972).
2. Therapist reinforcement techniques (Jeffrey, Christensen, and Pappas, 1973; Mann, 1972).
3. Nutritional information (McReynolds *et al.*, 1976).
4. Regular exercise program (Stuart, 1975).

Combining self-managed antecedent stimulus control techniques (self-monitoring of caloric intake, weight, and activity, self-initiated goal setting, self-initiated environmental planning) and self-initiated consequent control techniques (self-reinforcement, self-punishment, and self-initiated environmental reinforcement), with therapist reinforcement techniques (contingency contracting) early in treatment should result in maximal weight reduction and its maintenance over a long-term period. During treatment it is also important to convey nutritional information (e.g. Bennett and Simon, 1973; McReynolds *et al.*, 1976) and encourage a regular exercise program (e.g. Cooper, 1970; Stuart, 1975). A number of manuals and books (e.g. Christensen, Jeffrey and Pappas, 1973; Hagen, Wollersheim, and Paul, 1969; Mahoney and Jeffrey, 1974; Paulsen *et al.*, 1974; Stuart and Davis, 1972; Wollersheim, 1969) which incorporate some of these techniques are available. Many of the articles in this book contain specific techniques which will be helpful when developing a treatment program. For clients who are compulsive overeaters and have difficulty controlling their intake of specific forbidden high caloric food, the aversion techniques (electric aversive conditioning, noxious odors, covert sensitization) may be considered. For patients in mental hospitals, retardation centers, and other institutions, the operant therapist reinforcement techniques, such as the use of tokens, may be the most effective program.

Along with the advances that have been made, there are still many unanswered questions that require investigation. The major problems in the research to date include:

1. *Lack of adequate follow-up periods.* If behavior therapists are going to make a substantial contribution to combatting this problem the time is now at hand to begin reporting long term data regarding the maintenance of behavioral changes. As Atthowe (1973, p.40) has pointed out:

> Psychology and the applied behavioral sciences are presently on the witness stand. The credibility of our methods and their outcomes have been challenged. The point at which we are most vulnerable is in the persistence of our methods. We are building a technology of behavioral change, but we lack a technology of behavioral persistence.

This book is filled with studies demonstrating the short-term effectiveness of various weight-loss techniques. There is a critical need to assess which of these techniques, or which combination, seems most effective in maintaining losses over extended periods. Follow-up periods of both 6 months and 1 year are needed to begin to make conclusions regarding effectiveness, with periods of 2 to 10 years required to strengthen claims.

2. *Presence of uncontrolled variables.* It is difficult to attribute behavioral changes and weight losses in many studies to the behavioral treatments because of the presence of uncontrolled or poorly controlled variables. Demand characteristics of the study, therapist and subject expectations, and the presence of difficult to measure, nonspecific variables serve to confound treatment results. The use of placebo control conditions, along with therapists who have confidence in the placebo (they may not be so difficult to find judging from some of the research showing placebo treatments to be as effective as experimental treatment conditions) will help in untangling some of the confounding (e.g. Diament and Wilson, 1975; Foreyt and Hagen, 1973).

3. *Inability to generalize results.* Most of the behavioral research to date has been done with college age, mildly overweight females. There is a smaller number of studies investigating institutionalized psychiatric patients, but very few with individuals in the community (Hall *et al.*, 1974). Until a number of studies are reported using groups other than undergraduate females or chronic schizophrenics, it will be difficult to make statements regarding the effectiveness of the techniques on larger populations.

4. *Failure to report attrition data.* Almost all investigators are faced with the problem of subjects who drop out before the treatment is completed or disappear during follow-up. Some studies do not report the partial data they

have collected on such subjects. Such data are important for the interpretation of results and it is hoped that investigators include what information they have on their dropouts, even though it may not be used in the statistical analysis. Research is also needed into methods to reduce attrition (e.g. Hagen, Foreyt and Durham, 1976).

5. *Lack of standards for reporting results.* A cursory inspection of the behavioral studies will reveal the variety of ways results are presented, including number of pounds lost, percentage of weight lost, change in percentage of overweight, and rate of weight loss. Part of the problem is due to the fact that although the techniques treat specific behaviors the results are usually reported not in terms of whether or not the behaviors changed, but in terms of weight change. Indeed, few studies have attempted to measure behavior change in subjects along with the presumed result of those changes, weight loss (Stuart, 1973). At the very least, it is hoped that investigators report *individual* weight data, including pretreatment, posttreatment, and follow-up weights, along with number and length of treatment sessions. Percentage overweight, both pre- and posttreatment are also useful.

6. *Difficulty in determining effective treatment components.* Because most treatment programs use a combination of treatments, including a variety of self-control techniques, it is difficult to determine the relative effectiveness of each component of the program. The use of matched groups receiving different parts of a program, multiple baselines, minimal therapist involvement, and placebo controls will aid in evaluating the role of each of the components of a program.

The results of the research to date have generally shown the behavioral treatments to be superior to other forms of treatment at least during reported short term follow-up periods. The most effective overall approach to the obesity problem will probably involve different combinations of techniques for different individuals. There is a cautious optimism among many therapists that further significant advances will be made during the next few years and will help clarify why, when, and with whom the techniques work most effectively.

References

Abramson, E. E. A review of behavioral approaches to weight control. *Behaviour Research and Therapy*, 1973, **11**, 547–556.

Ashem, B., Poser, E., and Trudell, P. The use of covert sensitization in the treatment of overeating. In R. D. Rubin, H. Fensterheim, J. D. Henderson, and L. P. Ullman (Eds.), *Advances in behavior therapy*. New York: Academic Press, 1972. Pp. 97–103.

Atthowe, J. M., Jr. Behavior innovation and persistence. *American Psychologist*, 1973, **28**, 34–41.

Bennett, I. and Simon, M. *The prudent diet.* New York: David White, Inc., 1973.

Christensen, E. R., Jeffrey, D. B., and Pappas, J. P. *A therapist manual for a behavior modification weight reduction program.* Research and Development Report No. 37, Counseling and Psychological Services, University of Utah, 1973.

Cooper, K. H. *The new aerobics.* New York: Bantam Books, 1970.

Diament, C. and Wilson, G. T. An experimental investigation of the effects of covert sensitization in an analogue eating situation. *Behavior Therapy,* 1975, 6, 499–509.

Ferster, C. B., Nurnberger, J. I., and Levitt, E. E. The control of eating. *Journal of Mathetics,* 1962, 1, 87–109.

Foreyt, J. P. Control of overeating by aversion therapy. Unpublished doctoral dissertation, The Florida State University, 1969.

Foreyt, J. P. and Hagen, R. L. Covert sensitization: Conditioning or suggestion? *Journal of Abnormal Psychology,* 1973, 82, 17–23.

Foreyt, J. P. and Kennedy, W. A. Treatment of overweight by aversion therapy. *Behaviour Research and Therapy,* 1971, 9, 29–34.

Hagen, R. L. Group therapy versus bibliotherapy in weight reduction. *Behavior Therapy,* 1974, 5, 222–234.

Hagen, R. L., Foreyt, J. P., and Durham, T. W. The dropout problem: reducing attrition in obesity research. *Behavior Therapy,* 1976, 7 (in press).

Hagen, R. L., Wollersheim, J., and Paul, G. Weight reduction manual. Unpublished manuscript, University of Illinois, 1969.

Hall, S. M. Self-control and therapist control in the behavioral treatment of overweight women. *Behaviour Research and Therapy,* 1972, 10, 59–68.

Hall, S. M. Behavioral treatment of obesity: a two-year follow-up. *Behaviour Research and Therapy,* 1973, 11, 647–648.

Hall, S. M. and Hall, R. G. Outcome and methodological considerations in behavioral treatment of obesity. *Behavior Therapy,* 1974, 5, 352–364.

Hall, S. M., Hall, R. G., Hanson, R. W., and Borden, B. L. Permanence of two self-managed treatments of overweight in university and community populations. *Journal of Consulting and Clinical Psychology,* 1974, 42, 781–786.

Harris, M. B. Self-directed program for weight control: pilot study. *Journal of Abnormal Psychology,* 1969, 74, 263–270.

Harris, M. B. and Hallbauer, E. S. Self-directed weight control through eating and exercise. *Behaviour Research and Therapy,* 1973, 11, 523–529.

Jeffrey, D. B. A comparison of the effects of external control and self-control on the modification and maintenance of weight. *Journal of Abnormal Psychology,* 1974, 83, 404–410.

Jeffrey, D. B., Christensen, E. R., and Pappas, J. P. Developing a behavioral program and therapist manual for the treatment of obesity. *Journal of the American College Health Association,* 1973, 21, 455–459.

Kennedy, W. A. and Foreyt, J. P. Control of eating behavior in an obese patient by avoidance conditioning. *Psychological Reports,* 1968, 22, 571–576.

Kiell, N. *The psychology of obesity.* Springfield, Illinois: Charles C. Thomas, 1973.

Mahoney, M. J. Self-reward and self-monitoring techniques for weight control. *Behavior Therapy,* 1974, 5, 48–57.

Mahoney, M. J. and Jeffrey, D. B. A manual of self-control procedures for the overweight. Abstracted in the JSAS *Catalog of Selected Documents in Psychology,* 1974, 4, 129.

Mann, G. V. The influence of obesity on health. *The New England Journal of Medicine,* 1974, 291, 226–232.

Mann, R. A. The behavior-therapeutic use of contingency contracting to control an adult behavior problem: Weight control. *Journal of Applied Behavior Analysis,* 1972, 5, 99–109.

McReynolds, W. T., Lutz, R. N., Paulsen, B. K., and Kohrs, M. B. Weight loss from two behavior modification procedures with nutritionists as therapists. *Behavior Therapy,* 1976, 7, 283–291.

Meyer, V. and Crisp, A. H. Aversion therapy in two cases of obesity. *Behaviour Research and Therapy,* 1964, 2, 143–147.

Morganstern, K. P. Cigarette smoke as a noxious stimulus in self-managed aversion therapy for compulsive eating: technique and case illustration. *Behavior Therapy,* 1974, 5, 255–260.

Paulsen, B., McReynolds, W. T., Lutz, R. N., and Kohrs, M. B. Effective weight control through behavior modification and nutrition education: a treatment manual. Unpublished paper, Lincoln University, 1974.

Penick, S. B., Filion, R., Fox, S., and Stunkard, A. J. Behavior modification in the treatment of obesity. *Psychosomatic Medicine*, 1971, 33, 49–55.

Penick, S. B. and Stunkard, A. J. The treatment of obesity. *Advances in Psychosomatic Medicine*, 1972, 7, 217–228.

Rachman, S. and Teasdale, J. *Aversion therapy and behaviour disorders: an analysis.* Coral Gables, Florida: University of Miami Press, 1969.

Romanczyk, R. G., Tracey, D. A., Wilson, G. T., and Thorpe, G. L. Behavioral techniques in the treatment of obesity: a comparative analysis. *Behaviour Research and Therapy*, 1973, 11, 629–640.

Sachs, L. B. and Ingram, G. L. Covert sensitization as a treatment for weight control. *Psychological Reports*, 1972, 30, 971–974.

Stuart, R. B. Behavioral control of overeating. *Behaviour Research and Therapy*, 1967, 5, 357–365.

Stuart, R. B. A three-dimensional program for the treatment of obesity. *Behaviour Research and Therapy*, 1971, 9, 177–186.

Stuart, R. B. Behavioral control of overeating: A status report. Paper presented at the Fogarty International Center Conference on Obesity, Bethesda, Maryland, 1973.

Stuart, R. B. Exercise prescription in weight management: Advantages, techniques and obstacles. *Obesity and Bariatric Medicine*, 1975, 4, 16–24.

Stuart, R. B., and Davis, B. *Slim chance in a fat world*: Behavioural control of obesity. Champaign, Illinois: Research Press, Inc., 1972.

Stunkard, A. J. The management of obesity. *New York State Journal of Medicine*, 1958, 58, 79–87.

Stunkard, A. J. New therapies for the eating disorders: Behavior modification of obesity and anorexia nervosa. *Archives of General Psychiatry*, 1972, 26, 391–398.

Stunkard, A. J., and McLaren-Hume, M. The results of treatment for obesity. *A.M.A. Archives of Internal Medicine*, 1959, 103, 79–85.

Thorpe, J. G., Schmidt, E., Brown, P. T., and Castell, D. Aversion-relief therapy: a new method for general application. *Behaviour Research and Therapy*, 1964, 2, 71–82.

Tyler, V. O. and Straughen, J. H. Coverant control and breath holding as techniques for the treatment of obesity. *The Psychological Record*, 1970, 20, 473–478.

U.S. Public Health Service. Definitions and methods: Definitions of obesity and methods of assessment. In the U.S. Public Health Service Publication No. 1485, *Obesity and health: a sourcebook of current information for professional health personnel.* Washington, D.C.: U.S. Government Printing Office, 1966. Pp.5–17.

Wijesinghe, B. Massed electrical aversion treatment of compulsive eating. *Journal of Behavior Therapy and Experimental Psychiatry*, 1973, 4, 133–135.

Wollersheim, J. Therapist general orientation manual. Unpublished manuscript, University of Illinois, 1969.

Wollersheim, J. P. Effectiveness of group therapy based upon learning principles in the treatment of overweight women. *Journal of Abnormal Psychology*, 1970, 76, 462–474.

Wolpe, J. Reciprocal inhibition as the main basis of psychotherapeutic effects. *A.M.A. Archives of Neurology and Psychiatry*, 1954, 72, 205–226.

Wolpe, J. *The practice of behavior therapy.* New York: Pergamon Press, 1969.

PART I
OVERVIEW

Introduction

It is a fairly common belief that professionals gravitate toward some particular field like obesity research because they have a specific unresolved problem in that area, such as being obese themselves. Harris (1971), the author of our first article, was interested in whether such an idea might have some truth to it, so she sent a questionnaire to individuals who had written her asking for a reprint of her weight research. Perhaps not too surprisingly she found that the majority of people interested in weight research were indeed overweight themselves. However, being the clever investigator she is, she also sent her questionnaire to individuals doing research in other areas unrelated to weight control and when she looked at her responses, she found that she had gotten the same results — the majority of them were overweight too. Her study not only suggests the prevalence of the obesity problem but also points out one of the critical needs in this line of research, the necessity for adequate controls when generalizing about groups.

Our second article (U.S. Public Health Service, 1966) deals with the question of defining obesity, differentiates it from overweight (obesity refers to excess fat; overweight implies nothing about the amount of fat present) and describes various methods for measuring it. The article includes the popular height–weight tables of both average weights and desirable weights for men and women according to height and frame from the 1959 Build and Blood Pressure Study of the Society of Actuaries, used by many of the weight studies in this book for defining obesity. These tables have the practical advantage of allowing the researcher to calculate the percentage overweight (some use 10% above desirable weight as an operational definition of "overweight;" 20% above desirable weight as a definition of "obesity") before treatment and to assess how close subjects come to achieving their goal of reaching desirable weight. However, because the tables provide a range of weights for each of three frame sizes, small, medium, and large, they make it difficult for researchers to ascertain the true "desirable" weight for each subject since no criteria are given for determining frame size. Several investigators have followed the procedure Wollersheim (1970) used to determine desirable weights. She took the lowest weights given for persons of medium frame at heights 2 inches taller than her subjects (because her subjects had their height measured without shoes; the table is based upon height measurements of individuals wearing shoes). Her rationale for using the lower

11

end of the weight range was that her subjects were younger (median age = 19) than the women who made up the norms (age 25 and over).

Height—weight tables are obviously not the best method for determining overweight. All of the Green Bay Packers linemen, for example, would be considered obese by these standards, because the tables do not adequately reflect the relation of fat, muscle, and bone. The article discusses other more accurate methods for defining obesity but points out that most of them would be impractical for everyday use. The article does recommend the use of a skinfold caliper as a simple, reliable measure of body fat. Few studies have used the triceps skinfold measure in their research to date. In our experiences with the skinfold calipers, having used them in four studies, we have had considerable difficulty getting any reliability. Poor as they may be, the tables and the physician's balance scale continue to be the most practical instruments for use in obesity research.

Most articles on obesity research cite the classic review of the literature by Stunkard and McLaren-Hume (1959), our third article. They covered the obesity literature over a 30-year period and concluded that "The results of treatment for obesity are remarkably similar and remarkably poor". The authors found that most studies were so vague or difficult to interpret that it was impossible to meaningfully evaluate them. When they eliminated the vast majority of the studies with major shortcomings, they were left with just eight reports. With the exception of one, no researcher reported even the modest success of a 20 lb weight loss in more than 29% of his subjects, and the per cent losing 40 lb was far smaller, an average of 5%. Since these studies had been done by supposed experts in their field, Stunkard and McLaren-Hume concluded that these results were probably better than those obtained by the average physician.

The results of their own program using a dietary regimen, also reported in this article, were even poorer than those they reviewed. Only 12 out of 100 patients succeeded in losing more than 20 lb at any time during the two years of the program, and only 1 of these lost more than 40 lb. Maintenance of the weight loss was even more disappointing. Only 6 of the 12 persons who had lost at least 20 lb were still successful at a 1-year follow-up and only 2 of the 6 were successful at a 2-year follow-up.

Other reviewers of the obesity literature have come up with essentially the same conclusion as Stunkard and McLaren-Hume (1959). Glennon (1966), for example, reported that his review of the literature since 1958 did not reveal a single successful long-term study using a diet regimen by itself or in combination with drugs, psychotherapeutic treatment, or an exercise program. He concluded that the published long-term results of treatment programs agree with Astwood's (1962) proposal that it is incurable. Feinstein (1967), addressing a meeting of the American College of Physicians in New York, said, "The five-year cure rate for obesity is virtually zero — most people who lose excess weight soon gain it back." Strang (1968) has written, "The experience of a great many physicians is that the chance of obtaining an immediate adequate result in a patient with moderate obesity is not good, usually less than 20 percent. In the grossly obese, success is rare except in especially dramatized situations."

Some of the more recent reviews of obesity research (Penick and Stunkard, 1972; Stuart and Davis, 1972; Stunkard, 1972) have included evaluations of behavioral approaches and have concluded that these techniques appear to be the most successful to date. Stunkard (1972, p.398), for example, said, "Greater weight loss during treatment and superior maintenance of weight loss after treatment indicates that behavior modification is more effective than previous methods of treatment for obesity", and Stuart and Davis (1972, p.75) wrote, "The effectiveness of weight reduction, the absence of apparent untoward psychological side effects and the great probability of maintaining the overeater in treatment, all commend the energetic adoption of these [behavioral] techniques".

Our last two articles (Abramson, 1973; Hall and Hall, 1974) in this section are reviews specifically covering the behavioral treatments of obesity. Abramson (1973), reviewing aversive conditioning, covert sensitization, coverant conditioning, therapist reinforcement, and self-control studies concludes that the self-control procedures used in combination with therapist controlled reinforcement seem to hold the most promise for treating obesity.

Hall and Hall (1974) also review the behavioral literature but evaluate the studies in terms of their sophistication of design and the conclusions that the designs can support. They also compare the "experimenter-managed" with the "self-managed" treatment techniques. Of the studies reviewed, they conclude that only Wollersheim's (1970) (Part VI) is designed well enough to conclude unequivocally that the behavioral techniques used resulted in significant weight losses compared to the other treatments. All other studies evaluated, according to Hall and Hall, were not designed to permit clear conclusions, since they lacked adequate follow-up periods, attention-placebo controls, failed to include more than one therapist, or did not assign therapists in a way so that experimenter effects could be adequately measured. The authors clearly describe the many flaws in the behavioral research to date, particularly the failure to control for experimenter, non-specific, control, and subject variables.

One particularly relevant finding Hall and Hall (1974) reported is that studies which reported follow-up periods up to 12 weeks generally showed significant differences between treated experimental groups and untreated controls. However, the few controlled studies that reported longer follow-up periods found that the original differences between groups were no longer significant.

They conclude that combined self-managed techniques seem to be the most promising for effective long-term weight loss. They also mention that the use of experimenter-managed techniques (which generally result in fairly rapid weight loss) early in treatment, along with self-managed techniques which the subject is taught while undergoing the experimenter-managed program, should theoretically be the ideal combination.

To date, there are apparently no published reviews suggesting any techniques that are systematically effective with the obese except perhaps the behavioral therapies. Unfortunately, there are few studies evaluating the *long-term* effectiveness of behavioral techniques, but it is hoped that as these techniques become more popular, studies of this kind will be reported.

References

Abramson, E. E. A review of behavioral approaches to weight control. *Behaviour Research and Therapy*, 1973, 11, 547–556.

Astwood, E. The heritage of corpulence. *Endocrinology*, 1962, 71, 337–341.

Feinstein, A. Address to the American College of Physicians, New York, January 18, 1967. Cited in: More people should be fat. *Saturday Evening Post*, November 4, 1967.

Glennon, J. Weight reduction – an enigma. *Archives of Internal Medicine*, 1966, 118, 1–2.

Hall, S. M. and Hall, R. G. Outcome and methodological considerations in behavioral treatment of obesity. *Behavior Therapy*, 1974, 5, 352–364.

Harris, M. B. The portly psychologist, or, on the perils of using a control group. *Psychological Reports*, 1971, 29, 557–558.

Penick, S. B., and Stunkard, A. J. The treatment of obesity. *Advances in Psychosomatic Medicine*, 1972, 7, 217–228.

Society of Actuaries. *Build and blood pressure study*. Chicago: Society of Actuaries, 1959.

Strang, J. M. Obesity. In H. F. Conn (Ed.), *Current therapy 1968*. Philadelphia: W. B. Saunders Company, 1968.

Stuart, R. B. and Davis, B. *Slim chance in a fat world: Behavioral control of obesity*. Champaign, Illinois: Research Press, 1972.

Stunkard, A. J. New therapies for the eating disorders: behavior modification of obesity and anorexia nervosa. *Archives of General Psychiatry*, 1972, 26, 391–398.

Stunkard, A. J. and McLaren-Hume, M. The results of treatment for obesity. *A.M.A. Archives of Internal Medicine*, 1959, 103, 79–85.

U.S. Public Health Service. Definitions and methods: Definitions of obesity and methods of assessment. In the U.S. Public Health Service Publication No. 1485, *Obesity and health: a sourcebook of current information for professional health personnel*. Washington, D.C.: U.S. Government Printing Office, 1966, Pp. 5–17.

Wollersheim, J. P. Effectiveness of group therapy based upon learning principles in the treatment of overweight women. *Journal of Abnormal Psychology*, 1970, 76, 462–474.

CHAPTER 1

The Portly Psychologist, or,
on the Perils of using a Control Group

MARY B. HARRIS

University of New Mexico

Summary—A questionnaire was sent to people who had requested reprints of an article on weight control as well as to a control group of people who requested reprints of articles on other topics. Although a majority of people who requested the weight-control paper reported that they had a weight problem, were overweight, had an overweight friend or relative, etc., the control group reported an equal preoccupation with obesity; in fact, the two groups did not differ on any measure except frequency of openended comments. The results imply that adequate control groups should be used whenever possible in generalizing about characteristics of groups.

The Freudian theory of sublimation as well as many theories of occupational choice would predict that people might tend to enter professions in which they can deal with their own resolved or unresolved problems. Although the choice of a career may be more influenced by social and economic factors, specialization within a profession might be particularly susceptible to influences of personal problems. Specifically, psychologists interested in research on weight control might be expected to manifest problems in this area (operationally defined as excess poundage), which led to their interest in this area. Having confirmed this hypothesis on an N of 1 (herself), the author proceeded to perform a somewhat broader test by sending a questionnaire to the first 80 people to write in for a preprint or reprint of an article published on a self-control program for weight reduction (Harris, 1969). In addition, the questionnaire was sent to a control group of 50 people who had written other psychologists at the university for reprints of articles on other topics. An astounding 65 of the 80 persons requesting the weight-control article (81%) and 41 of the 50 persons requesting other articles (82%) responded to the questionnaire, plus one unimpressed soul who could not remember whether or not he had requested the study, for an over-all return rate of 82%. Since the questionnaire was completely anonymous, no follow-up letters were sent.

As may be deducted from the high return rate, the questionnaire was extremely brief. Respondents were asked to indicate their sex, height, weight,

Reprinted with permission from *Psychological Reports*, 1971, **29**, 557–558. © Psychological Reports 1971.

estimated degree of overweight or underweight, whether or not they had weight problems and watched their diets, how bothered they were by their weight, and whether they had a close friend or relative who was overweight, in addition to their area of specialization. In addition, those people who had requested the reprint were asked to indicate how long they had been interested in weight control, how overweight or underweight they were at the time they became interested, and whether their reason for requesting the reprint was personal or professional. Room was left for other information respondents wished to add.

For purposes of analysis, the questionnaires were divided into four groups: 57 men who requested the article, 33 men who did not request the article, 8 women who requested the article, 4 women who did not request the article, and 5 unclassifiable men, one of whom did not remember whether he had requested the article, 3 of whom had not previously requested it but now did, and one who would have requested it but owns the journal in which it appears. Table 1 presents the primary results for the questionnaire. Data on area of specialization and beginning of interest in the field of weight control are not reported, as most respondents left these questions blank.

TABLE 1. Responses of subjects to questionnaire

	Men		Women		Unclassifi-able Men
	Request	No Request	Request	No Request	
N^*	57	33	8	4	5
Mean weight (lb)	172.8	175.8	139.5	133.8	171.8
Mean height (in.)	70.8	71.3	64.4	65.8	70.8
M estimated overweight (lb)	5.3	9.3	16.0	8.8	8.0
% with weight problem	86	61	71	100	60
% watching their diet	34	27	25	25	60
M concern with weight†	.72	1.06	1.50	2.00	1.2
% with overweight friend or relative	57	73	75	100	80
% giving a weight ending in 0 or 5	63	73	37.5	50	80

*Because not all respondents answered all questions, some of the individual means and percentages are based on slightly smaller Ns. †0 is low; 4 is high.

Looking only at the data of those who requested the reprint, it appears that the hypothesis was confirmed: 56% of the 57 men and 71% of the 7 women who answered this question report having a weight problem; the men reported themselves a mean of 5.3 lb overweight and the women a mean of 16.0 lb overweight; 57% of the men and 75% of the women have a close friend or relative who is overweight, etc. Unfortunately, the data from the control group follow precisely the same pattern! None of the differences between the men requesting the reprint and those who did not or between the corresponding groups of women approach statistical significance, when tested by the appropriate t, χ^2, or exact test. Although more people who requested the reprint gave their weight as ending in a number other than 5 or 0, presumably indicating a greater attentiveness to their weight, this difference is also insignificant.

In short, although a majority of psychologists interested in weight control declare that they are overweight and have a weight problem, so do a majority of psychologists interested in other topics. Since only 2 of the 65 who requested the reprint said that their reasons for doing so were purely personal, it does appear that the respondents were a sample from the population of professionals rather than society at large. This is confirmed by the fact that almost all respondents gave their addresses as professional institutions, primarily universities, hospitals, and clinics.

The only difference which appeared between the groups was that those who requested the article and the unclassifiable group were much more likely to provide comments (54% and 100%, respectively) than those who did not request the article (18%). The comments ranged from the ridiculous ("no more questionnaires, please") to the sublimated "honest to consciousness (who knows about repression?) I wrote because I am interested in self control and behavior therapy." Several people commented on their own spare tires and beer bellies, several on their wives' overweight, and one on her delight at receiving the questionnaire in the middle of a successful diet. Even the more prosaic comments on the weight-control article and their own research were generally humorous and entertaining. Thus, although the idea that within a profession people gravitate to areas concerning their personal problems has not been substantiated, at least the stereotype of the jolly fat man has not completely withered away. The high return rate suggests also that psychologists are not averse to answering brief questionnaires and that using ourselves as an object of study may be very feasible. The data also suggest that the inclusion of an appropriate control group may often aid in interpretation of questionnaire data on the characteristics of a particular group.

Reference

HARRIS, M. B. A self-directed program for weight control: a pilot study. *Journal of Abnormal Psychology*, 1969, 74, 263–270.

B

CHAPTER 2

Definitions and Methods:
Definitions of Obesity and Methods of Assessment

U.S. Department of Health, Education, and Welfare, Public Health Service

Obesity, according to dictionary definition, is a "bodily condition marked by excessive generalized deposition and storage of fat". Weight, on the other hand, is defined as "a quantity of heaviness" or "relative heaviness". Overweight, then, would be simply "over-heaviness" and by definition does not carry any direct implication with regard to fatness.

Body weight is made up of a number of components. Those which cause greatest variation in weight at a given age, sex, and height in most normal individuals are fat, muscle, and bone. Because a number of components contribute to total weight, an individual may be overweight relative to some arbitrarily chosen standard on the basis of either his bony structure or musculature and yet not be obese or excessively fat. It is also true that an individual may be of average weight and yet excessively fat if he has relatively small musculature or bony structure.

Anyone who has had occasion to examine many individuals of the same sex and of approximately the same age is impressed with the need to consider each person's body structure on an individual basis. The ratio of bony structure, musculature and fat and the distribution of the fat are of far more importance in arriving at an assessment of weight status than the blind application of even the best height—weight table. There is no substitute for good clinical judgement in the determination of the desirable weight for an individual based on his actual weight, his appearance, and some idea of his subcutaneous fat pads as indicated by certain skinfolds.

Overweight vs. Obesity

All too often when weight reduction is recommended, no distinction is made between the obese and the overweight individual. The individual's weight is determined and compared with a height—weight standard. This standard may be based on either the average weight per height, age and sex or on the so-called

Reprinted with permission of the U.S. Public Health Service Publication No.1485, *Obesity and Health: A sourcebook of current information for professional health personnel.* Washington, D.C.: U.S. Government Printing Office, 1966, pp.5—17.

ideal, desirable, or best weights. The former represents average findings for insured populations in which weight increases with age. The latter, in general, have been considered more desirable as a standard of reference since presumably they are associated with lower mortality rates. Recently published data, however, suggest that when these data are viewed from the standpoint of body type rather than weight, the association of body fat and mortality below the level of frank obesity is not clear.

A comparison of actual weight to either average or desirable weight standards gives an estimate of degree of overweight or underweight but does not give any real index of fatness or of body composition unless the degree of overweight or underweight is excessive. There is no universal agreement on the degree of overweight which constitutes a presumption of obesity. Some consider a deviation of even 10 percent above the average or desirable weight to constitute such a presumption. Others use 20 percent as the outside limit of normality, and still others use even a higher percentage.

The definitions used in the oft-quoted insurance statistics on morbidity and mortality associated with excess weight are in terms of weight, not in terms of "fatness." In general, obesity and overweight are not differentiated in these or other studies, and it is not known which is the greater health hazard or, if both are involved, what their relative contributions are to morbidity and mortality. The urgent need at present is for studies that relate body composition *per se* and body fatness to morbidity and mortality. There seems to be little or no question that the markedly overweight individual is obese. The unanswered question, however, is to what extent excessive fat is a contributing factor in the moderately overweight person or in the small-boned or small-muscled person of average or desirable weight.

That part of excess weight which we desire to reduce is the fatty component. Very little can be done to constructively affect the bony or muscular components of the body or the state of hydration of a healthy individual over a prolonged period of time. Thus, the only possible attack on the relationship of excess weight to morbidity and mortality is the reduction of excess fat, if excess fat is present. In practice, one should be more interested in determining the relative fatness of an individual rather than in comparing his weight to the desirable weight for his height as given on a table.

In assessing the nutritional status of an individual, basic measurements are needed of his *height, weight,* and *relative fat content.* How may these be measured and how are they interpreted as measures of obesity?

Height–Weight Tables

Despite the limitations noted, the measurement of actual weight in relation to a selected average or desirable weight for age, sex, and height is still the most commonly used criterion of caloric overnutrition.

Average weight tables for men and women aged 15 to 69 years are found in the 1959 Build and Blood Pressure Study of the Society of Actuaries.[1] Table 1 is an adaptation of one of these tables. While it attempts to describe the adolescent and adult population in the United States and includes individuals in all weight categories, even those who are markedly overweight, it should not be used as a standard for desirable weight. Weights in the Build and Blood Pressure Study were recorded in ordinary indoor clothing, and heights were recorded with shoes. For men, the height in shoes was considered to exceed barefoot height by about an inch; for women, by an average of 2 inches. Nude weights for men were estimated to be 7 to 9 pounds less than those recorded in the table; for women, 4 to 6 pounds less.

TABLE 1. Average weight of Americans[1] (in pounds according to height and age range)

		Men							
		Age range							
Height		15-16	17-19	20-24	25-29	30-39	40-49	50-59	60-69
Feet	Inches								
5	0	98	113	122	128	131	134	136	133
5	2	107	119	128	134	137	140	142	139
5	4	117	127	136	141	145	148	149	146
5	6	127	135	142	148	153	156	157	154
5	8	137	143	149	155	161	165	166	163
5	10	146	151	157	163	170	174	175	173
6	0	154	160	166	172	179	183	185	183
6	2	164	168	174	182	188	192	194	193
6	4	–	176	181	190	199	203	205	204
		Women							
4	10	97	99	102	107	115	122	125	127
5	0	103	105	108	113	120	127	130	131
5	2	111	113	115	119	126	133	136	137
5	4	117	120	121	125	132	140	144	145
5	6	125	127	129	133	139	147	152	153
5	8	132	134	136	140	146	155	160	161
5	10	–	142	144	148	154	164	169	–
6	0	–	152	154	158	164	174	180	–

[1] Adapted from table on average weights and heights, *Build and Blood Pressure Study, 1959*, Society of Actuaries, Chicago, 1959. vol. 1.[1]

Desirable weight tables are based on the concept that once growth in height has ceased there is no biological need to gain weight and that the best health prognosis (as reflected by mortality and morbidity data) is found in individuals of average or less than average weight in their early 20s. The 1960 Metropolitan Life Insurance Company's Desirable Weight Tables are designed to be applied to individuals aged 25 and over; measurements are with indoor clothing and shoes.[2] Table 2 is adapted from the 1960 Metropolitan Life Insurance tables,

TABLE 2. Desirable weights for men and women aged 25 and over[1] (in pounds according to height and frame, in indoor clothing)

Height[2]		Small frame	Medium frame	Large frame
		Men		
Feet	Inches			
5	2	112-120	118-129	126-141
5	3	115-123	121-133	129-144
5	4	118-126	124-136	132-148
5	5	121-129	127-139	135-152
5	6	124-133	130-143	138-156
5	7	128-137	134-147	142-161
5	8	132-141	138-152	147-166
5	9	136-145	142-156	151-170
5	10	140-150	146-160	155-174
5	11	144-154	150-165	159-179
6	0	148-158	154-170	164-184
6	1	152-162	158-175	168-189
6	2	156-167	162-180	173-194
6	3	160-171	167-185	178-199
6	4	164-175	172-190	182-204
		Women		
4	10	92- 98	96-107	104-119
4	11	94-101	98-110	106-122
5	0	96-104	101-113	109-125
5	1	99-107	104-116	112-128
5	2	102-110	107-119	115-131
5	3	105-113	110-122	118-134
5	4	108-116	113-126	121-138
5	5	111-119	116-130	125-142
5	6	114-123	120-135	129-146
5	7	118-127	124-139	133-150
5	8	122-131	128-143	137-154
5	9	126-135	132-147	141-158
5	10	130-140	136-151	145-163
5	11	134-144	140-155	149-168
6	0	138-148	144-159	153-173

[1] Adapted from Metropolitan Life Insurance Co., New York. New weight standards for men and women. *Statistical Bulletin* **40**, 3, Nov.–Dec. 1959.[2]

which are derived from the 1959 Build and Blood Pressure Study. Three frame sizes are used, with a range of weights for each rather than a single weight. Unfortunately, no indication is given as to how to estimate frame size.

Desirable weights for heights are presented also in "Recommended Dietary Allowances."[3] The weights suggested were based on the weights of college men and women aged 25 to 29 and 20 to 24, respectively. A range of weights for heights is presented, but, again, no suggestion is made for estimating body build in order to determine where within the range the normal weight should be. One can only assume that it is the thick-chested, broad-shouldered, and broad-pelvised person who is large-framed, and that the small-framed person is one with a thin chest, narrow shoulders, and narrow pelvis, and that all those in between are considered to be medium-framed.

Recently, data on height, weight, and selected body dimensions have been published by the National Center for Health Statistics, Public Health Service.[4] These data, collected in 1960-62, were based on a nationwide probability sample. They are, therefore, more representative of the adult civilian, non-institutionalized population in the United States, than are the data from the Build and Blood Pressure Study, which represent an "insured" population.

Another important difference in the two studies is that standardized techniques were employed for making all measurements in the Public Health Service study. In the Build and Blood Pressure report, variations in procedure existed in measuring height and weight, and in some instances measurements were simply recorded as reported by the applicant.

Table 3 presents these new average weights for men and women, by age and height. More details regarding range of weights for age are presented in the published report.

Despite the fact that these new data may be considered more accurately descriptive of height—weight patterns in United States adults, it should again be noted that the use of these or other tables to define obesity (excess body fat) without more definitive assessments of "fatness" may well be not only misleading but inaccurate.

The Committee on Nutritional Anthropometry of the Food and Nutrition Board, National Research Council, has suggested that bi-cristal (bi-iliac) diameter is the best measure of skeletal laterality and that the next best measure is bi-acromial diameter, but there are no readily available percentile distributions by age and sex for these measurements.[5] The committee also suggests that upper-arm circumference be used as a measure of muscular development provided that the thickness of the subcutaneous layer is determined at the same level. Along with consideration of the laterality of the skeleton in the interpretation of body weights, the relative contribution of the trunk to total height should not be forgotten, since for any given height and skeletal width, the long-trunked, short-legged individual is usually heavier than his short-trunked, long-legged counterpart.

TABLE 3. Smoothed average weights[1] for men and
women (by age and height: United States 1960-62[2])

Height	Weight (in pounds)						
	18-24 years	25-34 years	35-44 years	45-54 years	55-64 years	65-74 years	75-79 years
Men							
62 inches	137	141	149	148	148	144	133
63 inches	140	145	152	152	151	148	138
64 inches	144	150	156	156	155	151	143
65 inches	147	154	160	160	158	154	148
66 inches	151	159	164	164	162	158	154
67 inches	154	163	168	168	166	161	159
68 inches	158	168	171	173	169	165	164
69 inches	161	172	175	177	173	168	169
70 inches	165	177	179	181	176	171	174
71 inches	168	181	182	185	180	175	179
72 inches	172	186	186	189	184	178	184
73 inches	175	190	190	193	187	182	189
74 inches	179	194	194	197	191	185	194
Women							
57 inches	116	112	131	129	138	132	125
58 inches	118	116	134	132	141	135	129
59 inches	120	120	136	136	144	138	132
60 inches	122	124	138	140	149	142	136
61 inches	125	128	140	143	150	145	139
62 inches	127	132	143	147	152	149	143
63 inches	129	136	145	150	155	152	146
64 inches	131	140	147	154	158	156	150
65 inches	134	144	149	158	161	159	153
66 inches	136	148	152	161	164	163	157
67 inches	138	152	154	165	167	166	160
68 inches	140	156	156	168	170	170	164

[1] Estimated values from regression equations of weights
for specified age groups.
[2] Adapted from National Center for Health Statistics:
Weight by Height and Age of Adults, United States,
1960-1962. *Vital Health Statistics*. PHS. Publication No.
1000–Series 11, No. 14. May 1966.

WEIGHT EVALUATION IN CHILDREN

The problems of evaluating weight status in children from height—weight
tables are more complex than for adults. Consideration must be given to rates of
growth and to the effects of sexual maturation. Children, like adults, show a
great diversity of body types. Sexual maturation and growth spurts do not occur
at the same chronological age in all children. Average tables for height and

weight for given ages, therefore, are often not representative of actual growth patterns.

Weight evaluation of children should take into account not only weight or fatness for height but also the history of the height—weight relationship which may be obtained from school health records.

We need also to keep in mind that an accumulation of fat at the pre-pubertal period in a hitherto normal child is not at all unusual. It is in fact a frequent occurrence and probably does not have the same significance as obesity that occurs in the early school years or after the adolescent growth spurt has taken place.

Falkner, in 1962, presented a collection of the best available data on physical growth standards for white North American children, with charts giving height and weight of children from birth to 18 years at the 5th, 50th, and 95th percentiles.[6] Table 4 presents this data in summary. This table simply gives a general picture for American children. When used as a standard, the individual variation in children's growth should not be overlooked. In most cases, the height—weight relationship is probably a more valid index of weight status than a weight-for-age assessment.

HEIGHT AND WEIGHT MEASUREMENTS

Care should be taken in making measurements of height and weight. As indicated, the adult average and desirable height—weight tables of the Metropolitan Life Insurance Company are for measurements obtained in usual indoor clothing with shoes, while the National Research Council height—weight tables are for measurements made without shoes or other clothing.[3] And for children, height—weight standards are for nude weights without shoes.[6]

Ideally, body weight should be reported as nude body weight, with an appropriate correction made for the clothing worn. The body weight estimate can be checked from time to time by actually weighing the clothes worn.

Height is the distance from the soles of the feet to the top of the head; it should be measured without shoes. The individual to be measured should stand erect, with heels and scapulae in contact with the wall or other flat vertical surface. The head should be held so that the line of sight is horizontal. Height is then measured from the soles of the feet to a lowered rectangular wood object or other suitable guide kept in contact with the vertical measuring scale until firm contact is made with the scalp.

When measuring a child's height, "lying-height" measurements should be made until the child is 2 or 3 years of age. For this purpose, the child lies recumbent on a rigid board with a right-angled foot support.

These, then, are some of the standards that may be used in evaluating weight status. In order to use weight as an assessment of obesity, one needs an estimate of fatness also.

TABLE 4. Physical growth standards for children
from birth to age 18 (at 5th, 50th, and 95th percentiles[1])

Age	Height (in inches)			Weight (in pounds)		
Month or year	5th P	50th P	95th P	5th P	50th P	95th P

			Boys			
Birth	18.4	19.8	21.1	5.9	7.5	9.1
1 mo.	19.9	21.4	22.9	7.3	9.4	11.1
3 mo.	22.6	24.0	25.4	9.8	13.4	16.0
6 mo.	25.1	26.7	28.3	14.7	18.0	21.3
9 mo.	27.2	28.7	30.2	16.8	21.4	25.1
1 yr.	28.4	30.2	32.0	18.7	23.3	27.8
2 yrs.	32.1	34.6	37.1	23.3	28.3	33.3
3 yrs.	35.3	37.8	40.3	27.1	32.5	37.9
4 yrs.	38.3	40.8	43.3	30.0	36.1	42.2
5 yrs.	40.3	43.4	46.4	33.0	40.3	47.6
6 yrs.	42.8	45.9	49.0	36.0	44.7	53.4
7 yrs.	44.8	48.1	51.4	40.3	50.9	61.5
8 yrs.	46.9	50.5	54.1	44.4	57.4	70.4
9 yrs.	48.8	52.8	56.8	48.0	64.4	80.4
10 yrs.	50.6	54.9	59.2	51.4	71.4	91.4
11 yrs.	51.9	56.4	60.9	53.3	78.9	102.5
12 yrs.	53.5	58.6	63.7	60.0	86.0	113.5
13 yrs.	55.2	61.3	67.4	65.3	98.6	131.9
14 yrs.	57.5	64.1	70.7	75.5	111.8	148.1
15 yrs.	61.0	66.9	72.8	88.0	124.3	160.6
16 yrs.	63.8	68.9	74.0	97.8	133.8	169.8
17 yrs.	65.2	69.8	74.4	106.5	139.8	174.0
18 yrs.	65.9	70.2	74.5	110.3	144.8	179.3

			Girls			
Birth	18.3	19.5	20.7	5.3	7.3	8.8
1 mo.	19.5	21.0	22.5	6.6	8.3	9.8
3 mo.	22.2	23.6	25.0	10.2	12.4	14.4
6 mo.	24.6	26.1	27.6	13.4	16.7	19.8
9 mo.	26.3	27.9	29.5	15.3	19.8	24.1
1 yr.	27.6	29.4	31.2	17.4	21.7	26.0
2 yrs.	31.6	33.8	36.0	22.3	27.1	31.9
3 yrs.	35.3	37.5	39.7	26.3	32.3	38.3
4 yrs.	38.1	40.7	43.3	28.8	36.1	43.4
5 yrs.	40.6	43.4	46.2	32.2	40.9	49.6
6 yrs.	42.8	45.9	49.0	35.5	45.7	55.9
7 yrs.	44.5	47.8	51.1	38.3	51.0	63.7
8 yrs.	46.4	50.0	53.6	42.0	57.2	72.4
9 yrs.	48.2	52.2	56.2	45.1	63.6	82.1
10 yrs.	49.9	54.5	59.1	48.2	71.0	95.0
11 yrs.	51.9	57.0	62.1	55.4	82.0	108.6
12 yrs.	54.1	59.5	64.9	63.9	94.4	124.9
13 yrs.	57.1	62.2	66.8	72.8	105.5	138.2
14 yrs.	58.5	63.1	67.7	83.0	113.0	144.0
15 yrs.	59.5	63.8	68.1	89.5	120.0	150.5
16 yrs.	59.8	64.1	68.4	95.1	123.0	150.1
17 yrs.	60.1	64.2	68.3	97.9	125.8	153.7
18 yrs.	60.1	64.4	68.7	96.0	126.2	156.4

[1] Adapted from Falkner, F. Some physical growth standards
for white North American children. *Pediatrics* **29**, 467-474,
1962.

Unusual Fat Deposits

Before we consider some of the practical and more scientific means of assessing fatness, a comment is in order about the problem of unusual fat depositions on the otherwise nonobese body. This is one of the most common and one of the most difficult problems treated in obesity.

The therapist needs to have a realistic point of view about this problem, and he should make it clear to his patient so that the patient will understand what he faces.

To a large extent the distribution of body fat is controlled genetically and hormonally. Except in treatable cases of endocrine abnormality, fat deposition patterns cannot be changed. Persons with abnormal fat deposits may be obese also, but as these people reduce, the abnormal fat deposits will still remain disproportionately large even though they do decrease.

Therapeutic efforts should concentrate on bringing understanding to the patient and helping him to live with the situation. This is particularly true for young women, for whom esthetic considerations are so important, because their lack of understanding may lead to unwarranted anxiety or unnecessary dieting.

The patient should be helped to understand that his disproportionate fat distribution is there to stay. He should be guarded against vain attempts to bring the offending fat deposits down to normal by excessive dieting. This can result in loss of the normal, essential protective and organ-supporting fat in the subcutaneous tissues and abdomen.

Gross Assessment

From a practical point of view, a determination of whether or not any one individual is too fat is rather simple and does not require scientific acumen.

An easy answer without weighing oneself on a scale is to look in the mirror. A realistic appraisal of the nude body is often a more reliable guide for estimating obesity than body weight.[7]

If sheer appearance fails to give a clear answer, there is the "pinch test". This test is particularly helpful for adults who are under 50. At least half of the body fat in young individuals is found directly under the skin. At many locations on the body (for example, the back of the upper arm, the side of the lower chest, the back just below the shoulder blade, to name a few), a fold of skin and subcutaneous fat can be lifted between thumb and forefinger so that it is held free of the underlying soft tissue and bony structure. One report states that for individuals with normal amounts of fat the layer beneath the skin should be one-fourth to one-half inch thick. The skinfold is of double thickness, one-half to one inch. In most cases, skinfolds thicker than one inch are an indication of excessive body fatness. Folds that are markedly thinner than one-half inch indicate abnormal thinness.[8] A pinch in several places on the body will tell whether the first skinfold attempted is characteristic of body fatness. It should be reemphasized that these foregoing statements refer to gross assessment, and that variations exist between women and men in terms of what may be considered excess fat. Specific criteria for measuring skinfold thickness are discussed on pages 30–32.

Another simple indicator of fatness is the so-called ruler test.[8] When one is lying flat on his back and is relaxed, the surface of the abdomen between the flare of the ribs and the pubis is normally flat or slightly concave. A ruler placed on the abdomen parallel with the vertical axis should touch both ribs and pubis.

Another test is to compare the circumference of the chest at the level of the nipples with the circumference of the abdomen at the level of the navel. Normally, the circumference of the chest exceeds abdominal circumference by a few inches. When abdominal girth approaches, equals, or exceeds the girth of the chest, it usually means an excess of abdominal fat.

Total Body Fatness

Other techniques, of a more scientific nature, are available for determining body fatness. Some are quite complex, others are fairly simple. In cases where both complex and simple measurements have been made in sequence on the same individuals, it has been possible to formulate relationships for use in predicting total fatness on the basis of the simpler techniques. Such studies have been made for both sexes in several age groups, but there is need for more studies of this type based on representative population samplings, particularly of children and adolescent girls.

Total fatness may be measured directly only in cadavers, unfortunately. One of the greatest needs in body composition studies is for more such basic analyses of essentially normal bodies of both sexes at all ages. In the living human, data on total body fatness for groups of people have come from densitometry studies, hydrometry studies, and, to a limited extent, from measurements of body electrolytes.[9–21] More recent information on total body fatness has come from measurement of whole body K^{40} content through the use of whole body counters.[22–23]

Available data, however, is insufficient to say that we have real norms for most population groups although the accumulated fragments from various laboratories tend to give a consistent picture with regard to age and sex trends.

Throughout the life span, from 9 years of age on, fat accounts for a higher percentage of total body weight in the female than in the male. Body fatness for both sexes increases with age, and, in adult life, increases at a faster rate for men than for women, yet, women at all ages above 9 are on the average fatter than men. This may be seen by comparing the obesity standards given in both sexes in Table 5.

Somatotyping, a technique involving anthropometry, is another method for assessing body composition. Somatotyping has been tested sufficiently for

TABLE 5. Obesity standards for Caucasian
Americans[1] (minimum triceps skinfold
thickness in millimeters indicating
obesity)[2]

Age (years)	Skinfold measurements	
	Males	Females
5	12	14
6	12	15
7	13	16
8	14	17
9	15	18
10	16	20
11	17	21
12	18	22
13	18	23
14	17	23
15	16	24
16	15	25
17	14	26
18	15	27
19	15	27
20	16	28
21	17	28
22	18	28
23	18	28
24	19	28
25	20	29
26	20	29
27	21	29
28	22	29
29	23	29
30-50	23	30

[1] Adapted from Seltzer, C. C., and Mayer, J. A
simple criterion of obesity. *Postgrad Med.* 38,[2] A
101-107, 1965.[24]

[2] Figures represent the logarithmic means of the
frequency distributions plus one standard
deviation.

validity and reliability to have earned a measure of approval from the scientific community. But, unfortunately, this method is not easily adapted to mass population surveys or to general clinic or office practice. Its reproducibility depends on application by trained somatotypists — individuals who are in short supply. And, the necessity of photographs "in the nude" further limits its usefulness.

Subcutaneous Fat

The indirect methods just described are too complex to be used for measuring body fat in field studies or in the offices of physicians. Simpler anthropometric methods can be used. Since a large proportion of adipose tissue is located under the skin, the measurement of subcutaneous fat yields an index of fatness which can be adapted to office use or to field conditions. The two measurements used are (1) thickness of the fat pad on soft-tissue X-ray and (2) measurement of skinfold thickness by a calibrated caliper.

SOFT-TISSUE X-RAY

An advantage to using the soft-tissue X-ray for measuring fat thickness is that the fat is not compressed during measurement. The technique offers an opportunity to measure muscle and bone mineralization as well as fat pads that are difficult to measure with a caliper.[25] The technique does require the use of X-ray equipment, however, and it is expensive and requires expert positioning.

Fairly extensive data on soft-tissue X-ray measurement of fat are available for children by sex and age, and more limited data are available on adult men and women.[10, 15, 16, 26 − 32] The trochanteric pad is the best single predictor of total fat in men, and the iliac fat pad, in women. Until recently, efforts to estimate total body fatness on the basis of soft-tissue X-ray were not cross validated with other more basic measures such as densitometry and hydrometry.[32]

SKINFOLD THICKNESS

Densitometry, hydrometry, radiography, and multiple anthropometric and skinfold regression formulas are desirable techniques used by researchers to further the development of more accurate body fat-content procedures. However, their use is too cumbersome, too complicated and time consuming for the professional lacking the training, who needs to judge whether a subject is obese and to estimate the extent of the obesity.[33 − 41]

For clinicians, family doctors, school physicians and school nurses, nutritionists, and physical educators, there is a pressing need for a simple and rapid procedure whereby a reasonably precise measurement of fat can be made with a minimum of time and effort and without discomfort and embarassment to the subject. Again, it is emphasized that the designation of obesity is a function of the amount of fat. When judging any one individual, judgement as to fatness should not be determined only by degree of relative overweight or by percentage of overweight.

Skinfold measurements appear to be the best single, simple, and eminently practical determination of adiposity. Skinfold measurements reflect the amount of subcutaneous fat.[5 ,9 ,13 , 15 − 17, 42 − 49] Skinfold thickness is measured by pressing a skinfold caliper on certain selected sites on the body. The validity of the measurement as an indicator of total body fat has been demonstrated by the extent of its correlation with results obtained by other, more specific methods for determining subcutaneous and total body fat.

The consensus is that skinfolds are of proven value as useful measures of total adiposity, particularly in young people. Furthermore, the techniques involved in making skinfold measurements are not difficult to master. It is not necessary to be a skilled anthropometrist. With proper direction and a minimum of demonstration from an experienced practitioner, one can acquire sufficient skill with a skinfold caliper to obtain satisfactory measurement reliability.

USING A CALIPER

Standardization of skinfold calipers has become a necessary requirement for universal comparability of fat-fold measurements and for conversion to total body fat.[5] The accepted national recommendation is to have a caliper so designed as to exert a pressure of 10 g/mm^2 on the caliper face. The contact surface area to be measured should be in the neighborhood of 20 to 40 square millimeters.

The skinfold measure to be obtained is the doubled thickness of the pinched, folded skin plus the attached subcutaneous adipose tissue.

The skinfold must be picked up in a standard fashion. The approved method is to pinch up a full fold of skin and subcutaneous tissue (between thumb and forefinger) at a distance of about one centimeter from the site on which the caliper is to be placed and then to pull the fold away from the underlying muscle. The fold is pinched up firmly and held during the full time the measurement is being taken.

The calipers are then applied to the fold about a centimeter below the fingers so that the pressure on the fold at the point measured is exerted by the faces of the caliper and not from the fingers. The handle of the caliper is released to permit the full force of the caliper arm pressure, and the dial is read to the nearest one-half millimeter. Caliper measurement should be made at least twice to obtain a stable reading. When skinfolds are extremely thick, dial readings should be made three seconds after application of the caliper pressure to provide for utmost accuracy.

SITES TO BE MEASURED

Triceps and subscapular skinfold measurements are recommended by the Committee on Nutritional Anthropometry as good methods for characterizing an individual's overall fatness.[5]

The triceps skinfold is measured midway at the back of the upper right arm flexed at 90°. It is critical that the midpoint between the tip of the acromion and the tip of the olecranon be located because of the gradation of subcutaneous fat thickness for the upper arm from elbow to shoulder. A steel tape is useful in locating and marking the midpoint. The arm of the subject should hang freely when the skinfold measurement is made.

The subscapular skinfold is measured just below the angle of the right scapula (shoulder and arm relaxed), with the fold picked up in a line slightly inclined in the natural cleavage of the skin. Because subcutaneous fat is fairly uniform in this region of the body, precision of location is less critical for this measurement.

SKINFOLDS IN DEFINING OBESITY

The triceps skinfold measurement is a single, easy, reasonably precise and reproducible yardstick, to be used in making a definition of obesity in an individual based on the fat content of his body as well as for gauging the degree of his obesity. The upper arm seems to be the most representative single site for estimating the overall deposition of fat in obese individuals, regardless of fat patterning. From a practical standpoint, the use of the triceps measurement alone is satisfactory, especially since the subscapular skinfold involves the attendant difficulties of further time and effort and the possible embarrassment of having the subject undress.[24] There is no appreciable advantage to using both the triceps and subscapular skinfolds although the use of both will give a somewhat more definitive measure of fatness.

As stated, obesity refers to fatness in contrast to overweight, which, by definition, does not carry any direct implication of fatness. The data on total body fatness or on fatness in relationship to health are insufficient to establish norms.

In like manner, valid standards for skinfold measurements are necessarily arbitrary at present. Nevertheless, whatever limits are defined, they should be based on a representative frequency distribution for an average healthy population, with a consideration for skewness in the distribution curve. In addition, differential factors of age and sex must also be taken into account.

Table 5 will aid in determining the existence of obesity. The table presents the upper limits of the normal range of fatness for the average healthy Caucasian American population.[24] Five of six persons have less fat than that indicated by the figures given. A triceps skinfold compared with these standards and used in conjunction with a clinician's assessment will be of assistance in determining whether a person should be considered obese.

References

1. *Build and Blood Pressure Study, 1959.* Society of Actuaries. Chicago, 1959. Vol. 1.
2. Metropolitan Life Insurance Co., New York. New weight standards for men and women. *Statistical Bulletin* 40, 3, Nov.–Dec. 1959.
3. *Recommended Dietary Allowances* (6th revised edition). National Academy of Sciences-National Research Council, Washington, D.C., 1964. Publication 1146.
4. National Center for Health Statistics: Weight by Height and Age of Adults, United

States, 1960–1962. *Vital and Health Statistics.* Public Health Service Pub. No. 1000–Series 11, No. 14. U.S. Gov. Printing Office. May, 1966.

5. Committee on Nutritional Anthropometry, Food and Nutrition Board, National Research Council (A. Keys, *chairman*). Recommendations concerning body measurements for the characterization of nutritional status. In *Body Measurements for Human Nutrition* (J. Brozek, Ed.) Wayne University Press, Detroit, 1956, p. 10.

6. Falkner, F. Some physical growth standards for white North American children. *Pediatrics* 29, 467–474, 1962.

7. Keys, A. Body composition and its change with age and diet. In *Weight Control.* Iowa State Press, Ames, Iowa, 1955, p. 18.

8. Jolliffe, N. *Reduce and Stay Reduced,* 3rd ed. Simon and Schuster, New York, 1963, p. 23.

9. Parizkova, J. Total body fat and skinfold thickness in children. *Metabolism* 10, 794-807, 1961.

10. Heald, F. P., Hunt, E. D., Jr., Schwartz, R., Cook, C. D., Elliot, O., and Vajda, B. Measures of body fat and hydration in adolescent boys. *Pediatrics* 31, 226-239, 1963.

11. Novak, L. P. Age and sex differences in body density and creatinine excretion of high school children. *Ann. N.Y. Acad. Sci.* 110, 545-577, 1963.

12. Brozek, J. and Keys, A. The evaluation of leanness–fatness in man: Norms and interrelationship. *Brit. J. Nutr.* 5, 194-206, 1951.

13. Pascale, L. R., Grossman, M. I., Sloane, H. S., and Frankel, T. Correlations between thickness of skinfolds and body density in 88 soldiers. *Human Biol.* 28, 165-176, 1956.

14. Chen, K. Report on measurement of total body fat in American women estimated on the basis of specific gravity as an evaluation of individual fatness and leanness. *J. Formosan Med. Ass.* 52, 271, 1953.

15. Young, C. M., Martin, M. E. K., Chihan, M., McCarthy, M., Manniello, M. J., Harmuth, E. H. and Fryer, J. H. Body composition of young women. *J. Amer. Diet Ass.* 38, 332-340, 1961.

16. Young, C. M. *et al.* Body composition studies of "older" women, thirty to seventy years of age. *Ann. N.Y. Acad. Sci.* 110, 589-607, 1963.

17. Fryer, J. H. Studies of body composition in men aged 60 and over. In *Biological Aspects of Aging* (N. W. Shock, ed.). Columbia University Press, New York, 1962, pp. 57-78.

18. Edelman, I. S. and Leibman, J. Anatomy of body water and electrolytes. *Amer. J. Med.* 27, 256-277, 1959.

19. Friis-Hansen, B. Body water compartments in children: Changes during growth and related changes in body composition. *Pediatrics* 28, 169-181, 1961.

20. Edelman, I. S. Body water and electrolytes. In *Techniques for Measuring Body Composition* (J. Brozek, and A. Henschel, eds.). National Academy of Sciences, Washington, D.C., 1961, p. 140.

21. Moore, F. D. Further comments on total exchangeable electrolyte and body composition. In *Techniques for Measuring Body Composition* (J. Brozek and A. Henschel, eds.). National Academy of Sciences, Washington, D. C., 1961, p. 155.

22. Anderson, E. C. and Langham, W. H. Average potassium concentration of the human body as a function of age. *Science* 130, 713-714, 1959.

23. Forbes, G. B., Gallup, J., and Hursh, J. B. Estimation of total body fat from potassium-40 content. *Science* 133, 101-102, 1961.

24. Seltzer, C. C. and Mayer, J. A simple criterion of obesity. *Postgrad. Med.* 38(2); A101-A107, 1965.

25. Stuart, H. C., Hill, P., and Shaw, C. *The Growth of Bone, Muscle and Overlying Tissues as Revealed by Studies of Roentgenograms of the Leg Area* (monograph). Society for Research in Childhood Development, Inc., Evanston, Ill., 1940, Vol. 5, No. 3, Serial No. 26.

26. Stuart, H. C., and Sobel, E. H. The thickness of the skin and subcutaneous tissue by age and sex in childhood. *J. Pediat.* 28, 637-647, 1946.

27. Reynolds, E. L., *Distribution of Subcutaneous Fat in Childhood and Adolescence.*

Society for Research in Childhood Development, Inc., Evanston, Ill., 1950, Vol. 15, No. 2, Serial No. 50.

28. Garn, S. M., and Haskell, J. A. Fat thickness and developmental status in childhood and adolescence. *AMA J. Dis. Child* **99**, 746-751, 1960.

29. Garn, S. M. and Harper, R. V. Fat accumulation and weight gain in the adult male. *Hum. Biol.* **27**, 39-49, 1955.

30. Brozek, J. and Mori, H. Some interrelationships between somatic, roentgenographic and densitometric criteria of fatness. *Hum. Biol.* **30**, 322-336, 1958.

31. Garn, S. M. Fat weight and fat placement in the female. *Science* **125**, 1091-1092, 1957.

32. Young, C. M., Tensuan, R. S., Sault, F. and Holmes, F. Estimating body fat of a normal young woman. Visualizing fat pads by soft-tissue X-rays. *J. Amer. Diet. Ass.* **42**, 409-413, 1963.

33. Behnke, A. R., Guttentag, O. E., and Brodsky, C. Quantification of body weight and configuration from anthropometric measurements. *Hum. Biol.* **31**, 213-234, 1959.

34. Behnke, A. R. The estimation of lean body weight from "skeletal" measurements. *Hum. Biol.* **31**, 295-315, 1959.

35. Young, C. M. and Blondin, J. Estimating body weight and fatness of young women. Use of "envelope" anthropometric measurements. *J. Amer. Diet. Ass.* **41**, 452-455, 1962.

36. Young, C. M. and Tensuan, R. S. Estimating the lean body mass of young women. Use of skeletal measurements. *J. Amer. Diet. Ass.* **42**, 46-51, 1963.

37. Miller, A. T., Jr., and Blyth, C. S. Estimation of lean body mass and body fat from basal oxygen consumption and creatinine excretion. *J. Appl. Physiol.* **5**, 73-78, 1952.

38. Behnke, A. R. The relation of lean body weight to metabolism and some consequent systematizations. *Ann. N.Y. Acad. Sci.* **56**, 1095-1142, 1953.

39. Ryan, R. J., Williams, J. D., Ansel, B. M., and Bernstein, L. M. The relationship of body composition to oxygen consumption and creatinine excretion in healthy and wasted men. *Metabolism* **6**, 365-377, 1957.

40. Young, C. M., McCarthy, M., Fryer, J. H., and Tensuan, R. S. Basal oxygen consumption as a predictor of lean body mass in young women. *J. Amer. Diet. Ass.* **43**, 125-128, 1963.

41. Sheldon, W. H., Stevens, S. S., and Tucker, W. B. *The Varieties of Human Physique.* Harper & Bros., New York, 1940.

42. Pett, L. B. and Ogilvie, G. F. The Canadian weight–height survey. *Hum. Biol.* **28**, 177-188, 1956.

43. Tanner, J. M. and Whitehouse, R. H. Standards for subcutaneous fat in British children. Percentiles for thickness of skinfolds over triceps and below scapula. *Brit. Med. J.* **5276**, 446-450, 1962.

44. Newman, R. W. Skinfold measurements in young American males. *Hum. Biol.* **28**, 154-164, 1956.

45. Brozek, J., *et al.* Skinfold distributions in middle-age American men: A contribution to norms of leanness-fatness. *Ann. N.Y. Acad. Sci.* **110**, 492-502, 1963.

46. Skerlj, B., Brozek, J., and Hunt, E. E., Jr. Subcutaneous fat and age changes in body build and body form in women. *Amer. J. Phys. Anthrop.* **11**, 577-600, 1953.

47. Young, C. M., Martin, M. E. K., Tensuan, R. S., and Blondin, J. Predicting specific gravity and body fatness in young women. *J. Amer. Diet. Ass.* **40**, 102-107, 1962.

48. Young, C. M. Predicting specific gravity and body fatness in "older" women. *J. Amer. Diet. Ass.* **45**, 333-339, 1964.

49. Rathbun, R. N. and Pace, N. Studies on body composition; the determination of total body fat by means of body specific gravity. *J. Biol. Chem.* **158**, 667-676, 1945.

CHAPTER 3

The Results of Treatment for Obesity

ALBERT STUNKARD,
Philadelphia,

and

MAVIS McLAREN-HUME[1]
New York

The current widespread concern with weight reduction rests on at least two assumptions: first, that weight-reduction programs are effective; second, that they are harmless. Recent studies indicate that such programs may be far from harmless.[1,2] This report documents their ineffectiveness. The results of treatment, as reported in the medical literature of the past 30 years, are first reviewed. The results of routine treatment of 100 consecutive obese persons in the Nutrition Clinic of the New York Hospital are then reported.

Review of the Literature

Hundreds of papers on treatment of obesity have been published in the past 30 years. Most, however, do not give figures on the outcome of treatment, and of those that do, most report them in such a way as to obscure the outcome of treatment of individual patients. Some authors, for example, report the total number of patients and the pounds lost without making clear how many patients achieved satisfactory results. Others report rates of weight loss of groups of patients for whom the duration of treatment was short or even unspecified. Still others use as their standard the percentage of excess weight lost, without noting the amount in pounds. Perhaps the greatest difficulty in interpreting the results of weight-reduction programs, however, is due to the exclusion from reports of

Reprinted with permission from the *A.M.A. Archives of Internal Medicine*, 1959, **103**, 79-85.

[1] From the Departments of Psychiatry and Medicine of the University of Pennsylvania School of Medicine and the Department of Nutrition of the New York Hospital.

This work was supported in part by the Research and Development Division, Office of the Surgeon General, Department of the Army, under Contract No. DA–19–007–MD–925.

patients who did not remain in treatment or were otherwise "uncooperative". Such patients probably represent therapeutic failures, and they certainly constitute an impressive part of any group. Reports which exclude them, therefore, are not useful in evaluating treatment. If papers with these shortcomings are omitted, the vast literature on treatment for obesity shrinks to just eight reports[3-10] These are summarized in Table 1.[2]

Interpretation of these results is complicated by two omissions: the method of selecting patients and their degree of overweight. The first of these factors is often difficult to ascertain; the second makes reporting so complex as almost to obviate comparisons between groups. To facilitate such comparison we have listed the per cent of patients in each series who lost 20 and 40 lb, irrespective of their original weights. Although these criteria may introduce a bias in favor of treatment of more severely obese persons (who have more weight to lose), they have the virtue of being sufficiently modest to be widely applicable. Twenty pounds is indeed a small weight loss for the grossly overweight persons who are the subjects of these reports.

TABLE 1. A summary of results of treatment for obesity as reported in medical literature during the past thirty years

Author	Type of treatment	Patients, No.	Weight loss, % of patients			
			Less than 10 lb	10-20 lb	More than 20 lb	More than 40 lb
Fellows (1931)	Employees clinic: individual instruction and self-selected diet	294	47	27	26	5
Evans (1938)	Private practice (internist): 600 Cal. diet	130	59	19	22	5
Gray and Kallenbach (1939)	Nutrition clinic: 900 Cal. diet and thyroid	314	52	20	28	8
Osserman and Dolger (1951)	Diabetes clinic: dextro amphetamine (Dexedrine)	55	35	36	29	2
Munves (1953)	Home economics research: interview or group discussion	48	61	27	12	4
Harvey and Simmons (1954)	Group psychotherapy project: 1000 Cal. diet	290	47	30	23	6
Young et al. (1955)	Experimental nutrition clinic: interview and diet	131	40	32	28	3
Feinstein et al. (1958)	Obesity research clinic: 900 Cal. formula diet	106	17	24	59	31

The review in Table 1 reveals two significant points. The results of treatment for obesity are remarkably similar and remarkably poor. Thus, with the exception of Feinstein, no author has reported even the modest success of a 20 lb weight loss in more than 29% of his patients. The per cent of patients losing 40 lb is far smaller. Furthermore, the results in six of the eight reports are within 7 percentage points of each other. This remarkable uniformity, despite the widely differing circumstances of the studies, increases the assurance with which these results may be regarded.

[2] The present study deals only with outpatient treatment of obesity. Inpatient treatment, with its far greater control over food intake, does not present the same problems.

These reports were all written by persons with a particular interest in obesity, by experts in the field. It is probable that their results, poor as they seem, are nevertheless better than those obtained by the average physician. To ascertain the results of treatment in routine clinic practice, a study was undertaken of the results of treatment for obesity of 100 consecutive obese persons in the Nutrition Clinic of the New York Hospital. These results follow.

Results in a Nutrition Clinic

One of the functions of the Nutrition Clinic of the New York Hospital is instruction of overweight persons in weight-reduction diets. Since there is no obesity clinic or other specialized weight-reduction agency in connection with the hospital, all reducing diets prescribed in every clinic are supervised in the Nutrition Clinic. The obese persons seen in this clinic thus represent a very large per cent and a relatively unbiased sample of the obese patient population of the hospital.

During a 3-month period, one of us (M. M.) interviewed each obese person admitted to the Nutrition Clinic. (Obesity was considered as a body weight which exceeded by 20% the ideal weight for a person of medium build as established by the tables of the Metropolitan Life Insurance Company[11].) Patients were referred from every clinic in the hospital, but the greatest number came from the General Medical Clinic. There was a wide variety of diagnoses in addition to obesity, but the health of most of the patients was good. Ninety-seven of the patients were women, and only three were men. Median age was 45, with a range from 20 to 67, while the median per cent of excess weight was 44, with a range from 21 to 119.

At their initial clinic visit the patients were instructed in balanced weight-reduction diets of from 800 to 1500 Cal. They were seen thereafter at intervals of from 2 to 6 weeks in the Nutrition Clinic, and they also continued treatment for their original complaints in the clinic from which they had been referred. No drug therapy was administered in the Nutrition Clinic, but anorexigenic drugs were prescribed for a few patients in other clinics.

Two and one-half years later the patients' charts were reviewed to determine the outcome of their efforts at weight reduction. The lowest weight reached after the first Nutrition Clinic appointment was considered the therapeutic effect, even though the weight had subsequently increased.

RESULTS OF TREATMENT

The results of treatment in the Nutrition Clinic were even poorer than those reported in the literature. Only 12 of the 100 patients succeeded in losing more than 20 lb at any time during the 2 years, and only one of these was able to lose more than 40 lb. Furthermore, 39 patients did not return to the Nutrition Clinic after their first visit, and, what is even more striking, 28 never returned to any clinic of the hospital. Since admission to the Nutrition Clinic occurs entirely by referral from other clinics, this represents the rupture of at least two therapeutic relationships.

MAINTENANCE OF WEIGHT LOSS

Maintenance of weight loss is even more difficult to appraise than its achievement. Five studies indicate,[5,8,10,13,14] however, that maintenance is no more successful than initial weight loss; a majority of persons regain a majority of the pounds lost. We also found this to be the case. Our results are summarized in Table 2. In this table any person who maintained a weight loss of 20 lb or more is classified as a "success"; any person whose weight was within 19 lb of the starting weight is a "failure". By these criteria, only six persons were still successful 1 year after treatment, and only two persons were successful 2 years after treatment. Four of the nine "failures" had regained all of the weight lost by the time of the 2-year follow-up. Of the remaining five "failures", one had lost a maximum of 51 lb and then had regained 35 of them; one had lost 32 lb and regained 18 of them. Three lost 21 or 22 lb; they regained, respectively, 13, 9, and 6 lb.

TABLE 2. Two-year follow-up of patients who
lost weight*

	Success	Failure	No Information
End of treatment	12	–	–
1 yr. later	6	5	1
2 yr. later	2	9	1

*Study covers 12 patients, in the Nutrition Clinic of New York Hospital, who achieved a 20 lb weight loss during treatment.

ILL EFFECTS OF DIETING

Attention has lately been drawn to the occurrence of emotional disturbances in obese persons in the course of attempts at weight reduction.[1] Such disturbances, occurring in one-third of the obese persons treated in a psychosomatic clinic, are the subject of a more detailed report by one of us.[2] This report, by a psychiatrist, is subject to the criticism that it is based on a highly selected group of patients. The present study permitted us to ascertain more nearly the true incidence of untoward effects of attempts at weight reduction among the obese population as a whole. During the initial interview by the dietitian, each patient was questioned as to any ill effects encountered during her most recent weight-reduction regimen and attributed by her to the regimen. This aspect of the study, then, was retrospective and provided information which is, not strictly comparable to that obtained in its other aspects. No diagnostic formulation of the patient's complaints was attempted, but the presence and the character of the symptoms were recorded.

Of the 100 patients referred for reducing diets, 72 reported that they had attempted dieting previously, several on more than one occasion. Of these 72 patients, 54% reported the presence of symptoms during at least one reducing regimen, and 55% of all such regimens were characterized by the presence of symptoms. The commonest complaints were "nervousness" and "weakness", each reported by 21% of the patients. Less frequent symptoms were "irritability" in 8%, "fatigue" in 5%, and "nausea" in 4%.

No attempt was made to study emotional disturbances which occurred in the course of the treatment prescribed in the Nutrition Clinic. Such information, however, became available during the investigation of four patients who had successfully reduced and had then discontinued treatment. One was a man who achieved the greatest weight loss of the study, from 241 lb to 190 lb. He reported that the reducing regimen had been associated with mounting tension which culminated in what was diagnosed as an acute schizophrenic reaction. He was treated with tranquilizers in a hospital for 4 months and was discharged much improved. He discontinued dieting shortly before hospitalization and gradually regained 35 lb. For the past 2 years his weight has remained stable and he has been in good health.

Evaluation of Possible Indices of Prognosis

In view of the ineffectiveness and ill effects of weight-reduction regimens, knowledge of factors influencing prognosis would be helpful. If it were possible to select in advance those patients most likely to benefit from such regimens, others could be spared suffering and fruitless effort and physicians could concentrate on those in whom their intervention might make the difference between success and failure. Furthermore, such information might provide a basis for differentiating different types of obesity and, ultimately, for understanding the causes of this disorder.

In the present study four factors were investigated for their usefulness as indices of prognosis. They were (1) sex of the patient, (2) presence of the "night-eating syndrome", (3) the outcome of previous attempts at weight reduction, and (4) response to the Taylor Test for Manifest Anxiety. Only the first of these indices, the sex of the patient, seemed of predictive value.

SEX OF THE PATIENT

Sex of the patient has not, to our knowledge, been previously suggested as a possible factor in the success of efforts at weight reduction. We were, therefore, surprised to discover that whenever results of treatment have been reported according to the sex of the patient, men have been shown to be more successful than women. These results, together with those of the present study, are summarized in Table 3.[4,9] It will be noted that in each study a far higher percentage of men than women were able to achieve the modest success of a 20 lb weight loss. These differences are significant at the 2% level (Feinstein), the 7% level (Munves), and the 2% level (present series), as determined by direct calculation of probability.

TABLE 3. Relation of sex of patient to outcome of attempts at weight reduction*

	Feinstein et al.		Munves		Present series	
	Success	Failure	Success	Failure	Success	Failure
Men	10	1	5	15	2	1
Women	50	45	1	27	10	87

*"Success" is defined here, as elsewhere in this report, as a 20 lb weight loss.

The discrepancy between results of treatment for men and for women is even more pronounced if 40 lb is considered as a criterion of success. Sixty-eight per cent of the men in Feinstein's report lost 40 lb as compared with 28% of the women. Furthermore, the only four subjects in Munves' study to lose 40 lb and the only one in the present study who lost this much, were all men. It is worthy of note that these differences are not a result of differences in age, per cent overweight, or pounds overweight between the men and the women.

A fourth study[12] reported in a somewhat different manner, also found men to be more successful than women in attempts at weight reduction. The mean percentage of excess weight lost by a group of 13 men was 46%, as compared with a value of 34% for 97 women.

THE NIGHT-EATING SYNDROME

A previous report has described a peculiar pattern of food intake characterized by morning anorexia, evening hyperphagia, and insomnia.[15] This "night-eating syndrome", which appears to be confined to obese persons, was found in 66% of those attending a psychosomatic clinic. Attempts at weight reduction by persons manifesting the syndrome were usually unsuccessful. An attempt was made to determine if this were also true of a less carefully selected population.

The results of the present study gave no support to the expectation that the night-eating syndrome might be of value in predicting inability to lose weight. Although 12 of the 14 persons manifesting the syndrome were indeed unsuccessful, 2 succeeded in losing more than 20 lb. This rate of failure is no higher than that among persons free of the syndrome.

There are at least two possible explanations of this finding. Presence of the night-eating syndrome may, indeed, be of no relevance to the outcome of attempts at weight reduction. On the other hand, the low incidence of persons manifesting the night-eating syndrome and of those successful in losing weight makes it unlikely that any but the closest association could be demonstrated.

OUTCOME OF PREVIOUS ATTEMPTS AT WEIGHT REDUCTION

It has been suggested that previous successful weight reduction increases the probability of successful weight reduction in any later effort, and, conversely, that failures in previous attempts bode ill for further trials.[16] No support for this hypothesis was obtained.

TABLE 4. Relation of outcome of previous attempts at weight reduction to outcome of current attempt*

	Previous outcome			
Current Outcome	Success	Failure	No attempt	Total
Success	2	8	2	12
Failure	14	32	14	60
Did not return	7	9	12	28
Total	23	49	28	100

*It will be noted that previous success or failure is not predictive of the outcome of later attempts at weight reduction.

Table 4 reveals that of the 23 persons who had reported any previous dietary success, only 2 were able to lose 20 lb. On the other hand, of the 49 who had failed in all previous attempts at weight reduction, 8 were successful in this one. The results were thus the antithesis of those predicted by the hypothesis: probability of success was actually slightly higher for persons with previous dietary failure.

TAYLOR TEST FOR MANIFEST ANXIETY

It is widely believed that emotional disturbances contribute to the pathogenesis of obesity as well as to the failure of attempts at weight reduction. An effort was made, therefore, to determine if an index of emotional disturbance could predict the outcome of attempts at weight reduction. For this purpose the Taylor Test for Manifest Anxiety was administered to each patient during the initial visit to the Nutrition Clinic. This test is a 50-item true–false questionnaire comprising those items of the Minnesota Multiphasic Personality Inventory which deal with manifest, or free, anxiety[17] One point is scored for each response indicating the presence of anxiety; the higher the score, the greater the anxiety. We postulated that subjects with higher scores should have a poorer prognosis for weight reduction. A corollary hypothesis, deriving from the purported relationship of emotional disturbances and obesity, was that obese persons should show higher scores than normal controls.

Only the corollary hypothesis was validated. The mean score of the 100 obese persons was 18.0±9.5. This contrasts with scores of 15.3±7.9 and 15.9±7.5 for two control groups of 750 and 414 subjects respectively,[18] a difference significant at the 1% level. These obese persons appear to show greater anxiety than normal, as anxiety is measured by the Taylor test. The test was not, however, predictive of the outcome of attempts at weight reduction. The subjects who reduced successfully actually had higher anxiety scores than those who failed, although the difference did not approach statistical significance.

Comment

In recent years the ill effects ascribed to excessive body weight have received wide attention, as have the benefits to be achieved by weight reduction. As a result many physicians and their patients, who had formerly looked upon weight reduction as a cosmetic conceit, have come to consider it a therapeutic imperative. A variety of lay institutions, notably the magazines for women, have seized upon this growing interest in weight reduction and have helped to magnify it to the proportions of a national neurosis. The influences responsible for this unfortunate development are not fully understood. The medical profession, however, must accept some responsibility. For underlying the extravagances of the miracle diets and the reducing salons are certain widely held medical attitudes.

Many years ago detailed metabolic studies demonstrated that human beings do not defy the second law of thermodynamics and that excessive body fat results from an excess of caloric intake over caloric expenditure. This not unreasonable finding was thereupon enshrined as the dictum that "all obesity comes from overeating", and the treatment of obesity lost its glamour. The physician's job, it seemed, was simply to explain that semistarvation reduces fat stores, to prescribe a diet for this purpose, and to sit by. If the patient lost weight as predicted, this merely confirmed the comfortable feeling that treatment of obesity was really a pretty simple matter. However, if, as so often happened, the patient failed to lose weight, he was dismissed as uncooperative or chastized as gluttonous. It was the rare physician who entertained the possibility that failure to follow a regimen might in itself be a medical problem. Rarely have physicians so readily surrendered a part of their domain to moralizing, indifference, and despair.

What have been the consequences of this surrender? First, the naive optimism of the medical profession about treatment for obesity has been widely accepted by the lay public. Most obese persons feel that they should be able to lose large amounts of weight in a short time and with little discomfort. When they find that these expectations are not realized and when they encounter the irritation of their physicians over this failure, they turn to any agency which promises results. The profusion of nonmedical agencies testifies to the extent of our patients' needs and to the magnitude of our failings.

How may the medical profession regain its proper role in the treatment of obesity? We can begin by looking at the situation as it exists and not as we would like it to be. We can acknowledge that treatment for obesity is a terribly difficult business, one in which our experts achieve only modest success, and the rest of us, even less. It is a treatment which can be fraught with danger, a treatment not to be undertaken lightly by any obese person and by some perhaps not at all. Certainly weight reduction is not a matter to be left to unqualified practitioners.

Lowering our level of aspiration may be far toward achieving our aims. If we do not expect weight reduction as a matter of course we may be able to accord due recognition to success. If we do not feel obliged to excuse our failures we may be able to investigate them. Learning to respect the complexities of their illnesses will help us to respect our patients. And the patient who has the respect of his physician has little reason to seek elsewhere for treatment.

Summary

A review of the literature on outpatient treatment for obesity reveals that the ambiguity of reported results has obscured the relative ineffectiveness of such treatment. When the per cent of patients losing 20 and 40 lb is used as a criterion of success, the reports of the last 30 years show remarkably similar results. Although the subjects of these reports are grossly overweight persons, only 25% were able to lose as much as 20 lb and only 5% lost 40 lb.

Routine treatment of 100 consecutive obese outpatients in the Nutrition Clinic of a large teaching hospital was even less successful. Only 12% were able to lose 20 lb and only 1 patient lost 40 lb. Furthermore, 28% of the patients never returned to either the Nutrition Clinic or the referring clinic after their first visit. Two years after the end of treatment only two patients had maintained their weight loss.

A search for criteria which might aid in predicting the outcome of attempts at weight reduction revealed only one: Men appear to be more successful than women.

Hospital of the University of Pennsylvania, Functional Disease Service, 3400 Spruce St. (4).

References

1. Bruch, H. *The Importance of Overweight*, New York, W. W. Norton & Company, Inc., 1957.
2. Stunkard, A. J.: The "Dieting Depression". *Am. J. Med.* **23**, 77-86, 1957.
3. Evans, F. A. Treatment of Obesity with Low Calorie Diets: Report of 121 Additional Cases. *Internat. Clin.* **3**, 19-23, 1938.
4. Feinstein, R., Dole, V. P., and Schwartz, I. L. The Use of a Formula Diet for Weight Reduction of Obese Out-patients. *Ann. Int. Med.* **48**, 330-343, 1958.
5. Fellows, H. H. Studies of Relatively Normal Obese Individuals During and After Dietary Restriction. *Am. J. M. Sc.* **181**, 301-312, 1931.
6. Gray, H. and Kallenbach, D. C. Obesity Treatment: Results on 212 Outpatients. *J. Am. Dietet. A,* **15**; 239-245, 1939.
7. Harvey, H. L. and Simmons, W. D. Weight Reduction: A study of the Group Method. *Am. J. M. Sc.* **227**, 521-525, 1954.
8. McCann, M. and Trulson, M. F. Long-term Effect of Weight-reducing Programs. *J. Am. Dietet. A,* **31**, 1108-1110, 1955.
9. Munves, E. D. Dietetic Interview or Group Discussion-decision in Reducing? *J. Am. Dietet. A,* **29**, 1197-1203, 1953.
10. Osserman, K. E. and Dolger, H. O. Obesity in Diabetes: a Study of Therapy with Anorexigenic Drugs. *Ann. Int. Med.* **34**, 72-79, 1951.
11. Cecil, R. L. and Loeb, R. F. *et al.. A Textbook of Medicine*, Ed. 9, Philadelphia, W. B. Saunders Co., 1955.
12. Young, C. M., Moore, N. S., Berresford, K., Einset, B. M., and Waldner, B. G. The Problem of the Obese Patient. *J. Am. Dietet. A,* **31**, 1111-1115, 1955.
13. Dole, V. P., Schwartz, I. L., Thaysen, J. H., Thorn, N. A., and Silver, L. Treatment of Obesity with a Low-protein, Calorically-unrestricted Diet. *Am. J. Clin. Nutrition* **2**, 381-390, 1954.
14. Rony, L. *Obesity and Leanness*, Philadelphia, Lea & Febiger, 1931.
15. Stunkard, A. J., Grace, W. J., and Wolff, H. G. The Night-eating Syndrome. *Am. J. Med.* **19**, 78-86, 1955.
16. Stunkard, A. J. and Reader, J. The Management of Obesity. *New York J. Med.* **58**, 78-87, 1958.
17. Taylor, J. A. A Personality Scale of Manifest Anxiety. *J. Abnorm. & Social Psychol.* **48**, 285-290, 1953.
18. Bechtoldt, H. P. Personal communication to the authors.

CHAPTER 4

A Review of Behavioral Approaches to Weight Control[1]

EDWARD E. ABRAMSON

California State University, Chico, U.S.A.

Summary—Forty case reports and experimental studies of behavioral approaches to weight control were reviewed. The treatments, categorized as: aversive conditioning, covert sensitization, coverant conditioning, therapist controlled reinforcement and self-control of eating, were evaluated in terms of their empirical support. It was suggested that self-control procedures may be the most promising treatment, particularly when used in conjunction with therapist controlled reinforcement. Methodological difficulties and implications for future research were discussed.

It has been estimated that there are currently between 40 and 80 million obese individuals in the U.S. alone (Stuart and Davis, 1972). The magnitude of the problem has led the U.S. Public Health Service to classify obesity as "one of the most prevalent health problems in the United States today" (U.S. Public Health Service, undated). Traditional treatments for this problem have included medication (e.g. Penick, 1970), psychotherapy (e.g. Bruch, 1957) and therapeutic starvation (e.g. Swanson and Dinello, 1969). Several hundred published reports of outpatient treatment for obesity were reviewed by Stunkard and McLaren-Hume (1959). Taken together, the eight studies that met their criteria for acceptable research design indicated that only 25 per cent of the grossly obese were able to lose 20 lb, while fewer than 5 per cent lost 40 lb or more. The discouraging outcomes of traditional treatments have been summarized by Stunkard (1958): "Most obese persons will not remain in treatment. Of those that remain in treatment, most will not lose weight, and of those who do lose weight, most will regain it" (p. 79).

Recently, attention has focused upon behavioral approaches to weight reduction. The purpose of the present article will be to review the various behavioral treatments, evaluate their empirical support and suggest possible directions for future research.

A variety of behavioral techniques have been applied to the problem of obesity. Although many of the studies to be reviewed make use of several

Reprinted with permission from *Behaviour Research and Therapy*, 1973, 11, 547-556.

[1] An abbreviated version of this paper was presented at the meeting of the Western Psychological Association, Anaheim, California, April 1973.

procedures, for the sake of convenience the treatments can be categorized as: aversive conditioning, covert sensitization, coverant conditioning, therapist reinforcement of weight loss, and self-control of eating. For each treatment, case reports and experimental studies will be reviewed.

AVERSIVE CONDITIONING

Moss (1924) provided one of the first examples of aversive conditioning used to modify eating behavior. After several trials in which a clicking noise was paired with vinegar consumption, the single S rejected orange juice when it was presented with the clicking noise.

Electric shock has been used by several investigators in the treatment of obesity. Wolpe (1954) paired shock with images of desirable foods, Meyer and Crisp (1964) with approach to temptation foods, and Thorpe et al. (1964) with verbalizations of a stimulus word ('overeating'). Three of the four Ss did not remain in treatment (Wolpe's died from unrelated causes), while the fourth exhibited a considerable weight loss which was maintained for at least 20 months.

Kennedy and Foreyt (1968) paired the smells of desirable foods with the noxious odor of butyric acid. Although S lost 30 lb, treatment had the effect of increasing consumption of non-target foods; the reported weight loss was attributed to other techniques (e.g. increased exercise). In an experimental study, the authors (Foreyt and Kennedy, 1971) compared the effectiveness of this treatment with a control procedure. Experimental Ss averaged a 13-lb weight loss which was significantly greater than 1 lb loss of control Ss. Although a 48-week follow-up revealed that experimental Ss maintained an average loss of 9 lb the authors felt that the relationship that developed with the therapist was "vital in achieving the initial weight loss" (p. 33).

Stollak (1967) compared the effectiveness of an aversive conditioning technique similar to Wolpe's with two control and three treatment groups. The aversive treatment did not result in significant weight loss after 8 weeks of treatment.

It appears safe to conclude that despite some early enthusiasm, there is little evidence to indicate that aversive procedures are an effective treatment for obesity. The reported outcomes of the case studies are equivocal, at best. The most optimistic conclusion that can be drawn from the two experimental studies is that ". . . combined with other procedures it may help the patient lose weight more easily . . ." (Foreyt and Kennedy, 1971, p. 33).

COVERT SENSITIZATION

In two early articles describing covert sensitization, Cautela (1966, 1967) presents the rationale and procedures used in the application of this technique to the treatment of obesity. Typically, the patient is taught to relax, and the therapist vividly presents scenes in which the patient approaches forbidden foods, becomes nauseous and vomits. Interdispersed with these scenes are scenes in which the patient approached the target food, felt nauseous, retreated and immediately felt a sense of relief. Fortunately, Cautela notes that there is no generalization of treatment response to acceptable eating behavior. More recently, Cautela (1972) outlined a treatment program for overeating which adds covert reinforcement to the covert sensitization program.

In the first experimental test of covert sensitization, Meynen (1970) compared the effects of eight weekly group covert sensitization sessions with a modified systematic desensitization treatment, a relaxation treatment and a control group. All treatments resulted in significant weight losses, however there were no significant differences between treatments. Negative findings were also reported by Lick and Bootzin (1971). Two covert sensitization groups (differing in the explanations for treatment that were given *S*s) were compared to a no-treatment control. While all groups exhibited weight losses, the authors judged the losses to be trivial. Furthermore, no relationship was found between discomfort during treatment and weight loss. The authors note, however, that some *S*s changed their food preferences but did not lose weight because of their increased consumption of non-target foods.

More encouraging results were reported by Janda and Rimm (1972) and Manno and Marston (1972). Janda and Rimm compared covert sensitization to a no-treatment control and a placebo treatment. At a 6-week follow-up, the covert sensitization group showed a mean loss of 11.7 lb, which was significantly greater than the two other groups. Unlike the Lick and Bootzin (1971) study, a significant relationship ($r = 0.53$) between subjective distress and weight loss was found. This would suggest that the covert conditioning, rather than non-specific factors was responsible for the weight reduction. Manno and Marston found that both covert sensitization and covert reinforcement treatments were significantly more effective than a minimal treatment group, although the two covert treatments produced similar weight losses.

Several investigators have attempted to assess the relative importance of the various component factors in covert sensitization. Manno (1972) compared five treatments, including two that made use of covert imagery without aversive scenes. These treatments were significantly more effective than the typical covert sensitization treatments which made use of aversion. Sachs and Ingram (1972) found that backward conditioning (*S*s visualized unpleasant scenes first, then the target food) was as effective as forward conditioning; both treatments resulted in significant decrements in consumption of target foods. The results were interpreted as suggesting that motivational factors, rather than aversive conditioning are responsible for the effectiveness of covert sensitization.

Despite some favorable outcomes with covert sensitization, several difficulties must be considered. Of the studies reporting actual weight losses, the largest was an average of 11.7 lb. More typically, losses averaged between 4 and 5 lb. These findings may be partially explained by the tendency of some Ss to increase consumption of non-target foods while decreasing consumption of target foods. Since the effects of covert sensitization are very specific (Cautela, 1967) the therapeutic application of this technique conceivably could require conditioning a wide range of foods.

If covert sensitization is viewed as a technique for reducing consumption of specific problematic foods or decreasing eating in specific situations, it would be reasonable to assess its efficacy by measuring consumption of target foods rather than weight loss. By this criterion, it is probably a success, although the reason why is still unclear. It appears unlikely however, that covert sensitization used exclusively will result in the modification of generalized patterns of inappropriate eating.

COVERANT CONDITIONING

In an article presenting the technique and rationale for coverant control, Homme (1965) describes its applicability to weight control. Essentially, coverant conditioning is an extension of the Premack Principle (Premack, 1965) to private mental events. Thus low probability thoughts (or covert operants, coverants) which are incompatible with eating are reinforced by high probability behavior. Studies reported by Tyler and Straughan (1970) and Horan and Johnson (1971) yielded discouraging results. The utility of coverant conditioning for the treatment of obesity remains to be demonstrated.

THERAPIST REINFORCEMENT OF WEIGHT LOSS

In an early case study, Ayllon (1963) described a straightforward environmental manipulation which resulted in a significant weight loss on the part of an institutionalized psychotic. Treatment consisted of removing S from the dining room when she approached tables other than her own or when she picked up unauthorized food. Following the elimination of food stealing (after 2 weeks) Ss weight gradually declined to 180 lb, a 17 per cent loss from her original weight. Two later case studies demonstrated the treatment of obesity within the context of a token economy (Bernard, 1968; Upper and Newton, 1971). In both studies Ss were placed on a restricted diet and were reinforced for weight loss with tokens and social approval. Similar procedures were used by Moore and Crum (1969) with a schizophrenic patient in a traditional psychiatric institution, and by Dinoff, Rickard and Colwick (1972) with a 10-yr-old emotionally disturbed boy attending a summer camp. All of the case reports indicated that significant weight loss was accomplished.

In the first experimental study of therapist reinforcement of weight loss, Harmatz and Lapuc (1968) compared the effectiveness of behavior modification, group therapy and diet-only treatments using 21 hospitalized schizophrenic males. Behavior modification Ss were deprived of a portion of their $5.00

weekly allotment if they did not exhibit a weight loss at the weekly weighing. At the end of 6 weeks the group therapy and behavior modification groups had lost significantly 'more weight than the control group, although there was no difference between these two treatments. However, a follow-up 4 weeks later revealed that the behavior modification group weighed less than the other two groups, which did not differ significantly.

Therapist controlled reinforcement presents practical problems when applied outside of an institutional setting. In typical outpatient treatment, the therapist may be able to control reinforcing contingencies for one hour per week. Tighe and Elliott (1968) described a technique involving threatened loss of money as a method of establishing therapist controlled reinforcers in the natural environment. Although the authors applied the technique to modifying smoking behavior, they suggested that it could be applied to overeating and other undesirable behavior.

In a single subject, reversal design experiment, Mann (1972) evaluated a program in which personal possessions (e.g. clothes and money) were surrendered to *E* to be used as reinforcers. A contract was signed which specified *S*s terminal weight reduction goal as well as the number of pounds to be lost during each 2 week period during the study. All eight *S*s maintained or increased their weight during the baseline, lost weight during the first treatment period, regained weight during the reversal period, and finally lost weight during the second treatment period. A second experiment was conducted which revealed that the punishing contingencies (i.e. permanently losing personal possessions) were an essential component of treatment. Although treatment was successful (five *S*s reached their goal, the remaining *S*s achieved reductions ranging from 40 to 70 per cent of their goal) there were several problems. Since the target was weight, rather than actual eating behavior, several *S*s made use of extreme measures such as taking laxatives or diuretics to promote rapid weight loss. No follow-up data were reported, and hence the long-term effects of treatment are unknown. However, an indication of the long-term effects of this type of treatment was provided by Jeffrey *et al.* (1972). Although the four *S*s in this study exhibited a mean weight loss of 27 lbs by the end of treatment, at the 6 month follow-up one *S* returned to his baseline weight, while a second regained 14 of the 32 lb he had lost.

While the application of therapist reinforcement is relatively straightforward in an institutional setting, outpatient treatment may present problems. Unless the therapist is willing to assume the costs of reinforcers, the requirement that patients surrender possessions prior to treatment may have the effect of excluding potential patients lacking the necessary affluence, motivation or both. Of greater importance is the question of the long-term effects of treatment. Specific eating behavior is not modified directly, only weight losses are reinforced. Presumably, for treatment to result in permanent change, *S*s have to devise their own techniques for altering eating patterns. If these techniques are aversive to *S*s, the reinforcers occurring in the natural environment may not be sufficient to maintain the loss after treatment has concluded. The follow-up data reported by Jeffrey *et al.* (1972) strongly suggest that for some *S*s, natural reinforcers are inadequate to maintain the reduction.

SELF-CONTROL OF EATING

The first behavioral self-control program for overeating was described by Ferster *et al.* (1962). It was theorized that the act of putting food into one's mouth is reinforced by its immediate pleasurable consequences, while the negative consequences (i.e. getting fat) are postponed to some indefinite time in the future. The goal of treatment, then, was to make the negative consequences more immediate so that they would become more potent as determinants of eating behavior.

The early group sessions were devoted to training the participants to accurately record their food consumption, and reviewing the unpleasant consequences of their obesity. Suggestions were offered for environmental manipulations intended to promote the acquisition of self-control. Although the results of treatment were not reported, Ferster was later quoted by Penick *et al.* (1971) as characterizing the outcome as 'disappointing'. Goldiamond (1965) presented a similar rationale for a self-control treatment with a brief illustrative example.

Stuart (1967) reported the results of a program similar to that of Ferster *et al.* (1962). The program, comprised of between 19 and 41 sessions, was outlined in detail and impressive treatment results for eight female patients were provided. In subsequent reports Stuart (1971; Stuart and Davis, 1972) expanded his program to include dietary planning and increased energy expenditure.

Three experimental studies demonstrated the effectiveness of self-control procedures in treating obesity. In the first, Harris (1969) compared a no-treatment control with a behavioral group treatment comprised of three techniques: training *S*s to reinforce themselves for appropriate eating behavior, reducing the number of stimuli eliciting eating and lengthening the chain of responses involved in eating (e.g. chewing food slowly and taking short breaks during meals). After 2.5 months, experimental *S*s were divided into two groups for a continuation of group treatment or individual covert sensitization sessions. The results indicated significant differences between treatment and control groups and between sexes (men lost more than women) but no additional weight loss could be attributed to covert sensitization.

In the most thoroughly controlled study, Wollersheim (1970) compared three group treatments (behavioral self-control, positive expectation-social pressure, and non-specific therapy) with a no-treatment control. *S*s in the behavioral group were taught deep muscle relaxation to be used in situations where tension would have typically resulted in eating, and discussed their food consumption records in order to provide a functional analysis of their eating behavior. The functional analysis included the development of stimulus control of eating, self-reinforcement for control of eating and establishing alternative behavior incompatible with eating. The positive expectation-social pressure treatment was an attempt to replicate the procedures of weight reduction clubs such as TOPS, while the non-specific therapy was devoted to the discussion of 'underlying motives' and 'personality make-up' that are related to obesity. Although Ss in all three treatment groups lost significantly more than controls, *post hoc* comparisons revealed that the behavioral treatment was more effective than the other treatments. Sixty-one per cent of the behavioral group lost 9 lb or more as contrasted with 6 per cent of the controls, 25 per cent of the social pressure group and 40 per cent of the non-specific treatment group. At the 8-week follow-up 50 per cent of the behavioral Ss still met this criterion.

Penick *et al.* (1971) contrasted the effectiveness of a group behavioral treatment with traditional group therapy. Unlike earlier studies, experimenter expectancy (Rosenthal, 1966) was partially controlled by using therapists who strongly believed in the procedures they were using. The behavioral treatment (similar to that of Stuart, 1967) resulted in weight losses significantly greater than those produced by the traditional group treatment, although within treatment variability was greater for the former group.

Studies comparing therapist controlled reinforcement with self-control procedures were conducted by Harris and Bruner (1971) and Hall (1972). In the first of two experiments reported by Harris and Bruner both the self-control and the therapist reinforcement treatments resulted in significant weight losses; the therapist reinforcement procedure being significantly more effective. However, a 10-month follow-up revealed no significant differences between pre-treatment and follow-up weight for any group. The second experiment was originally intended to be a replication of the first, however, all Ss assigned to the therapist reinforcement group refused to participate. There was no difference in weight loss between the two remaining groups (self-control and attention placebo). The authors note that the lack of positive findings may be partially attributed to the extremely sporadic attendance of Ss.

Using a single subject, cross-over design, Hall (1972) compared self-control and therapist reinforcement treatments. Fourteen female Ss received 5 weeks of each treatment. Unlike previous studies of therapist reinforcement, the therapist supplied the reinforcement ($20.00). This treatment resulted in weight losses averaging 1 lb per week while the self-control treatment was judged to be relatively ineffectual. In contrasting her results with those of similar studies, the author notes that her self-control procedures achieved results comparable to those of Harris (1969) but somewhat lower than those reported by Stuart (1967) and Wollersheim (1970). It was suggested that the comparatively poor showing of self-control may have been due to age differences (Hall's Ss were older), the short duration of treatment or variations in treatment techniques.

Jeffrey and Christensen (1972) combined therapist controlled reinforcement with self-control techniques and compared the results with no-treatment control and "will power" groups. Ss in the experimental group completing treatment lost an average of 16.31 lbs, while "will power" and control Ss lost 5.09 and 1.70 lb respectively. The losses of the behavioral group were maintained 12 weeks after treatment. The results compare favorably with earlier studies (e.g. Penick *et al.*, 1971) despite the comparatively modest amount of patient contact (14 vs. 54 hr).

Finally, Hagen (1970) compared the effectiveness of a no-treatment control with a group treatment using Wollersheim's (1970) group procedures, a no-contact bibliotherapeutic treatment using Wollersheim's materials and a combination of both treatments. All treatments were significantly more effective than the control, but did not differ significantly from each other thus suggesting that bibliotherapy may be as effective as group treatment.

Discussion

Although two of the studies cited above reported discouraging results using self-control procedures, the preponderance of favorable outcomes suggests that this approach may hold the most promise. Unlike therapist controlled reinforcement, specific skills are taught to control eating behavior. Unlike covert sensitization, the target is a broad range of eating behavior rather than specific foods or situations. Unfortunately, self-control is also unlike the other two treatments in that the therapist merely presents a series of suggestions to the patient. The degree to which the patient makes use of the various suggestions is likely to be a function of non-specific and extra-therapeutic factors operating during treatment. It is suggested that the addition of therapist controlled reinforcement would increase the likelihood of the newly learned self-control techniques being implemented. The findings of Jeffrey and Christensen (1972) suggest, if nothing else, that the combination of procedures results in a more efficient treatment program. Likewise, it is suggested that covert sensitization appears to have some utility in helping patients to deal with particularly difficult eating behavior (Stuart, 1967).

While the studies previously cited justify cautious optimism, several problems become apparent. On the most basic level, much of the methodology used by investigators in this field has been inadequate. Many of Bernstein's (1969) criticisms of smoking research are equally applicable to obesity research (e.g. lack of controls for experimenter bias). Jeffrey (1972) identified several additional methodological problems that characterize obesity research. Criteria for determining improvement following treatment are too diverse to permit direct comparisons between studies. The criteria used have included mean weight loss, percentage of Ss losing more than a predetermined amount, and average weekly weight loss. Furthermore, the reported statistical significance of treatment outcomes is no guarantee of clinical utility. For example, an average weight loss slightly greater than 4 lb resulted from Manno and Marston's (1972) covert sensitization treatments. Although this was significantly greater than control group weight losses, it is hardly an impressive amount. Other problems include different methods of dealing with data from *S*s who drop out prior to the completion of treatment and the frequent failure to provide follow-ups.

Further progress will require that future research move beyond the demonstration stage. Specifically, it is suggested that future research should be directed towards devising methods for predicting success in treatment. Several investigators (e.g. Wollersheim, 1970; Jeffrey and Christensen, 1972) have attempted to use various psychometric instruments for this purpose, generally without much success. The non-behavioral literature may offer worthwhile leads for developing prediction strategies. For example, it has been demonstrated (Glucksman and Hirsch, 1968; Glucksman *et al.*, 1968; Grinker *et al.*, 1973) that the age of onset of obesity may determine the affective responses to weight reduction. It could be hypothesized that the success of behavioral treatment may also be affected by this variable.

Additional factors that may influence treatment outcome include sex, age and external source of reinforcement. The majority of studies reviewed used female *S*s exclusively. The findings reported by Harris (1969) suggest that further research exploring sex differences in response to treatment would be warranted. Likewise, Hall's (1972) results point to the possible effects of age as a determinant of treatment effectiveness. Finally, Stuart (1972) noted that his treatment program is rarely successful if the patient's family does not provide sufficient reinforcement to take the place of the gratification associated with eating. In light of these findings, it is suggested that future research should consider some or all of these variables as possible predictors of success in treatment.

Another problem that warrants further investigation relates to the role of the therapist. The two studies making use of no-contact bibliotherapy (*S*s were given self-control literature and told to apply the techniques by themselves) yielded conflicting results. Hagen (1970) found that this approach was as effective as a group self-control treatment, while Jeffrey and Christensen (1972) reported insignificant weight losses for their "will power" (i.e. bibliotherapy) group. However, in the latter study it was noted that successful *S*s in this group were significantly more internal (Rotter, 1966) than unsuccessful *S*s. In light of the potential benefits of this type of program, research devoted to the development of selection criteria for participation in bibliotherapy would be worthwhile.

A final consideration is suggested by the findings of the extensive research program conducted by Schachter (1971). In several ingenious studies he provides evidence to demonstrate that obese individuals regulate their food consumption on the basis of external cognitive and social cues rather than the internal physiological cues (e.g. gastric motility and hypoglycemia) that determine the eating behavior of normals. While there has been some reluctance on the part of behavior therapists to investigate problems couched in terms of cognition, Ullmann (1970), among others, has suggested that activities called cognitions can be dealt with in the same manner as other behavior. It is suggested therefore that future research might be profitably directed towards the modification of the externality of obese individuals' food consumption.

In summary, it has been demonstrated that several behavioral procedures are effective in treating obesity, at least on a short-term basis. It is suggested that future research, making use of standardized criteria, should attempt to assess the long term effects of treatment and predict which treatment will be effective for a given individual. It is further suggested that behavioral treatments be expanded to include the direct modification of the externality of obese individuals.

References

AYLLON, T. (1963) Intensive treatment of psychotic behavior by stimulus satiation and food reinforcement. *Behav. Res. & Therapy* 1, 53–61.

BERNARD, J. L. (1968) Rapid treatment of gross obesity by operant techniques. *Psychol. Rep.* 23, 663–666.

BERNSTEIN, D. A. (1969) Modification of smoking behavior: an evaluative review. *Psychol. Bull.* 71, 418–440.

BRUCH, H. (1957) *The Importance of Overweight.* W. W. Norton, New York.

CAUTELA J. R. (1966) Treatment of compulsive behavior by covert sensitization. *Psychol. Rec.* 16, 33–41.

CAUTELA, J. R. (1967) Covert sensitization. *Psychol. Rep.* 20, 459–468.

CAUTELA, J. R. (1972) The treatment of over-eating by covert conditioning. *Psychotherapy: Theory, Research and Practice* 9, 211–216.

DINOFF, M., RICKARD, H. C., and COLWICK, J. (1972) Weight reduction through successive contracts. *Am. J. Orthopsychiat.* 42, 110–113.

FERSTER, C. B., NURNBERGER, J. I., and LEVITT, E. E. (1962) The control of eating. *J. Mathetics* 1, 87–109.

FOREYT, J. P. and KENNEDY, W. A. (1971) Treatment of overweight by aversion therapy. *Behav. Res. & Therapy* 9, 29–34.

GLUCKSMAN, M. L. and HIRSCH, J. (1968) The response of obese patients to weight reduction: a clinical evaluation of behavior. *Psychosom. Med.* 30, 1–11.

GLUCKSMAN, M. L., HIRSCH, J., McCULLY, R. S., BARRON, B. A. and KNITTLE, J. L. (1968) The response of obese patients to weight reduction: II. A quantitative evaluation of behavior. *Psychosom. Med.* 30, 359–373.

GOLDIAMOND, I. (1965) Self-control procedures in personal behavior problems. *Psychol. Rep.* 17, 851–868.

GRINKER, J., HIRSCH, J. and LEVIN, B. (1973) The affective responses of obese patients to weight reduction: a differentiation based on age at onset of obesity. *Psychosom. Med.* 35, 57–63.

HAGEN, R. L. (1970) Group therapy versus bibliotherapy in weight reduction. *Diss. Abstr. Int.* 31(5-B), 2985–2986 (Abstract).

HALL, S. M. (1972) Self-control and therapist control in the behavioral treatment of overweight women, *Behav. Res. & Therap.* 10, 59–68.

HARMATZ, M. G. and LAPUC, P. (1968) Behavior modification of overeating in a Psychiatric population. *J. Consult. Clin. Psychol.* 32, 583–587.

HARRIS, M. B. (1969) Self-directed program for weight control: a pilot study. *J. Abnorm. Psychol.* 74, 263–270.

HARRIS, M. B. and BRUNER, C. G. (1971) A comparison of a self-control and a contract procedure for weight control. *Behav. Res. & Therapy* 9, 347–354.

HOMME, L. E. (1965) Perspectives in psychology: XXIV. Control of coverants, the operants of the mind. *Psychol. Rec.* 15, 501–511.

HORAN, J. J. and JOHNSON, R. G. (1971) Coverant conditioning through a self-management application of the Premack Principle: Its effect on weight reduction. *J. Behav. Therapy Exp. Psychiat.* 2, 243-249.

JANDA, L. H. and RIMM, D. C. (1972) Covert sensitization in the treatment of obesity. *J. Abnorm. Psychol.* 80, 37–42.

JEFFREY, D. B. (1972) Some methodological issues in obesity research. Paper presented at the meeting of the Association for Advancement of Behavior Therapy, New York.

JEFFREY, D. B. and CHRISTENSEN, E. R. (1972) The relative efficacy of behavior therapy, will power and no-treatment control procedures for weight loss. Paper presented at the meeting of the Association for Advancement of Behavior Therapy, New York.

JEFFREY, D. B., CHRISTENSEN, E. R. and PAPPAS, J. P. (1972) A case study report of a behavioral modification weight reduction group: treatment and Follow-up. (Research and Development Report No. 33) University of Utah Counseling Center, Salt Lake City, Utah.

KENNEDY, W. A. and FOREYT, J. P. (1968) Control of eating behavior in an obese patient by avoidance conditioning. *Psychol. Rep.* 22, 571–576.

LICK, J. and BOOTZIN, R. (1971) Covert sensitization for the treatment of obesity. Paper presented at the meeting of the Midwestern Psychological Association, Detroit, Michigan.

MANN, R. A. (1972) The behavior-therapeutic use of contingency contracting to control an adult behavior problem: Weight control. *J. Appl. Behav. Anal.* 5, 99–109.

MANNO, B. (1972) Weight reduction as a function of the timing of reinforcement in a covert aversive conditioning paradigm. *Diss. Abstr. Int.* 32(7-B), 4221 (Abstract).

MANNO, B. and MARSTON, A. R. (1972) Weight reduction as a function of negative covert reinforcement (sensitization) versus positive covert reinforcement. *Behav. Res. & Therapy* 10, 201–207.

MEYER, V. and CRISP, A. H. (1964) Aversion therapy in two cases of obesity. *Behav. Res. & Therapy* 2, 143–147.

MEYNEN, G. E. (1970) A comparative study of three treatment approaches with the obese: relaxation, covert sensitization and modified systematic desensitization. *Diss. Abstr. Int.* 31(5-B), 2998 (Abstract).

MOORE, C. H. and CRUM, B. C. (1969) Weight reduction in a chronic schizophrenic by means of operant conditioning procedures: a case study. *Behav. Res. & Therapy* 7, 129–131.

MOSS, F. A. (1924) Note on building likes and dislikes in children. *J. Exp. Psychol.* 7, 475–478.

PENICK, S. B. (1970) The use of amphetamines in obesity. *Psychiatric Opinion* 1, 27–30.

PENICK, S. B., FILION, R., FOX, S. and STUNKARD, A. J. (1971) Behavior modification in the treatment of obesity. *Psychosom. Med.* 33, 49–55.

PREMACK, D. (1965) Reinforcement theory. In *Nebraska Symposium on Motivation* (Ed. D. LEVINE), University of Nebraska Press, Lincoln, Neb.

ROSENTHAL, R. (1966) *Experimenter Effects in Behavior Research*, Appleton–Century–Crofts, New York.

ROTTER, J. B. (1966) Generalized expectancies for internal versus external control of reinforcement. *Psychol. Monogr.* 80, (1, Whole No. 609).

SACHS, L. B. and INGRAM, G. L. (1972) Covert sensitization as a treatment for weight control. *Psychol. Rep.* 30, 971–974.

SCHACHTER, S. (1971) Some extraordinary facts about obese humans and rats. *Am. Psychol.* 26, 129–144.

STOLLAK, G. E. (1967) Weight loss obtained under different experimental procedures. *Psychotherapy: Theory, Research and Practice* 4, 61–64.

STUART, R. B. (1971) A three-dimensional program for the treatment of obesity. *Behav. Res. & Therapy* 9, 177–186.

STUART, R. B. (1972) Behavioral control of obesity. Paper presented at the Fourth Annual Southern California Conference on Behavior Modification, Los Angeles.

STUART, R. B. (1967) Behavioral control of overeating. *Behav. & Res Therapy* 5, 357–365.

STUART, R. B. and DAVIS, B. (1972) *Slim Chance in a Fat World: Behavioral Control of Obesity.* Research Press, Champaign, Ill.

STUNKARD, A. J. (1958) The management of obesity. *N.Y. St. J. Med.* 58, 79–87.

STUNKARD, A. J. and MCLAREN-HUME, M. (1959) The results of treatment for obesity. *Archs. Intern. Med.* 103, 79–85.

SWANSON, D. W. and DINELLO, F. (1969) Therapeutic starvation in obesity. *Dis. Nerv. Syst.* 30, 669–674.

THORPE, J. G., SCHMIDT, E., BROWN, P. T. and CASTELL, D. (1964) Aversion-relief therapy: A new method for general application. *Behav. Res. & Therapy* 2, 71–82.

TIGHE, T. J. and ELLIOTT, R. (1968) A technique for controlling behavior in natural life settings. *J. Appl. Behav. Anal.* 1, 263–266.

TYLER, V. O. and STRAUGHAN, J. H. (1970) Coverant control and breath holding as techniques for the treatment of obesity. *Psychol. Rec.* 20, 473–478.

ULLMANN, L. P. (1970) On cognitions and behavior therapy. *Behav. Ther.* 1, 201–204.

UPPER, D. and NEWTON, J. G. (1971) A weight-reduction program for schizophrenic patients on a token economy unit: Two case studies. *J. Behav. Therapy Exp. Psychiat.* 2, 113–115.

U.S. Public Health Service (undated) *Obesity and Health.* U.S. Government Printing Office, Washington, D.C.

WOLLERSHEIM, J. P. (1970) Effectiveness of group therapy based upon learning principles in the treatment of overweight women. *J. Abnorm. Psychol.* 76, 462–474.

WOLPE, J. (1954) Reciprocal inhibition as the main basis of psychotherapeutic effects. *Archs. Neurol. Psychiat.* 72, 205–226.

CHAPTER 5

Outcome and Methodological Considerations in Behavioral Treatment of Obesity

SHARON MARTINELLI HALL[1],[2]

The University of Wisconsin—Milwaukee

and

ROBERT GLENN HALL[3]

Wood Veterans Administration Center and The Medical College of Wisconsin

Summary— Studies determining the efficacy of behavioral treatment of obesity are divided into self and experimenter managed categories and reviewed with respect to outcome and adequacy of design. Methodological factors are considered, conclusions with regard to outcome and suggestions for research are offered.

Obesity has been considered a disorder most difficult to ameliorate. Traditional attempts to modify it have been varied, but generally unsuccessful (Stunkard and McClaren-Hume, 1959). However, within the past 15 years, behavior modification procedures have been used to effect weight loss in the obese, often with encouraging results. Behavior modifiers have based their treatment of obesity on several premises:

(1) That in otherwise healthy individuals, excess body fat results from excess food ingested for the energy requirements of the individuals.

(2) Decreases in food ingestion or increases in activity, or both, produce weight loss.

(3) Behaviors leading to food ingestion, or those involved in activity, can be modified by correct programming of the environment and the individual.

Reprinted with permission from *Behavior Therapy*, 1974, 5, 352–364. Copyright © 1974 by Academic Press, Inc.

[1] Requests for reprints should be sent to Sharon M. Hall, Department of Psychology, The University of Wisconsin—Milwaukee, Milwaukee, Wisconsin 53201.

[2] A more detailed version of this paper can be obtained from the APA's *Journal Supplement and Abstract Service*.

[3] Portions of work on this paper were completed while the authors were at the Behavior Therapy Institute, Sausalito, California and the Palo Alto Veterans Administration Hospital, respectively.

Here, the pertinent literature is examined with two points in mind: first, the relative sophistication of the design employed to study outcome of treatment, and the conclusions the design can support; second, comparisons of Experimenter-managed (EM) and Self-managed (SM) approaches to treatment, and maintenance of weight loss.

Emphasis is placed upon consideration of experimenter, nonspecific, control and subject variables (Paul, 1969). Studies are also examined with respect to follow-up data. Optimal treatment requires additional weight loss if ideal weight has not been reached, or maintenance if ideal weight is attained. Another variable of interest in evaluating treatment of obesity is premature termination rates. Traditionally, these are quite high: 20—80% (Stunkard, 1972).

This paper is also organized around a division of techniques, depending upon the locus of control over the stimuli and reinforcers used to effect change (Hall, 1972). Behavior modification techniques can be divided into two classes: Experimenter-managed (EM) and Self-managed (SM) (Mahoney, 1972). These two are not totally dichotomous categories, rather, they emphasize relative differences in experimenter activities (director vs. teacher), subject activities (passive vs. active), and location (therapy hour vs. natural environment). A variety of learning paradigms are incorporated within EM and SM categories, and these, too, are considered.

Case Studies (Table 1)

The earliest attempts to treat overeating through behavior modification were uncontrolled case studies. Studies reported vary greatly in techniques, amount of information supplied (e.g. subject characteristics, treatment procedures, pre and posttreatment weights, and the inclusion of follow-up periods). The techniques employed have suggested methods which have since been assessed, and, in some cases, proven fruitful in controlled studies of weight reduction.

Controlled Studies (Table 2)

With respect to Table 2, three points should be noted: First, sex of subject is included because there is some evidence that males lose more weight in traditional treatments (Stunkard and McClaren-Hume, 1959) and behavioral treatments (Harris, 1969). Second, in at least one instance (Manno and Marsten, 1972) the premature termination rate reported in the table may not accurately reflect the rate to be expected in an actual treatment situation, as the experimenter required a deposit returned contingent upon the completion of treatment. Higher premature termination rates might be expected with identical procedures and populations without such restraint upon the subjects. Third, population from which the subject sample was drawn is considered because treatment effects may well vary as a function of age, degree of obesity and population source, as will be discussed below.

TABLE 1. Case Studies: Control of Overeating and Obesity

Author(s)	Initial weight (lb)	No.	Sex	Age	Treatment method	Treatment period	Weight change in treatment (lb)	Follow-up period	Weight change at follow-up (lb)
Wolpe (1958)	—	1	F	36	Classical conditioning (US = shock; CS = food images)	5 sessions	—	—	—
Ferster et al. (1962)	—	10	F	—	Self-management techniques	—	5 to −20 (mode = −10)	—	—
Cautela (1964)	200	1	F	49	Covert sensitization (imaginal movement toward food paired with imaginal vomiting)	16 weeks	−66	7 months	−66
Meyer & Crisp (1964)	205 241	2	F	26 51	Punishment (shock contingent upon reaching for food)	6 weeks 1 session	−30 −10	20 mo. 12 mo.	−72 +25
Thorpe et al. (1964)	—	1	F	21	Aversion relief therapy (US = shock; CS = overeating; normal eating = no shock)	8 days	—	—	—
Goldiamond (1965)	—	1	M	—	Subject instructed in enhancement of stimulus control	2 sessions	—	—	—
Homme (1965)	—	—	—	—	Coverant conditioning	—	—	—	—
Stuart[1] (1967)	170–222	10	F	21–43	Self-management techniques + covert-sensitization in cases with cravings	12 months	−26 to −47	—	—
Bernard (1968)	407	1	F	mid-20's	Paid tokens for each lb lost + restrictions on food	20 weeks	−89	1.5 months	−102
Jeffrey et al. (1968)	154–292	4	F	29–45	Contingency contracting	24 weeks	$\bar{X}$ = 27	6 months	—
Kennedy & Foreyt	322	1	F	29	Classical conditioning (US = butyric acid gas; CS = odor of food)	22 weeks	−30	—	—
Moore & Crum (1969)	170	1	F	24	Social reinforcement	6 months	−35	—	—
Wolpe (1969)	—	2	—	—	Classical conditioning (US = asafetida; CS = smell, taste of food)	—	—	—	—
Upper & Newton (1971)	263 201	2	M	36–45	Reinforcement & punishment via tokens	28 weeks 26 weeks	−63 −31	—	—

[1] Premature termination rate = 20%.
[2] From termination of treatment.
[3] From pretreatment weight.

TABLE 2. Experimental Studies: Behavioral Control of Obesity

Author(s)	Subjects		Treatment methods	Premature termination (%)	Treatment period (weeks)	Follow-up period (weeks from termination of treatment)	Outcome[1]	
	No.	Sex					Post-treatment	Follow-up
Stollak[5,6] (1967)	140	M, F	Classical conditioning	33	8	8–10	AP > EM = NT	AP > EM = NT
Harmatz[4] & Lapuc (1968)	21	M	Negative reinforcement	0	6	4	EM = OT > NT	EM > OT > NT
Harris[5] (1969)	24	M, F	Complex self-management; Complex self-management + covert sensitization	14,	16	—	SM = SM + EM > NT	—
Wollersheim[5] (1970)	79	F	Complex self-management	10	12	8	SM > AP = OT > NT	SM > AP = OT
Hagen[5] (1970)	90	F	Complex self-management via manual, manual + contact, contact only	0	11	4	All SM = All SM > NT	All SM = All SM > NT
Tyler[6] & Straughan (1970)	57	F	Coverant conditioning	0	9	—	OT1 = OT2 EM = AP = OT	—
Foreyt[6] & Kennedy (1971)	12	F	Classical conditioning	0	9	48	EM > NT	EM ≧ NT
Harris[5] & Bruner (1971)	18	F	Complex self-management	25	16	—	SM = AP	—

Study	N	Sex	Treatment					
Harris[5] & Bruner (1971)	32	F	Complex self-management	83	12	28	EM > SM	EM = SM = NT
Horan[5] & Johnson (1971)	96	F	Contingency contracting	58.1	8	–	SM = OT SM > NT	–
(1971)			Coverant conditioning	16.6				–
Jeffrey[5] et al. (1971)	43	M, F	Complex self-management	18	18	12	EM + SM > OT = NT	(SM + EM > OT[3])
Penick[6] et al. (1971)	32	M, F	Complex self-management + positive reinforcement	7	12	12–24	Mixed	–
Shulman[5] (1971)	36	M, F	Decreasing bites + increasing eating time	0	10	16	SM > AP = NT	–
Stuart[6] (1971)	6	F	Complex self-management	0	15	12–24	(SM > AP[3])	(SM > AP[3])
Hall[6] (1972)	12	F	Complex self-management	14	5	4	(EM > SM > NT[3])	–
Janda[5] & Rimm (1972)	18	M, F	Covert sensitization	0	6	6	EM ≧ AP > NT	EM > AP = NT
Mann[6] (1972)	9	M, F	Contingency contracting	22	variable	–	(EM > NT[3])	–
Manno[5] & Marsten (1972)	41	M, F	Covert sensitization, covert positive reinforcement	0	4	12	Both EM = Both EM > NT	Both EM = Both EM > NT
Mahoney[5] et al. (1973)	53	M, F	Self-reward, self-punishment, self-reward + self-punishment, self-monitoring	—	4	16	Reward monitoring = control	Reward reward + punishment control

[1] Group designations are abbreviated, where SM = Self-management, EM = Experimenter Management, AP = Attention Placebo, NT = No Treatment, OT = Other Treatment. Significant differences designated by >; no differences by =.

[2] From termination of treatment.

[3] Statistics not computed, authors' conclusions.

[4] The subjects were hospitalized chronic schizophrenics.

[5] The subjects were college students and/or staff.

[6] Non-college, non-institutionalized population.

Methodological Issues

Paul (1969) has proposed that an adequate test of a treatment procedure should include control for therapist characteristics and expectations, and for nonspecific and placebo effects. Also, Paul has proposed that the characteristics of the sample to which procedures are employed should be considered, as effects might vary as a function of the population characteristics. The conclusions drawn from the studies reviewed are considered in light of these criteria. Of the studies listed in Table 2, only that of Wollersheim (1971) is sufficiently well designed to allow the conclusion that behavior modification techniques resulted in a weight loss (in young, mildly overweight college students) other than that resulting from attention, situational expectations, and a particular therapist. The most common shortcomings among the studies cited are the lack of an attention-placebo condition, lack of adequate follow-up, and failure to include more than one experimenter or to assign experimenters in such a way that experimenter effects could be assessed.

Three studies had used single-subject designs, either of the reversal (Mann, 1972) or cross-over type (Stuart, 1971; Hall, 1972). The value of individual subject research designs is evident because of the large intersubject variability frequently found in this area (Penick, et al., 1971; Hall, 1972). Such designs allow a precise determination of the effects of treatments upon the subject over time, and actual behavioral changes are not obscured by averages obtained from a sample with a large variance. This feature of these designs can be extremely informative in studying weight reduction because a steady weight loss is considered superior to a rapid, erratically patterned loss for reason of both physical health and habit training (Stuart and Davis, 1972). Although studies reviewed using single-subject designs have not controlled for as many variables as desirable, a research program using these designs which would do so is conceivable.

In general, but particularly with regard to SM techniques, both singly and in combination, it is worth noting that studies using non-college student populations have produced less striking results than studies using college students. For example, in two studies where experimental operations were similar enough to permit some comparisons, testing coverant conditioning (Horan & Johnson, 1971; Tyler & Straughan, 1970) Horan and Johnson, using a college population, found at least limited superiority for the coverant group; Tyler and Straughan, with older subjects, did not. Young (as quoted in Mayer, 1969) has suggested the existence of a population of overweight individuals who usually do not come in contact with health professionals because they are able to reduce independently. Only the most intractable cases come to the professional's attention, therefore, the results of traditional studies have shown high premature termination and little success. Studies which solicit subjects from a population of mildly overweight young people may, in fact, be tapping those who are able to lose independently and with whom the effectiveness of any technique may be exaggerated. These observations suggest caution in generalizing between populations, as well as increased research using "clinical" populations. A similar problem exists with respect to excessively rigid criteria, particularly with respect to motivation, which have sometimes been employed for acceptance into the experimental sample. Such carefully selected populations vitiate comparisons with earlier nonbehavioral studies which have less stringent criteria, often requiring only that a patient be referred from other departments in hospitals to the obesity clinic.

Direct comparisons of results between studies are difficult because of sample differences, as well as use of different measures of weight change (absolute pounds versus percent of body weight). Since neither absolute pounds nor percent is ideal, careful reporting of both measures, particularly for individuals, is helpful. In otherwise well-designed and reported studies, a precise sample description was often lacking. Minimal description should include: number, sex, mean, and range of percentage overweight, mean and age range, socioeconomic level, and method used to determine percentage overweight. All of these are variables which have either been shown to influence the outcome of weight treatment (Harris, 1969; Stunkard & McClaren-Hume, 1959), or psychotherapy in general (Hollingshead and Redlich, 1958). Some studies have used a self-report as criteria for inclusion in the experimental sample. This is questionable, both methodologically and ethically, for solicitation of subjects for weight loss studies may result in replies from many subjects who are not objectively overweight by any criterion.

Follow-up assessment has been included in 14 of the 18 studies presented. In general, those studies with follow-up periods of 12 weeks or shorter (Harmatz & Lapuc, 1968; Wollersheim, 1970; Hagen, 1970; Hall, 1971; Manno & Marsten, 1972; Janda & Rimm, 1972) find that differences between experimental and control groups remain significant, while the few controlled studies including longer follow-up periods have generally found that the originally observed differences between experimental and control groups were no longer significant (Foreyt & Kennedy, 1971; Harris & Bruner, 1972; Shulman, 1971). This may indicate that differences found at shorter follow-up periods exist because subjects simply have not had sufficient time to regain the weight lost during treatment and that no effective behavior change has been made which would allow the subjects either to retain the weight loss or to continue losing weight. Clearly, there is a need for longer follow-up periods in well-controlled studies, and for an increased emphasis on procedures which would aid participants in keeping weight off.

Premature termination rates have ranged from 0 to 83%. Considerable variability in premature termination is noted both within EM (0–58%) and SM (6–83%). Differences seem to be due neither to subject variables, nor to specific treatment procedures, nor to reported experimenter variables. Although the possibility of expectational and attentional variables may explain differences in termination rates, sufficient information was not provided within the reports to pinpoint these variables as contributors to variability in premature termination rates.

Efficacy of SM and EM Procedures

EXPERIMENTER-MANAGED PROCEDURES

One consistent finding of studies employing EM procedures has been the relatively rapid weight loss obtained when these techniques were successful. The findings are particularly encouraging with respect to methods which do not use aversive stimuli.

The status of EM aversive stimuli, particularly electric shock and noxious odors, is unclear. Studies employing such stimuli in a classical conditioning paradigm (Kennedy & Foreyt, 1968; Foreyt & Kennedy, 1971; Stollak, 1968) have failed to take into account the optimal CS—US interval; the interval used was not reported in any study and the operations employed appear to have resulted in longer intervals. These studies also failed to recognize the nature of eating among obese persons. Such individuals generally are not troubled by cravings for particular foods, rather, they tend to snack even though satiated, overeat at the end of meals (Mayer, Monello & Seltzer, 1965; Harvey & Simmons, 1954) and, in general, are more aware of external cues as opposed to internal cues of hunger (Schacter, 1971). Aversive conditioning aimed at these characteristics might be of greater value. To label these aversion procedures ineffective is premature, for such a statement fails to acknowledge these difficulties as well as problems involved in the application of aversive stimulation to any problem behavior (Rachman & Teasdale, 1968). Although covert sensitization does appear to have some effect on weight loss, controlling factors are not clear.

SELF-MANAGED PROCEDURES

The usefulness of complex combinations of SM techniques in obesity treatment is indicated by controlled studies (Wollersheim, 1970; Harris, 1969; Hagen, 1970; Stuart, 1971), although difficulties remain. Self-management combinations *have* produced greater weight losses than those obtained under no-treatment conditions, in every case where such comparisons were conducted (Harris, 1969; Wollersheim, 1970; Hagen, 1970; Stuart, 1971; Hall, 1972). When compared with other treatments or other attention-placebo conditions, the studies are fewer and the findings less consistent, although still promising (Wollersheim, 1970; Penick et al., 1971; Harris & Bruner, 1971).

Wollersheim (1970) found self-control treatment superior to an attention placebo, and to other treatment, Harris and Bruner (1971) and Hall (1972) found contracting procedures more effective.

Follow-up periods have ranged in length from 1–3 months after termination of treatment. Assessment at follow-up has indicated treatment via combinations of SM techniques results in either a stabilization in weight (Wollersheim, 1970; Hagen, 1970) or continuing losses (Stuart, 1971). In light of the tendency of obese people to regain weight loss (Stunkard & McClaren-Hume, 1959; Mayer, 1968), this latter finding is encouraging. However, the goal of SM is to teach clients *self*-management, and one would expect continued loss (if needed) after the termination of formal treatment rather than stabilization. A consistent finding is the relatively slow weight loss resulting from SM combinations. The only instances where mean weight loss approximated 1 lb or more per week were the studies of Wollersheim (1970) and Hagen (1970). Although moderate weight loss (1–2 lb per week) is healthy, such extremely slow losses may be discouraging to the client. One solution is to combine SM and EM techniques, and some evidence indicated that this combination will produce more rapid losses (Penick *et al.*, 1971). Theoretically, the most promising combination should be EM procedures early in treatment to produce relatively rapid weight loss, while the client is learning and practicing SM techniques, which will be thus reinforced by their association with weight loss and whose acquisition will result in maintained or continued loss following treatment.

With respect to simpler SM procedures, studies are fewer, findings are more tenuous, and further work is needed before conclusions can be drawn about their effectiveness. At present, Shulman's (1971) and Fowler's (1971) approaches appear promising, but further tests are needed to determine their usefulness for extended periods of time, with more clinically appropriate populations, and independent of therapist effects.

Assessment of Success in Treatment

Prediction of individual differences in weight loss has not been at all successful. Clinical intuition, MMPI, MPI, weight prior to treatment, general anxiety, situation specific anxiety, PAS, EPQ, I-E Scale, body image measures, attitudinal measures, and the 16 PF questionnaire have all failed to predict success in treatment. Closer attention to fairly gross variables, such as age, SE status, weight loss during first week of treatment, may be more fruitful than assessment of personality variables. Such evaluations may , of course, necessitate inclusion of more heterogeneous populations than usually employed.

Suggestions for Further Research

The SM techniques, particularly SM combinations appear to be the most promising, but further work is necessary in refining the technology, in separating the effective from ineffective components in SM packages, in attempts to apply these techniques to more heterogeneous and/or seriously obese populations, as well as development of methods which will allow the prediction of success in treatment and, if possible, remedial measures for those who lack a good prognosis. With regard to EM techniques, refinement of positive reinforcement paradigms is called for, particularly in developing methods for management of reinforcement so that steady, moderate (1–2 lb per week) losses are produced and maintained or continued during follow-up periods of some length. Research on EM techniques using aversive stimuli could focus on improvement on the mechanics of the conditioning situation, and on more appropriate conditioned stimuli. Research is needed to determine the maximally effective combination of EM and SM techniques for weight loss that is both of moderate speed and which can be continued or maintained after the termination of formal treatment. Finally, *long-term* evaluations (six months or more) are needed.

References

BERNARD, J. L. Rapid treatment of gross obesity by operant techniques. *Psychological Reports*, 1968, 23, 663–666.

BERNE, E. *Games people play*. New York: Grove Press, 1964.

CAUTELA, J. R. The treatment of compulsive behavior by coverant sensitization. *Psychological Record*, 1966, 16, 33–41.

CHAPMAN, R. F., SMITH, J. W., & LAYDEN, T. A. Elimination of cigarette smoking by punishment and self-management training. *Behavior Research and Therapy*, 1971, 9, 255–264.

FERSTER, C. B., NURNBERGER, J. I., & LEVITT, E. E. The control of eating. *Journal of Mathetics*, 1962, 1, 87–109.

FOREYT, J. P., & KENNEDY, W. A. Treatment of overweight by aversion therapy. *Behaviour Research and Therapy*, 1971, 9, 29–34.

FOWLER, R. S. *The mouthful diet*, unpublished manuscript, 1971.

GOLDIAMOND, I. Self-control procedures in personal behavior problems. *Psychological Reports*, 1965, 17, 861–868.

HAFFEY, V. A., SOROKO, M. L., & McCORMACK, J. H. Use of modeling and of operant reinforcement procedures in a group weight reduction program. *Newsletter for Research in Psychology*, 1972, 14, 17–22.

HAGEN, R. L. Group therapy versus bibliotherapy in weight reduction. Unpublished Doctoral Dissertation, University of Illinois, 1970.

HALL, S. M. Self-control and therapist control in the behavioral treatment of overweight women. *Behaviour Research and Therapy*, 1972, 10, 59–68.

HARMATZ, M. G. & LAPUC, P. Behavior modification of overeating in a psychiatric population. *Journal of Consulting and Clinical Psychology*, 1968, 32, 583–589.

HARRIS, M. B. Self-directed program for weight control: A pilot study. *Journal of Abnormal Psychology*, 1969, 74, 263–270.

HARRIS, M. S. & BRUNER, C. G. A comparison of self-control and a contract procedure for weight control. *Behavior Research and Therapy*, 1971, 9, 347–354.

HARVEY, J. I. & SIMMONS, W. D. Weight reduction: A study of the group method. *American Journal of Medical Science*, 1954, 227, 521–525.

HOLLINGSHEAD, A. B. & REDLICH, F. C. *Social class and mental illness: A community study*. New York: Wiley, 1958.

HOMME, L. E. Perspective in psychology: XXIV. Control of coverants, the operants of the mind. *Psychological Record*, 1965, 15, 501–511.

HORAN, J. J. & JOHNSON, R. G. Covenant conditioning through a self-management application of the Premack principle. Its effect on weight reduction. *Journal of Behavior Therapy and Experimental Psychiatry*, 1971, 2, 243–249.

JANDA, L. H. & RIMM, D. C. Covert sensitization in the treatment of obesity. *Journal of Abnormal Psychology*, 1972, 80, 37–42.

JEFFREY, D. B., CHRISTENSEN, E. R., & PAPPAS, J. P. A case study report of a behavioral modification weight reduction group: Treatment and follow-up. *Research and Development Report No. 33*, University of Utah Counseling Center, 1972 (a).

JEFFREY, D. B., CHRISTENSEN, E. R., & PAPPAS, J. P. Developing a behavioral program and therapist manuals for the treatment of obesity. *Research and Development Report No. 34*, University of Utah Counseling Center, 1972 (b).

KENNEDY, W. A. & FOREYT, J. Control of eating behavior in an obese patient by avoidance conditioning. *Psychological Reports*, 1968, 22, 571–576.

MAHONEY, M. J. Research issues in self-management. *Behavior Therapy*, 1972, 3, 45–63.

MAHONEY, M. J., MOURA, N. G. M., & WADE, T. C. The relative efficacy of self-reward, self-punishment and self-monitoring techniques for weight loss. *Journal of Consulting and Clinical Psychology* 1973, 40, 404-407.

MANN, R. A. The behavior-therapeutic use of contingency contracting to control an adult behavior problem: Weight control. *Journal of Applied Behavior Analysis*, 1972, 3, 99–109.

MANNO, B. & MARSTON, A. R. Weight reduction as a function of negative covert reinforcement (sensitization) versus positive covert reinforcement. *Behavior Research and Therapy*, 1972, 10, 201–207.

MAYER, J. *Overweight: Causes, cost and control.* Englewood-Cliffs, New Jersey: Prentice Hall, 1968.

MAYER, J., MONELLO, L. F., & SELTZER, C. C. Hunger and satiety sensations in man. *Postgraduate Medicine*, 1965, 97–100.

MEYER, V. & CRISP, A. H. Aversion therapy in two cases of obesity. *Behaviour Research and Therapy*, 1964, 2, 143–147.

PAUL, G. L. Behavior modification research: Design and tactics. In C. M. Franks (Ed.), *Behavior therapy: Appraisal and status.* New York: McGraw-Hill, 1969. Pp. 39–62.

PENICK, S. B., FILION, R., FOX, S., & STUNKARD, A. Behavior modification in the treatment of obesity. *Psychosomatic Medicine*, 1971, 33, 49–55.

RACHMAN, S. & TEASDALE, J. *Aversion therapy and behavior disorders: An analysis.* Coral Gables, Florida: University of Miami Press, 1969.

SCHACTER, S. *Emotions, obesity and crime.* New York: Academic Press, 1971.

SHULMAN, J. M. The behavioral control of overeating. Unpublished master's thesis, University of Montana, 1971.

SIDMAN, M. *Tactics of scientific research.* New York: Basic Books, 1960.

STOLLAK, G. E. Weight loss obtained under different experimental procedures. *Psychotherapy: Theory, research and practice*, 1967, 4, 61–64.

STUART, R. B. Behavioral control of overeating. *Behavior Research and Therapy*, 1967, 5, 357–365.

STUART, R. B. A three dimensional program for the treatment of obesity. *Behaviour Research and Therapy*, 1971, 9, 177–186.

STUART, R. B. & DAVIS, B. *Slim chance in a fat world: Behavioral control of overeating.* Champaign, Illinois: Research Press, 1972.

STUNKARD, A. & McCLAREN-HUME, M. The results of treatment of obesity. *Archives of Internal Medicine*, 1959, 103, 79–85.

THORPE, J. G., SCHMIDT, E., BROWN, P. T., & CASTELL, D. Aversion relief therapy: A new method for generation application. *Behaviour Research and Therapy*, 1964, 2, 71–82.

TYLER, V. O. & STRAUGHAN, J. H. Coverant control and breath holding for the treatment of obesity. *Psychological Record*, 1970, 20, 473–478.

UPPER, D. & NEWTON, J. G. A weight reduction program for schizophrenic patients on a token economy unit: Two case studies. *Journal of Behavior Therapy and Experimental Psychology*, 1971, 2, 113–115.

U.S. Department of Health, Education and Welfare. *Obesity and health: A source-book of information for professional health personnel.* Arlington, Virginia: U.S. Government Printing Office, 1966.

WOLLERSHEIM, J. P. Effectiveness of group therapy based upon learning principles in the treatment of overweight women. *Journal of Abnormal Psychology*, 1970, 76, 462–474.

WOLPE, J. *Psychotherapy by reciprocal inhibition.* Stanford, California: Stanford University Press, 1958.

WOLPE, J. *The practice of behavior therapy.* New York: Pergamon Press, 1969.

PART II

AVERSIVE TECHNIQUES

Introduction[1]

RICHARD A. FROHWIRTH

Psychometric Associates, Inc., Greenwich, Connecticut

Most discussions of the aversive control of behavior distinguish between classical and operant or instrumental conditioning techniques. In the former, the aversive unconditioned stimulus (UCS) is applied immediately following the conditioned stimulus (CS), regardless of the organism's response, while in the latter, the onset of noxious stimulation is contingent, according to a predetermined schedule, upon that response.

Aversive techniques in the treatment of obesity predominantly fit into the classical conditioning paradigm, and claim classical conditioning as their theoretical rationale, although elements of operant conditioning may be included as well. In the classical model, food or food imagery serves as the CS, while electric shock, offensive odors, or unpleasant images are used as the UCS. By repeated pairing of the CS and UCS, it is hoped that the patient will acquire an aversion, or at least a diminished liking, for attractive, high-caloric foods, and thereby learn to avoid them.

Wolpe (1954) appears to have been the first to attempt to treat overeating with classical aversion methods. Although he referred to his technique as "avoidance conditioning", a term usually reserved for the operant conditioning paradigm in which the subject's behavior may be instrumental in avoiding the onset of the noxious stimulus, the application of electric shock was clearly contingent upon the presentation of the target stimulus, food imagery. Wolpe reported a marked diminution in his patient's food obsessionality, although she died (from unrelated causes) soon after the completion of the treatment sessions. Had she not died, it would have been interesting to follow her eating behavior over a long period of time and her retention of the conditioned aversion responses to thoughts of "delectable food". In using imaginal rather than actual CS, Wolpe took direct aim at the patient's target symptom, obsessional thinking about food. In doing so, he also provided a precedent to Cautela's (1966) covert sensitization (Part III), in which both the CS and the UCS are presented in imagination.

---

[1] This introduction was written especially for this book.

Meyer and Crisp (1964) provide two case examples of what can be conceptualized as instrumental avoidance conditioning. Approach behavior toward attractive, high caloric food was punished with electric shock, while eating permitted foods was not punished. It is, of course, necessary to provide for alternative behavior whenever punishment is used and Meyer and Crisp met this requirement by providing a low calorie diet. One difficulty with avoidance conditioning is the possibility that the subjects will avoid the noxious stimulus entirely by refusing to engage in the punished behavior. This is precisely what happened in their second case when the subject simply refused to approach the target foods during the treatment sessions, and thereby avoided all shocks except for one initial practice trial. Her weight progress suggests that she did not avoid these foods at other times, however, which is not surprising in view of her having never been "conditioned" to avoid them. Their other subject was more cooperative and certainly must be regarded as a treatment success. The gradual phasing out of the shock apparatus may have facilitated generalization of the avoidance response to everyday settings.

Wijesinghe (1973) also employed electric shock as the UCS, but unlike Meyer and Crisp (1964), his procedure better fits into a classical conditioning model. His two subjects were requested to exhibit approach behavior toward tempting foods, and while doing so, were shocked. This procedure helps to preclude unwanted avoidance behavior during conditioning sessions, as was encountered by Meyer and Crisp, although it is certainly possible that subjects will resist making the required approach responses. One patient did quite well after this extremely brief (one day) treatment program. Unfortunately, weight data for the other patient are not reported, although she is said to have ceased her compulsive eating and to have made a better social adjustment.

Thorpe, *et al.* (1964) describe an "aversion-relief" treatment, which combines classical aversive conditioning using faradic shock for undesired behavior with relief from anxiety, which is presumably rewarding, for desired behavior. Stimuli were presented as words describing the deviant behavior (e.g. "sodomy" or "overeating") and the desired behavior (e.g. "girlfriend" or "normal eating"). In a series of eight patients, one was treated with this method for overeating. Although a cessation of eating bouts and a diminution of food obsessionality were obtained, the patient discontinued treatment. Unfortunately, no weight data or follow-up investigation of eating behavior were reported.

Many of the methodological objections to single-case study investigations can be surmounted by multiple-baseline designs, in which problematic behaviors are sequentially attacked and eliminated, thus demonstrating experimental control over these behaviors. A novel application of this design was employed in our fourth article in which cigarette smoking served as the unconditioned stimulus (Morganstern, 1974). Morganstern argued that since inhalation of cigarette smoke usually produces unpleasant reactions of gagging, nausea, and even vomiting in nonsmoking individuals, then smoking could serve as a practical and effective overt aversive stimulus for such persons. Over a period of 18 weeks cigarette smoking was paired with each of three target foods in three distinct phases. Meticulous food consumption records as well as weight-loss data were kept, thus providing direct information as to the effect of the aversive contingency on eating behavior. The subject was an 180-lb young woman who continually ate great quantities of high-caloric, snack foods, such as cookies, candy and doughnuts. Aversive conditioning was carried out by asking the subject to first chew a favorite food, then take a long "drag" on a lit cigarette and spit out the food saying, "Eating this junk makes me sick". She repeated this procedure ten times per session and was asked to practice it at home twice a day.

Results were striking both in terms of food consumption and body weight. As the aversive contingency was applied to each target food, the rate of consumption for that food rapidly fell to zero and was maintained there throughout treatment and follow-up at 24 weeks. Consumption of foods to which the aversive contingency had not yet been applied remained at baseline, indicating that experimental control over eating behavior had been achieved. A total weight loss of 53 lb over the 24 weeks provided some indirect check on the subject's honesty in reporting food consumption, which can be a great problem in weight-loss research (Kennedy and Foreyt, 1968). Even with this highly suggestive evidence of the effects of aversive conditioning, the author pointed out that "cognitive-symbolic processes" may have played an important role in the subject's weight loss. During the course of treatment as she eliminated the consumption of her favourite foods, the subject apparently recognized that eating behavior could come under her own control, and was thus able to institute dietary changes to produce further weight loss. In this context, aversive conditioning may be viewed as a means of inducing reappraisal of the self, and particularly of one's ability to exercise self-control.

In contrast to the single case studies previously mentioned, Stollak (1967) employed an experimental design, an adequate number of subjects, and a follow-up period. While these features are elementary for any scientific investigation of treatment for weight loss, they are far from typical in the weight reduction literature, especially in studies using aversion therapy. One of Stollak's groups, "Contact-Dairy-Shock-Food Association", fits into a classical aversion therapy paradigm. Overall, the results were disappointing, and clearly the addition of stimulus-contingent electric shock did nothing to increase the effectiveness of treatment. In his discussion of these results, Stollak offers the interesting speculation that the shock disrupted the therapeutic relationship between experimenter and subject or that it obliterated some components of the CS, effectively precluding conditioning.

In the article by Foreyt and Kennedy (1971), a classical conditioning procedure involving the pairing of food odors as the CS and foul-smelling odors as the UCS was used. Because food taste and odor are so intimately related and since organisms are likely to avoid foods which smell bad or make them nauseous, the use of noxious odors seems to be a logical choice of UCS in aversion therapy of overeating (Lazarus, 1971; Rachman and Teasdale, 1969). An earlier paper by the authors (Kennedy and Foreyt, 1968) described a 30 lb weight loss in a very obese woman. This was followed by an experimental study (Foreyt and Kennedy. 1971), which achieved a clinically modest but statistically significant initial weight loss in a group of women treated with aversion therapy, compared with a group of control subjects. Unfortunately, one-half of the experimental group and all of the control subjects were also members of a local weight loss club, TOPS (Take Off Pounds Sensibly). Further, as the authors noted, there was a great deal of interaction between the therapist and subjects, in addition to the conditioning procedure. These methodological problems make it difficult to assess the role that conditioning *per se* might play in modifying eating behavior. Frohwirth (1974) attempted to clarify this issue by using subjects not involved in other treatment programs, minimizing therapist–subject interaction, and using an appropriate placebo control group. The experimental group received classical aversion conditioning sessions, involving the pairing of noxious odors with odors of favorite, high caloric foods; a placebo group received the same number of sessions but in which pleasant rather than noxious odors were paired with food odors. Results suggested that there was no difference in outcome between the two groups, emphasizing the significant role that such variables as "suggestion" and "expectancy" play in studies of this type.

It is difficult to evaluate the efficacy of aversion therapy in obesity, but overall the results do not appear to be promising. Isolated cases of improvement must be weighed against cases of treatment failure and dropping out of treatment. Also to be considered are negative findings which do not find their way into publication. Foreyt and Kennedy (1971) suggested that aversion therapy might be useful as an adjunct to a comprehensive weight reduction program but in the absence of long-term follow-up data even this conservative statement may be too optimistic. Further, aversion therapy is often a difficult-to-administer, time-consuming technique which may be painful or frightening to the subject and unpleasant for the therapist. Considering the evidence at this time, aversive techniques for obesity cannot be recommended for general application.

Reference

Cautela, J. R. Treatment of compulsive behavior by covert sensitization. *The Psychological Record*, 1966, **16**, 33–41.

Foreyt, J. P. and Kennedy, W. A. Treatment of overweight by aversion therapy. *Behaviour Research and Therapy*, 1971, **9**, 29–34.

Frohwirth, R. A. Aversive conditioning treatment of overweight. Unpublished doctoral dissertation, The Florida State University, 1974.

Kennedy, W. A. and Foreyt, J. P. Control of eating behavior in an obese patient by avoidance conditioning. *Psychological Reports*, 1968, **22**, 571–576.

Lazarus,.A. A. *Behavior therapy and beyond*. New York: McGraw-Hill, 1971.

Meyer, V. and Crisp, A. H. Aversion therapy in two cases of obesity. *Behaviour Research and Therapy*, 1964, 2, 143–147.

Morganstern, K. P. Cigarette smoke as a noxious stimulus in self-managed aversion therapy for compulsive eating: Technique and case illustration. *Behavior Therapy*, 1974, 5, 255–260.

Rachman, S. and Teasdale, J. *Aversion therapy and behavior disorders: An analysis*. Coral Gables, Florida: University of Miami Press, 1969.

Stollak, G. E. Weight loss obtained under different experimental procedures. *Psychotherapy: Theory, Research and Practice*, 1967, 4, 61–64.

Thorpe, J. G., Schmidt, E., Brown, P. T., and Castell, D. Aversion-relief therapy: A new method for general application. *Behaviour Research and Therapy*, 1964, 2, 71–82.

Wijesinghe, B. Massed electrical aversion treatment of compulsive eating. *Journal of Behavior Therapy and Experimental Psychiatry*, 1973, 4, 133–135.

Wolpe, J. Reciprocal inhibition as the main basis of psychotherapeutic effects. *A.M.A. Archives of Neurology and Psychiatry*, 1954, 72, 205–226.

CHAPTER 6

Aversion Therapy in Two Cases of Obesity

V. MEYER and A. H. CRISP

Academic Psychiatric Unit, Middlesex Hospital, London, W.1

Summary–Two cases of obesity associated with overeating are described in relation to their differing responses to aversion therapy directed as the eating behaviour.

There have been frequent comments in the literature regarding the apparent importance of patients' motivation, personality type, level of anxiety and presence of other symptoms for the outcome of aversion therapy (Beech, 1960; Eysenck, 1960, Oswald, 1962). In general we do not know how these variables may influence the outcome of treatment and how we might usefully modify treatment methods to accommodate them (Beech, 1963; Thorpe, 1964). Aversion therapy is most commonly used in an attempt to modify various undesirable but pleasurable activities. Thus it has been used, with modifications, in the treatment of various sexual behaviour disorders, alcoholism and addiction to other drugs. The treatment method appears at first sight to be equally applicable to the problem of overeating.

The basis of overeating, as a determinant of simple obesity is a complex one. Constitutional (Parnell, 1958; Quaade, 1955) and biochemical (Lancet, 1964; Mayer, 1955; Paswan, 1963) factors are well recognized. Overeating has also been studied clinically as a culturally (Quaade, 1955) and neurotically (Bruch, 1940; Hamburger, 1951; Leavell and Clark, 1958) based habit. It is sometimes seen as characteristic of people with a certain personality type embodying fixed and excessive (oral) dependency needs. It is suggested that such people, particularly when experiencing separation, rejection or loss, feel excessively insecure, become readily apprehensive and depressed, and may compensatorily and defensively overeat–a so-called addiction to food (Fenichel, 1946). The dependence on overeating and the resistance to stopping the behaviour, implicit in this concept of addiction, is presumably provided, from a psychological viewpoint, by a continuing threatened emergence or re-emergence of the excessive and intolerable anxiety and depressive feelings in the individual. If such a mechanism is present then obese subjects should show less evidence of overt depression than a non-obese group of subjects. This observation has been confirmed in a phenomenological study by Simon (1963). Others (Dunbar, 1954;

Reprinted with permission from *Behaviour Research and Therapy*, 1964, **2**, 143–147.

Weiss and English, 1957) see the condition as a psychosomatic one in which the probable constitutional tendency to overeat is evoked in an emotionally unstable childhood. This behavior tends to emerge thereafter, as a form of latent visceral conditioning, during periods of similar stresses throughout the subject's life (Shorvon and Richardson, 1949). Overeating has also been commented on clinically in relation to such factors as boredom, sexual frustration and the menopause, and it has been studied systematically in connexion with the pre-menstrual period (Bruce and Russell, 1962). Attention has sometimes been drawn to the possible symbolic significance of eating and obesity for sexual indulgence and its repercussions both with reference to the clinical state of obesity and to that of anorexia nervosa (Fenichel, 1945; Waller et al., 1940). The treatment of obesity by simple dieting is rarely successful (Strang, 1959). Psychotherapy has sometimes been reported as being successful (Bruch, 1958; Nicholson, 1946; Shorvon and Richardson, 1949). In some studies, especially where dieting measures only have been used, the majority of patients have been observed to become depressed and anxious during treatment (Bruch, 1952; Hamburger, 1951; Stunkard, 1957).

This paper describes some of the contrasting features of two patients suffering with obesity, both apparently motivated towards treatment and both subjected to similar aversion therapies. Their responses to treatment were different.

Case 1

A 26-year-old woman was admitted to hospital in 1961 in a state of chronic amphetamine addiction and intoxication. She had been taking amphetamine periodically since 1955 ostensibly to help her to reduce weight. She nevertheless weighed 15 stone on admission. The patient's mother was a critical, rejecting figure. There was no family history of obesity. The patient had been plump as a child but was later slim for a time. She was involved in minor recurrent delinquency, had no regular employment and was sexually promiscuous. She suffered with a physical disorder in which her legs were disfigured by fatty deposits; she was very sensitive about this and had become depressed when rejected sexually on this account. She was not paranoid or overtly depressed on admission. She was pleasant and friendly on the ward and was very popular with other patients; she had a tendency to clown. It was considered that she was a psychopath. Her history indicated that she was an emotionally deprived person, basically depressed but clowning, constantly seeking for closer relationships with people and needing to be accepted by them, and with little sense of guilt. To this end she consorted indiscriminately with men socially more outcast than herself and minimally critical of her physical appearance. She was treated initially by withdrawal of amphetamine and psychotherapy. She did quite well in a strongly supportive therapeutic relationship and her weight fell to 12 stone. However, when the therapist left the hospital and social rehabilitation was attempted the patient relapsed immediately. She reverted to taking amphetamine and over-eating and her weight went up to 16 stone. The patient's conscious need remained that of losing weight and of being slim and attractive. It was agreed that if this could be achieved her general interpersonal relationships might improve; otherwise she was considered practically untreatable except by com-pulsory detention. A behaviour therapy approach to the problem of the overeating was made.

Case 2

A 51-year-old woman was referred because of her complaint of backache due to spinal arthritis which was considered to be exacerbated by obesity due to overeating. The obesity had proved unresponsive to dietetic control. Both her parents were obese at intervals throughout their lives. One of the patient's fourteen siblings suffered from a recurrent depressive illness. The patient, who was one of the elder siblings, was plump and anxious as a child. She did well at school. Subsequently she worked as a cashier in a food store. She married at the age of 19 "to escape from home". Sex relations had initially been satisfactory and there were five children; the youngest was 9-years-old, a plump girl. When she was pregnant with this child she discovered that her husband was being unfaithful to her. He has continued in this way ever since. In personality the patient was considered to be an anxious, obsessional, hypochondriacal person given to episodes of depression and superficial denial of emotional difficulties. Overtly she maintained a jolly appearance and was regarded as the "mother figure" of the street. At the time of admission she weighed over 18 stone. She had always tended to be mildly plump, i.e. up to 12–13 stone, but her real weight increase had occurred 9 years previously during the time of the last pregnancy and puerperium. At that time she had become aware of her husband's infidelity and had become depressed. She began to overeat, found some pleasure in this, and had been overeating ever since. She had grown into the image of a jolly and fat woman and was no longer overtly depressed. Her particular craving was for ice cream, cakes and nuts. Several previous attempts at dieting under in-patient hospital supervision had failed; on these occasions it had been discovered that the patient was eating secretly and she discharged herself.

Treatment Method

The nature of the treatment was discussed with each patient separately; they were told that they would be subjected to punishing electric shocks which would be sufficiently painful to inhibit their immediate behaviour.

The patient was put on a basic 1000 calorie diet and placed in an isolation room containing a one-way screen. Her weight chart was placed on the wall with a photograph of an obese subject at the level of the upper weight range and a slim, attractive subject at the level of the therapeutically desired weight level (10 stone). A transformer, connected to the mains with secondary winding designed to give electric shocks of varying voltages, was placed outside the room. Two electrodes were attached to the patient's left arm. The specific procedure for treatment was as follows. The "temptation food" (food for which the patient had most craving) was displayed for increasing periods of time, initially under constant observation. Any approach by the patient towards the food was punished by shocking to prevent eating (the strength of the shock was set at an uncomfortable level for the patient arrived at by increasing the voltage slightly above the level initially selected by the patient as being unpleasant but tolerable. The therapist always tested himself with this shock first. It was of the order of 80–90 V). The patient was never shocked whilst eating her prescribed diet. From the time that the patient ceased showing approach behaviour towards the "temptation food" the possibility of receiving immediate shocks was progressively reduced; firstly by disconnecting plugs, then by removing the electrodes on the patient's arm and finally by removing all electrical appliances from the room. At the same time she was told that she would not be constantly observed in the presence of the "temptation food". Finally she was told of the specific occasions when she would not be observed. The "temptation food" was by this time being kept in the treatment room for long periods of time, care being taken to keep it appetizing. Eventually the patient was given increasing social and dietary freedom under part-observation. The weight was plotted daily and diuretics were administered appropriately when there was a plateau in the rate of weight loss. Any obvious relapse by the patient so far as eating behaviour was concerned would lead to a re-institution of the early treatment procedure.

PROGRESS IN TREATMENT AND FOLLOW-UP

Case No. 1 was an in-patient from 7 November 61 to 4 April 63. She received treatment for her overeating from 4 June 62 until 16 July 62. In the first treatment session she required five shocks. During approximately thirty subsequent sessions she frequently made no approach to the "temptation food"; on the five occasions when she did, she immediately received further shocks which were always terminated on cessation of the approach behaviour. During the latter part of this time (from 11th treatment session onwards) when she was not actually connected up to the shocking apparatus she, in fact, made no approaches to the "temptation food". If she had done so the plan was to immediately reconnect the apparatus and revert to the earlier treatment procedure again. During the 6 weeks treatment period the patient lost weight (from 205 to 185 lb). During the next 6 months she continued to steadily lose weight. At the time of discharge her weight had been constant for 2 months at between 130 and 125 lb. Following treatment she had persisted with the low calorie diet and had become less reluctant to eat even this at times. Menstruation, however, remained regular throughout treatment and subsequently. Following discharge she failed to attend regularly for follow-up. She was last seen briefly on 17 March 64 (20 months after treatment). At that time she weighed 133 lb and she said that her weight had not fluctuated greatly. Otherwise her behaviour was unchanged, she was not depressed and she was taking the same amount of amphetamine as before.

Case No. 2 was an in-patient from 31 October 62 until 7 December 62 and again from 7 March 63 to 29 March 63. Following admission the patient began to lose weight without specific treatment. She attributed this to "being away from home" and added that, under such favourable circumstances, she had always been able to lose weight to 17 stone. She was put in the treatment situation at a time when she weighed 17 st. 3 lb. She was subject to one initial practice shock and became very concerned not to have it repeated. During subsequent treatment sessions with the electrodes attached she made no approach to the "temptation food" and ate only the prescribed diet. She therefore avoided further shocks. Her weight continued to fall very gradually during the next 5 weeks down to 16 st. 4 lb. During this period the patient became increasingly hypochondriacal and depressed. At a ward meeting she suddenly became aggressive, critical and suspicious and insisted on leaving the hospital. She was subsequently seen at intervals as an out-patient during the next 3 months. She rapidly gained weight to 17 stone and became less depressed. During this period she received brief interpretative psychotherapy and drug treatment. She agreed to enter the hospital again. On admission her weight was 16 st. 7 lb. The aversion procedure was reinstated. She again avoided receiving shocks. Her weight fell to 16 stone and her hypochondriacal and depressive symptoms returned. She started gaining weight even whilst ostensibly dieting and again insisted on discharge. She said at this time "I would rather be happy and healthy than slim". One month later she weighed 17 stone. During the past year her weight has gradually increased to 19 stone.

This case is discussed elsewhere in relation to measurements of some "transference" changes during therapy (Crisp, 1964).

Discussion

The number of variables which might be relevant in accounting for the difference in response to treatment of these two patients cannot be clearly determined or evaluated. However, some of the differences between the two cases which may be important were obvious. Thus, in the therapeutic situations, one patient entered into the conditioning treatment and the other avoided it; both experienced anxiety in this situation but only the former experienced it specifically in relation to her early approach behaviour towards the "temptation food" and therefore in some accordance with the theoretical requirements of

D

aversion therapy. The latter case could not specifically associate the early approach behaviour with actual experience of pain. This difference between the cases indicates the necessity of precise and absolute pairing of unconditioned and conditioned stimuli. Case No. 1 experienced an emotionally deprived childhood and had always "acted out" in a psychopathic indulgent way in many areas of pleasurable activity, one of which was overeating. After treatment she continued to actively derive pleasure in areas other than overeating and her more attractive figure may have been an advantage to her in this. Case No. 2, a psychoneurotic person with a family history of obesity due to overeating, began to overeat in a state of depression when a pleasurable relationship with her husband was denied her. Eating was her only pleasurable experience and was probably reinforced by the gratifying social role that her obesity conferred upon her. This proposition finds some support in that, every time her eating was curtailed, she became anxious and depressed. However, these latter symptoms may equally well have derived from her physical state of hunger or from her being an anxious person in a treatment involving punishment and need not necessarily have been related to her need to overeat. Another evident factor was that of the difference in age between the two cases. Thus it is usually more socially acceptable to be obese in later life than in your adulthood; it is certainly more common. Also Case No. 2 has a strong positive family history of obesity; this was not so with Case No. 1. As far as personality variables are concerned, clinically Case No. 1 had predominantly psychopathic traits while Case No. 2 was considered to have a neurotic character disorder. On the M.P.I., Case No. 1 scored E28, N20; and Case No. 2 scored E24, N9. This latter N score of 9 could be explained by denial on the part of Case No. 2 and this would be consistent with many of her clinical comments including her statements about her eating.

Acknowledgment—The authors are indebted to Professor Denis Hill for referring these patients to them for treatment and for his encouragement.

References

BEECH H. R. (1960) The symptomatic treatment of writer's cramp, in *Behaviour Therapy and the Neuroses* (Ed. H. J. Eysenck). Pergamon Press, London.
BEECH H. R. (1963) Some theoretical and technical difficulties in the application of behaviour therapy. *Bull. Brit. Psychol. Soc.* 16, 23–25.
BRUCE J. and RUSSELL G. F. M. (1962) Premenstrual tension. *Lancet* i, 267–271.
BRUCH H. (1940) Obesity in Childhood. III. Physiologic and psychologic aspects of the food intake of obese children. *Amer. J. Dis. Child.* 59, 739–781.
BRUCH H. (1952) Psychological aspects of reducing. *Psychosom. Med.* 14, 337–346.
BRUCH H. (1958) Obesity. *Ped. Clin. N. Amer.* 5, 613–627.
CRISP A. H. (1964) An attempt to measure an aspect of "Transference" *Brit. J. med. Psychol.* 37, 17–30.
DUNBAR F. (1954) *Emotions and Bodily Changes.* Columbia University Press, New York.
EYSENCK H. J. (1960) Introduction to Part IV of *Behaviour Therapy and the Neuroses.* Pergamon Press, London.
FENICHEL O. (1946) *Psychoanalytic Therapy of the Neuroses.* Routledge & Kegan Paul, London.

HAMBURGER W. W. (1951) Emotional Aspects of Obesity. *Med. Clin. N. Amer.* 35, 483–499.

Leading article (1964) Nothing to eat but food. *Lancet* i, 593–594.

LEAVELL H. R. and CLARK E. G. (1958) *Preventive Medicine for the Doctor in his Community.* McGraw-Hill, New York.

MAYER J. (1955) The physiologic basis of obesity and leanness. *Nutr. Abstrs Rev.* 25, 597–611, 871–883.

NICHOLSON W. M. (1946) Emotional factors in obesity. *Amer. J. med. Sci.* 211, 443–447.

OSWALD I. (1962) Induction of illusory and hallucinatory voices with consideration of behaviour therapy. *J. ment. Sci.* 108, 196–212.

PARNELL R. W. (1958) *Behaviour and Physique.* Arnold, London.

PASWAN G. L. S. (1963) *Metabolism in Obesity.* Final report in the symposium on obesity. William Warn, England.

QUAADE F. (1955) *Obese Children: Anthropology and Environment.* Danish Science Press, Copenhagen.

SHORVON H. J. and RICHARDSON J. S. (1949) Sudden obesity and psychological trauma. *Brit. med. J.* 2, 951–955.

SIMON R. I. (1963) Obesity as a depressive equivalent. *J. Amer. med. Ass.* 208–210.

STRANG J. M. (1959) *Diseases of Metabolism* (Ed. G. G. Duncan). W. B. Saunders, Philadelphia.

STUNKARD A. J. (1957) The dieting depression. *Amer. J. Med.* 23, 77–86.

THORPE J. G. (1964) Therapeutic failure in a case of aversion therapy. *Behav. Res. Ther.* 1, 293–296.

WALLER J. V., KAUFMAN M. R. and DEUTSCH F. (1940) Anorexia nervosa: a psychosomatic entity. *Psychosom. Med.* 2, 2–16.

WEISS E. and ENGLISH O. (1957) *Psychosomatic Medicine.* W. B. Saunders, Philadelphia.

CHAPTER 7

Massed Electrical Aversion Treatment of
Compulsive Eating

B. WIJESINGHE

Claybury Hospital, Woodford Bridge, Essex.

Summary– Two patients with long-standing compulsive eating problems were treated with massed electrical aversion therapy. Both patients when followed up 1 yr after treatment remained free from their compulsions and had made satisfactory adjustments to their life situations.

Aversion therapy has been one of the principal techniques used in the treatment of patients who are over-weight due to compulsive eating. While the studies of Wolpe (1958) and Foreyt and Kennedy (1971) have reported positive results, those of Meyer and Crisp (1964) and Kennedy and Foreyt (1968) were either equivocal or showed only temporary gains. Thus even though it is recognised that electrical aversion has the advantage that the timing, intensity and duration of the stimulus can be precisely controlled (Rachman, 1965), variations in the design of reinforcement schedules may lead to equivocal results. Of course, if over-eating is maintained by anxiety it is necessary to treat the anxiety before considering aversion (Wolpe, 1969).

This paper concerns the treatment of two patients with longstanding compulsive eating problems that were brought under control by massed electrical aversion, enabling satisfactory adjustments to their life situations.

Treatment

The treatment of both patients was carried out by the use of electric shock as the aversive stimulus in a classical conditioning paradigm. The shock was administered from an apparatus which had a voltage range of 80–140 V, induced from a 6 V power pack. A buzzer was paired with the shock, but could be sounded without the shock. The duration of the signal (buzzer/shock) could be carried by a timer which had 10 settings ranging between 0.1–2.5 sec.

The patient was requested to bring samples of all food for which she had a compulsion. These were placed on a table at which she sat. The electrodes were attached to her left hand. The therapist sat behind her in a position from which

Reprinted with permission from *Journal of Behavior Therapy and Experimental Psychiatry*, 1973, **4**, 133–135.

her movements could be observed. Before the aversion trials commenced a subjective shock range between slightly unpleasant to very unpleasant was established. The patient was then requested to pick up any item of food on the table, bring it gradually to her mouth and nibble at it. The shock and buzzer or the buzzer alone was activated by the therapist at varying stages in handling the food, touching it, bringing it half-way to the mouth, and nibbling at it, in random order. The intensity and duration of the stimuli were also varied randomly.

Altogether six sessions were held on a single day — three in the morning and three in the afternoon. In the first two sessions the buzzer/buzzer-and-shock ratio was 1 : 3, in the next two 1 : 1, and in the final two 3 : 1. Each session lasted approximately 30 min, the morning and afternoon sessions separated by a 2-hr interval, and the others by 20 min intervals. In each session 40–50 trials were given.

Case Data

PATIENT 1

A 37-yr-old woman, separated from her husband, was referred to the clinic with a 6-yr history of compulsive eating, that had become progressively worse in the previous 2 yr. It had started after her husband had left her, but even before that when she was depressed or frustrated she used to find solace in eating biscuits or chocolates. Some marked depressive symptoms had been successfully treated by anti-depressants, but the compulsive behaviour had persisted. There was a regular pattern of "binges" two or three times a week. At the beginning of an episode she would have sensations which she described as "feverish excitement" which would compel her to go to the nearest baker's shop and buy large quantities of sweet, starchy foods, — cakes, biscuits, chocolates — and either drive out in her car to some secluded place or take the food home. She would then set about consuming this food in a voracious manner, "making a pig of myself" as she put it. This would continue for an hour or two, by which time she would feel "bloated, tired and sick". This would usually be followed by loss of appetite for a day or two, while she would feel extremely guilty. The abstinence from food after a compulsive eating episode kept her weight within bounds. Nevertheless it seriously disrupted her work as an outdoor supervisor for a firm of dress machinists, and also her social life.

Following aversion therapy there was a complete cessation of the compulsive eating, with a marked change in her general behaviour. She was able to deal with her work satisfactorily and developed new social interests. She was seen on a supportive basis at fortnightly intervals for a period of 3 months. One year after treatment, complete control had been maintained without further treatment.

PATIENT II

A 20-yr-old graphic art student was referred as an out-patient because she had a compulsive habit of eating sweet starchy food between meals. This had started soon after her mother's sudden death when she was aged 12. She had been very close to her mother and her death had been a great shock to her. She weighed 190 lb at the initial interview. The patient described herself as "bitchy, rude, coarse and I swear too much". She dressed rather dowdily as if to emphasise her gracelessness. She did not have any boy friends or social interests.

Following aversion therapy she was seen at fortnightly intervals, when she was weighed and her weight recorded on a weight chart. No special diet was advocated. The compulsive eating stopped immediately after the treatment. After a fortnight her weight was down to 184 lb, and a steady decline was observed from then onwards till the sixth month when it was 165 lb. Meanwhile, she changed her outlook on life, took greater care over her appearance, became much more outgoing and sociable and entered into a relationship with a boy which she described as "serious". When she was followed up 1 yr later, the control in her eating was being maintained, and without any dietary restrictions her weight had levelled off at 162 lb. She had completed her course of studies, found satisfactory employment and was engaged to be married.

Discussion

The two cases reported here illustrate the effectiveness of massed electrical aversion in controlling a compulsive eating behaviour, which had gained at least partial autonomy. Aversion is an effective way of releasing the patient from the constraining forces of such a habit. The massed aversion treatment used here seemed to achieve marked change with economy of time and effort. Possibly, the good effects were enhanced by varying the nature, intensity and duration of stimulation. It is felt that support and guidance for some time after treatment may have been of considerable importance in helping the patients to readjust.

Acknowledgement—The author wishes to thank Dr. D. H. Irwin, Consultant Psychiatrist, Claybury Hospital for permission to publish the case material.

References

FOREYT J. P. and KENNEDY W. A. (1971) Treatment of overweight by aversion therapy, *Behav. Res. & Therapy* 9, 29–34.

KENNEDY W. A. and FOREYT J. P. (1968) Control of eating behaviour in an obese patient by avoidance conditioning, *Psychol. Rep.* 22, 571–576.

MEYER V. and CRISP A. H. (1964) Aversion therapy in two cases of obesity, *Behav. Res. & Therapy* 2, 143–147.

RACHMAN S. (1965) Aversion therapy: chemical or electrical, *Behav. Res. & Therapy* 2, 289–299.

WOLPE J. (1958) *Psychotherapy by Reciprocal Inhibition*, Stanford University Press, Stanford, California.

WOLPE J. (1969) *The Practice of Behavior Therapy*, Pergamon Press. New York.

CHAPTER 8

Aversion–Relief Therapy:
a New Method for General Application

J. G. THORPE, E. SCHMIDT, P. T. BROWN and D. CASTELL

Banstead Hospital, Sutton, Surrey

Summary– A new technique named Aversion–Relief Therapy is described. It appears to be suitable for general application in the field of neurosis and greatly simplifies the normal requirements of the treatment situation. Cases are presented in which the technique has been applied and the therapeutic results are so far encouraging. Some of the theoretical issues involved are discussed.

Introduction

"The fact that the present (behaviour therapy) procedures, crude as they are, yet appear to have some effect is the best justification for believing that the time spent in seeking for improvements will be well spent" (Eysenck, 1960, p. 464). Work at this hospital has been directed towards the production of such improvements. As the bulk of our earlier work was concerned with aversion therapy we were not happy with the idea of giving aversion to anxious patients. Secondly, we experienced considerable difficulty in reproducing the actual behaviour to be treated, and thirdly, we were looking for some method which would enable us not only to extinguish a particular pattern of behaviour but which would, in addition, facilitate the acquisition of new behaviour. Out of these problems a new technique has been developed which will be presented here. Examples of its application will be given and some of the theoretical implications discussed.

Before presenting this technique, the above problems will be pursued in more detail.

The most important one arises from Eysenck's assertion that ". . . psychoanalysts show a preoccupation with psychological methods involving mainly *speech*, while behaviour therapy concentrates on actual *behaviour* as most likely to lead to the extinction of the unadaptive conditioned responses" (Eysenck, 1960, p. 11). As a result of this assertion, behaviour therapists have gone to great lengths to produce the behaviour in question prior to the commencement of behaviour therapy—a task often requiring considerable ingenuity and effort (Jones, 1955, 1960; Lavin *et al*, 1961; Blakemore *et al.*,

Reprinted with permission from *Behaviour Research and Therapy*, 1964, **2**, 71–82.

1963a.) Appropriate stimuli are also of great concern, and again tremendous effort is expended in order to acquire them (Raymond, 1956; Meyer, 1957; Walton and Black, 1958; Bevan, 1960; Freund, 1960; Clark, 1963; Walton and Mather, 1963; Schmidt, 1964.) It would probably be true to say that more time is spent in satisfying these requirements than in carrying out the behaviour therapy itself. If one considers the richness of human experience, it is inevitable on this argument that many years will elapse before any conditioning laboratory is adequately equipped to deal with even a small fraction of neurotic maladaptations.

In our own experience at this hospital, the preparation of the conditioning situation has been costly both in time and in money. Our first patient, a transvestite, had to be photographed while in female attire and the photographs processed before treatment could begin (Lavin et al., 1961). Our second transvestite had to be provided with literally dozens of pairs of nylons which were torn to shreds as he cross-dressed dozens of times a day (Blackmore et al., 1963a). A homosexual patient required a large number of photographs of his male partners which, fortunately, he was able to provide (Thorpe et al., 1964). Lastly, a phobic patient had to be photographed in a number of anxiety-evoking situations which were, during treatment, presented as relief stimuli.

It is interesting to note that we have not, in these cases, been concerned with the behavioural maladaptation itself, but rather with a symbolic representation of it. It is also fairly obvious that in some cases the *actual* behaviour is not available for use in the behaviour therapy setting—for example in the case of the homosexual patient. What, moreover, could be used for the alcoholic patient who, if faradic aversion were to be employed, would slowly but surely become intoxicated as he imbibed his alcohol?

Once the necessity for obtaining real rather than symbolic behaviour is removed, however, the treatment situation is simplified considerably, and, at its simplest, permits the use of appropriate *words* to represent the maladaptive behaviour or appropriate stimuli for each individual patient. Whether behaviour therapy conceived in this way will produce changes in behaviour will be dealt with in a later section. Whether such a technique can be called behaviour therapy at all is debatable. It does, however, provide us with facilities for the treatment of any maladaptation whatever.

The new technique employs verbal representations of behaviour as a substitute for actual behaviour. It also employs verbal representations of stimuli instead of the stimuli themselves. In this respect it is to some extent similar to Wolpe's "symbolic" method of systematic desensitization in which relaxation responses are produced to mental images of stimuli which normally evoke anxiety (Wolpe, 1954). As he observes, however, this method is not applicable if the imaginary stimuli do not themselves evoke anxiety. In these cases, recourse has to be made to the production of real stimuli rather than imaginary ones (Clark, 1963).

The second problem arises out of a quotation from the Introductory section to Part IV of Eysenck's book. It is that "Aversion therapy should be preceded by careful diagnostic assessment of the degree of neuroticism of the patient" (p. 277). Evidence is cited that a high degree of neuroticism easily leads to a condition in which symptoms may be worsened rather than abolished through the use of aversion techniques. Presumably as a result of this statement, it is now accepted that aversion therapy will succeed only in making the anxious patient worse.

The work of Liversedge and Sylvester (1955), Raymond (1956) and Freund (1960), however, does not lead to this conclusion, nor does our own experience. We have treated patients who had high anxiety scores with aversion therapy, and no exacerbation of symptoms was observed (Blakemore *et al.*, 1963a, 1963b; Thorpe and Schmidt, 1964).

It was therefore decided to employ our new technique to patients irrespective of their degree of neuroticism or apparent anxiety. This step appeared to be fully justified in the light of the above examples.

The third problem is from the same source as the second. "It is likely", wrote Eysenck, "that aversion therapy by itself will be found useful in only a limited and carefully selected number of cases; it is probable that it will be found useful in many more cases if it can be combined with treatment by reciprocal inhibition" (p. 277). This means that two separate courses of treatment should be embarked upon. The new technique embodies the second treatment in the first, and is a necessary part of it. This is made possible by the fact that the termination of aversion conditioning is invariably followed by relief. The only problem therefore, is to select an appropriate stimulus—in this case a word, which can be expected to become the conditioned stimulus for the relief response which will follow. It is for this reason that we have named our technique "Aversion—Relief" conditioning.

Apparatus

To this end we constructed an apparatus by means of which words could be presented to the patient. This is a wooden box 15×15×3 in. containing a gramophone turntable geared to revolve at the rate of one revolution in four minutes. Into the side directly above the turntable is an aperture 2×2 in., near the edge and radial to the turntable. A small lamp is fixed above the aperture in order to illuminate it when required.

Appropriate words are typed on to a cardboard disk which is sellotaped on to the turntable top. Twenty-four words with equal distances between each can be used, and when the turntable motor is started each word appears in the aperture for about 2½ sec with 10 sec between the words. Twenty-four electrical contacts behind the disk enable an electrical circuit to be completed when each word is central in the aperture, and as each word appears one of a panel of 24 lamps is illuminated in the psychologist's room adjoining the treatment room. In this way we know what is appearing in the aperture at any moment. A microphone is also attached to the wall alongside the aperture, while the amplifier is in the psychologist's room. The psychologist is in control of the turntable, can tell what words are in the aperture at any moment, can control the illumination of the aperture, and can hear the subject. He also has control of another piece of apparatus by means of which electric shocks can be delivered to the subject. The electricity is provided by a G.P.O. hand operated generator delivering 120 V a.c. or by an apparatus described by McGuire and Vallance (1964) modified to give up to 150 V pulsed d.c. In both cases the shock is delivered through specially prepared shoes which the subject wears.

Method

For each patient a disk is prepared which has typed upon it up to twenty-three appropriate words, e.g. "homosexual" and its synonyms for the homosexual patient, "cross dressing" for the transvestite, "fear of clouds" for the cloud phobia, and so on. The twenty-fourth (or last) word is a different one in all cases. In our earlier work it became obvious that whenever a patient who was receiving aversion received a signal that the aversive session was over, he experienced tremendous relief. The signal might have been the opening of a door, or the statement "that is all" or something of the sort. We have been able to utilize this relief response by making the last word on each disk the signal that the patient has received his last shock. Thus we rapidly produce a relief response to whatever relief word we chose. In the case of the homosexual patient a word such as "heterosexual" would be used; in the case of the transvestite "normal dressing"; in the case of the cloud phobia "clouds" and so on. Patients quickly learn to look forward eagerly to the appearance in the aperture of this word they have been told signifies "no more shock".

The patient is ushered into the treatment room which is in darkness and is told to put on the shoes and to read out the words aloud as they appear in the illuminated aperture. If he fails to read a word he will receive an even more intense shock. He is told what the relief signal will be on each occasion. As each vocalization is heard through the speaker a shock is delivered as quickly as possible. The delay is seldom greater than 0.5 sec. Immediately after the relief word is read out the turntable motor is stopped, and the patient left in the room in which only the relief word is visible for 2 minutes. The aperture light is then switched off and the patient responds to this by coming out of the treatment room and spending five minutes in the rest room near by. The disk is then changed for a similar one, but having a different number and order of words again with a relief word at the end. This is to prevent the rote learning of the disk in which case the relief response would be expected to be less pronounced.

Five such trials constitute a session, and sessions are usually given at the rate of one per day. On average sixty shocks are delivered each session.

It is quite a common experience for patients receiving this treatment to show marked signs of anxiety between sessions. No drugs have been given for this anxiety for the simple reason that they may mask the effects of treatment which are necessary in evaluating its progress. The homosexual, for example, will become hostile and aggressive in his attitude to homosexuals; the transvestite will have a changed reaction to women's clothes; the phobic anxiety state will no longer show anxiety responses to his phobic object and so on. If the patients are not receiving sedatives they attribute these changes directly to the treatment and, although treatment is extremely unpleasant for them they are eager to continue with it.

Sessions are continued until there is some evidence that such changes have occurred, and that the patient himself feels that he is "cured". We have been fortunate in obtaining patients with a variety of psychiatric diagnoses for this treatment and details of the patients treated so far will follow.

It has been suggested that our method can best be regarded as a refinement and improvement on Wolpe's anxiety–relief technique. Wolpe's method requires that a continuous shock is delivered to the subject who is told to bear it until the desire to have it removed becomes very strong, then to say aloud the word "calm". As soon as he says the word the current is switched off. Most subjects report that after a few sessions, using the word in disturbing situations decreases their disturbed feeling (Wolpe, 1954). We would hold that any resemblances between this and our own method are superficial on the following grounds. In the first place Wolpe's method is used as an adjunct to some other form of therapy, whereas aversion–relief therapy is used by itself. Secondly, Wolpe's method requires that the subject can bear the shock for some time before the current is switched off, whereas in our method the shock is well above pain threshold. Thirdly the aversive stimulus is controlled by the subject in Wolpe's method, whereas in our own it is under the control of the operator. Finally, our method is designed to produce both aversive *and* relief responses. For these reasons we regard our own method as a development of aversive conditioning in which the relief response which inevitably follows the cessation of aversive conditioning is utilized. Further consideration of the relationship between our method and the methods of reciprocal inhibition in general is given in the discussion.

Cases Treated

CASE 1

Male homosexual aged 31. Admitted for treatment of a recurrent reactive depression. He attributed all his present symptoms of anxiety, tension and irritability to his sexual practices of which he was deeply ashamed. Following the successful treatment of his depression by drugs, the patient was referred to the Psychology Department for treatment of his homosexuality.

From the age of 12 he had been aware of his "unnatural emotional attachment to boys and lack of interest in girls". He had his first homosexual experience at 16 with an older man. Since the age of 25 he had been living in London where he worked as a receptionist, and had indulged in frequent homosexual activity with male prostitutes picked up in certain public houses. This had occurred at roughly fortnightly intervals but masturbation which was accompanied by homosexual fantasies occurred every 3 days. He had on rare occasions introduced females into his fantasy as well, though he had never had any heterosexual experience, and had never been emotionally or sexually attracted to women. For the first time in his life, while in hospital, he became friendly with a female patient.

Results of psychological tests showed him to be highly anxious, his score on the MAS (Taylor, 1953) falling at the 98th percentile. On the MPI (Eysenck, 1959) his score on the N-scale placed him at the 86th percentile, but his E-score was low (10th percentile). His performance on the Osgood Semantic Differential (Osgood *et al.*, 1957) revealed a very negative attitude both to himself and to women.

In this case, treatment was undertaken in two stages. During the first stage the patient was given photographs of attractive females and instructed to use them in his masturbation fantasy. He was to masturbate as often as possible using heterosexual fantasies only. Thus women would become associated with sexual reinforcement. At first, though masturbation was successful, he took a long time to reach orgasm, his fantasy was brief and the girl "just a body not a person". By the seventh session he reported a definite change—his fantasy now involved more prolonged and more satisfying sexual activity and the time taken to reach emission had decreased considerably.

At this point aversion therapy was introduced. Throughout this second stage, masturbation sessions continued with heterosexual fantasies which were becoming increasingly exciting. Aversion stimuli were words he connected with his homosexual practices, e.g. "gay pub", "sodomy", "in bed with a male", "flapping wrists", etc. For this patient the relief stimuli were at different times "sex with a woman", "women", "girl friend", and "female breasts".

In the course of treatment, the patient developed depression and various gastric ailments. However, he persisted and completed treatment because he felt it was doing him good and really changing his sexual orientation. He had observed that his reaction to the homosexuals he met both in and out of hospital was now one of aggression and disgust rather than pleasure. Also he was claiming great satisfaction from his heterosexual masturbation fantasies and from seeing and kissing his girl friend. He soon felt confident enough to leave hospital. He had had 30 aversion sessions, at the rate of 1 session per day, and 38 masturbation sessions.

On discharge psychological assessment showed a drop from the 98th to 88th percentile on the MAS. On the Osgood SD his attitude to himself had changed. He now saw himself as "manly" and "domineering", while women were now regarded as "desirable sexual partners". His own assessment of the treatment was "I never think about homosexuals now and when I meet one, all I feel is aggression and disgust. On the other hand for the first time in my life I am considering sex with a woman as a possibility and an enjoyable one too."

CASE 2

Male aged 27. The patient had strong homosexual feelings, although he was not an overt homosexual, but was anxious about becoming one and about his inability to form emotional relationships with girls. He had one homosexual experience at the age of 12 (mutual masturbation), but has had none since. At the age of 15 he felt emotionally attracted towards boys and thought he was different. At the age of 18 he had his first heterosexual experience, and since has had 7–8 girl friends with whom he had intercourse, which he enjoyed physically but not emotionally. He masturbated about once a fortnight, using homosexual and heterosexual fantasy in equal proportions. He had received no previous treatment.

The aversion stimulus was a single word "homosexual" and the relief stimulus "girl friends". The patient had 16 sessions at the rate of one session per day. He was instructed to masturbate as often as he could in order that we could assess changes in his sexual fantasy. After the 1st and 2nd sessions, he reported having nightmares, the content of which was a situation where the patient was being chased by homosexuals; to escape he ran into a wood and the dream finished by his having intercourse with a girl. The nightmares lasted for a week, after which he started having two nocturnal emissions a night associated with heterosexual dreams. He stated that he was thinking about girls nearly all the time. Thinking about homosexuality he found "frightening and sickening".

During the treatment the patient became anxious and apprehensive. Despite this apprehension he was quite willing to continue the treatment. Prior to discharge he reported feeling much happier about his future. He did not want even to think about boys, and he had formed a fairly strong relationship with a female patient. His MAS scores pre- and post-treatment had shown no change, falling at the 92nd percentile. On the other hand two psychometric attempts to assess change, Osgood's SD and Kelly's Repertory Grid (Bannister, 1963), showed a more assertive and positive response towards women and heterosexuality. The patient was seen 3 weeks after discharge in out-patients where he reported that he was still having a good relationship with the girl, and had had no problems about homosexual feelings.

CASE 3

American male, aged 40, MAS score at the 25th percentile, referred with a diagnosis of latent homosexuality. He had had no previous psychiatric treatment. Behaviourally he was concerned that when under the influence of alcohol he felt extremely attracted towards men; and also that when he masturbated he had fantasies of fellatio with men. Prior to admission his overt sexual activity had been entirely heterosexual except for his only homosexual experience at the age of 19. His range of heterosexual experience was wide, and he had been married at the age of 32 but separated from his wife after 6 months and divorced 18 months later. During his 18 months in England prior to admission he had had no prolonged heterosexual and no homosexual contacts.

Treatment started on an out-patient basis, and consisted of the patient's writing 3 essays a week all with the title "the Merits of Heterosexuality". Essays were marked on a random basis, the patient's task being to discover the marking system. It was considered that this might help to effect some cognitive change in the patient's homosexual attitude, and it was also seen as a device by which the patient could be kept in weekly contact with the hospital until his studies allowed him time for in-patient treatment. At the end of 6 weeks the patient was available for in-patient treatment. No behavioural change was apparent as a result of the essay writing. A fortnight's in-patient treatment followed. The aversion stimulus was "homosexual" and the relief stimulus "girl friends". With only a fortnight available for treatment, words were presented at a maximum of 35 per trial instead of 23 as described above. No sexual activity took place during treatment, as he preferred not to masturbate; two dreams were reported which could be construed as having heterosexual significance. Throughout treatment he felt "very positive about this kind of treatment" in that it had given the boost he needed to his own efforts to control his homosexual feelings.

Follow-up 4 weeks after discharge found him firmly maintaining that the treatment had worked. Behaviourally he had found no homosexual desires whilst well under the influence of alcohol during the kind of party situation when he would normally have experienced homosexual thoughts. He had, on the contrary, begun a heterosexual association one week after discharge, and had had intercourse. He reported that he felt much more sexually orientated towards women and since treatment found long standing acquaintances with women much more attractive as likely to lead to sexual activity, than at any time before treatment. Treatment thus appears to have resulted in a behavioural change in the desired direction — at least in the immediate post treatment period. Long-term follow-up is in progress.

CASE 4

Male patient aged 21 who came from Australia. Since the age of 16 he had indulged in transvestism (about thrice weekly), and occasionally in animal intercourse. He masturbated and ejaculated whilst in female attire, and on the occasions when he masturbated without female attire his fantasy was always concerned with cross dressing and gave rise to considerable guilt.

He had been advised in Australia to take a long trip abroad which would help him to get out of the habit, but soon after his arrival in England he cross dressed again and sought psychiatric help. In England he had met an Australian girl of whom he was fond, but he could not pursue the relationship because it would not be fair to her.

The aversion stimuli for this patient were: "sex with animals", "woman in mirror" (which he always used), "self as woman", "brassiere in mirror", "animal intercourse", "cross dressing", "sex with cow" and several variations. The relief stimulus used throughout was "masturbating". He was instructed to masturbate whenever he was sexually aroused and to report on this.

The patient received eleven sessions at the rate of one per day and reported considerable anxiety at the thought of coming for treatment. After 2 days he reported that his masturbation fantasy had changed completely—he now used images of his girl friend, and also that the quality of his masturbation had changed. It was accompanied by intense sensual pleasure and was not followed by guilt. At the end of 2 weeks he was convinced that he would never cross dress again, and was now pursuing his girl friend whom he was considering in terms of marriage. He was seen in the out-patients department 2 weeks after discharge and reported that everything was fine. He returned to Australia, promising to write at intervals and immediately if his previous behaviour recurred. This was in order to obtain similar treatment in Australia. He has not written to date—3 months after treatment.

CASE 5 (IN TREATMENT AT PRESENT)

Male, unmarried, aged 32, diagnosed as a motor-cycle fetishist and latent homosexual. A brief experiment (Brown, 1964) confirmed that his sexual interest was homo- rather than heterosexually orientated. Pre treatment MAS score was at the 87th percentile, with MPI scores N at the 89th percentile and E at the 18th percentile.

Behaviourally his practice was to steal a motor-cycle, drive it away, and at speed obtain an erection and emission. He then returned the motor-cycle. This behaviour pattern started in 1951, but he had first realised its abnormal sexual aspects in 1957 while undergoing 18 months group psychotherapy elsewhere. In the 10 months immediately prior to admission here in October 1963 he had stolen a motor-cycle once every 10 days on average. Associated with the fetishistic behaviour was dressing up in motor-cycle clothing which increased the pleasure derived.

Apart from the motor-cycle behaviour, it became apparent before treatment began that the patient was extremely ignorant regarding sexual information, and that he had a history of blacking out when the subject of female genitalia was discussed or when he read sexual material. It was also established that he had had no overt heterosexual experience, no satisfactory masturbation, and nocturnal emissions were commonly associated with a fantasy of his rescuing an unidentified man from some dangerous situation. Aversion stimuli were words such as "motor-cycles", "leather jackets", and "ton-up", while relief stimuli, which changed as treatment progressed, were (a) "masturbating", (b) pictures and words presenting basic sexual information, and (c) pictures of female nudes. After three months' treatment the patient now (a) feels no arousal at, or interest in, the sight or idea of motor-cycles; (b) can read about and discuss sexual material with ease; and (c) is actively pursuing heterosexual relationships. He has not yet masturbated successfully, but nocturnal emissions have begun to be associated with heterosexual fantasies for the first time in his life.

Overall, treatment appears to be progressing in the behavioural directions required — as evidenced by the patient's lack of interest in motor-cycles, increasingly more adequate heterosexual behaviour and absence of homosexual fantasies.

CASE 6

Male aged 43. He complained of phobic anxiety responses to clouds, lifts and tunnels. The fear of lifts was of some 10 years' duration. Four years ago the patient experienced a panic attack in a train which stopped in the Severn Tunnel; since then he has avoided tunnels. Fourteen months ago his attention was drawn to the oppressive effect of low clouds and this thought preyed on his mind until he experienced severe anxiety whenever clouds were low and thick. All these conditions were aggravated by the fact that the patient had rheumatic fever at the age of 21, and although he recovered completely he was afraid that a panic attack would cause heart failure. He had had 3 months' out-patient treatment on tranquillizers with little result. Initially, a treatment schedule involving the writing of essays about the positive aspects of lifts and clouds was followed. The tunnel symptom was left as a control. The patient wrote three essays a week on clouds and three on lifts for a period of 3 months (September to December). Initially an improvement was noticed on the cloud phobia, but as the weather worsened so the symptom worsened. He was still afraid of lifts. At this point it was decided to abandon this form of treatment as it induced only temporary change. Thus a treatment procedure based on aversion—relief was introduced. Separate sessions were given for each of the two symptoms. For the phobic anxiety of clouds the aversion stimulus was "fear of clouds", and the relief stimulus "clouds". For the phobic anxiety of lifts the aversion stimulus was "fear of lifts", and the relief stimulus "myself". The patient has had four sessions on each symptom at the rate of one per week on an out-patient basis. Before this treatment started the patient described himself as continually having to fight his fear of clouds, and although he rarely panicked he was continually aware of the presence of clouds. After four sessions the patient reported feeling much better about clouds. Although occasionally ideas about clouds occurred, he coped with them immediately. He stated that he considered himself much better than he was at the beginning of treatment. On the phobic anxiety for lifts he had noticed no improvement. This differential response to treatment can be explained by the differing duration of the symptoms. The fear of clouds has lasted only 14 months, but fear of lifts has lasted 10 years and tunnels 4 years. The treatment, in this case, is continuing.

CASE 7

Female patient aged 33, diagnosed as obsessive—compulsive neurosis. Symptoms were compulsive hand washing, touching her hip, saying a fictitious person's name to herself on numerous occasions, and many others. These symptoms had all developed during the past three and a half years following a particular incident. She had worked as a G.P.'s receptionist in New Zealand at which time one of the Doctor's patients had died. Our patient blamed herself for this although she was clearly not implicated. The name of the deceased patient was always in her mind and relief could be obtained only by going through the elaborate rituals of which she was complaining. She was not able to do any housework, and had, on occasions, sexual intercourse with men other than her husband because during these periods, she imagined that her husband had become the husband of the deceased patient. She could not walk past a mirror or shop window without having to go back and convince herself that she was herself, and not the deceased patient. On Monday mornings she believed she actually became the deceased patient until mid-day when she reverted to herself. She had received a wide variety of treatments for her condition including E.C.T., L.S.D., and hypnosis.

Psychometric testing produced scores falling at the 86th percentile on the MAS, 84th on the N-scale of the MPI and 62nd on the E-scale.

It was decided to avert her to the deceased patient by using her name on the disk. The relief stimulus was "myself". She was treated at the rate of two sessions per day. After a few days her hand washing disappeared and she was reporting that the treatment was already working. She was apprehensive between sessions and cried frequently. She complained that she could not sleep and felt tired all the time. After a week, however, she reported that she had been to a ward dance the night before and knew she was now herself.

After 2 weeks she stated that she could go on no longer. She simply "could not go in and say that girl's name again". She wept bitterly, but unconvincingly, and declined further treatment.

The psychiatric diagnosis had, in the meantime, changed to hysteria which was more appropriate to the behaviour which had been observed while she was receiving treatment. Treatment was discontinued.

CASE 8

A single Irish girl aged 21. Diagnosed as a case of recurrent depression. Referred for treatment of intermittent compulsive over-eating. She had been treated with tranquillizers and appetite suppressants without apparent change in her condition. This behaviour pattern had appeared 4 years ago following a very strict diet which had lasted 2 months. At first the over-eating bouts occurred every 6 weeks but recently their frequency had doubled. The patient reported that during these bouts her mind went blank to everything except food. She would stock up with food, particularly the starchy and sweet items forbidden during her diet, shut herself in her room and eat continuously for 2 to 3 days. By the end of this period she would have put on about a stone in weight and would be physically exhausted. This was accompanied by intense feelings of depression and inadequacy. During the interval between bouts, she still felt she wanted to eat continuously but could restrain herself with the help of drugs. However, she thought about food for "the best part of the day" and dreamed about it every night.

The pre-treatment psychological assessment showed the patient to be highly anxious, falling at the 82nd percentile on the MAS. On the MPI she was found to have a high N-score (88th percentile) but a very low E-score (14th percentile).

A single aversion stimulus was used for this patient — "over-eating" — with "normal eating" as the relief stimulus. Her reaction to the first aversion trial was very strong. She burst into tears and refused to go on with the further four trials that would have constituted her first session. However, she returned for treatment the following day, though complaining of headaches and depression, but again burst into tears and insisted on a one trial session.

By the fourth session, she was reporting a change — "I felt I wanted to start on an over-eating bout but something which wasn't there before held me back." By the sixth session she reported that the time she spent thinking about food was now approximately an hour a day whereas previously it had been as much as 10 to 11 hours. Also she was no longer dreaming about food.

Depression recurred following the eighth treatment session and was accompanied by violent gastric pains. She claimed she could not face any more treatment, preferring drugs. At this point her diagnosis was changed by the psychiatrist in charge from one of "recurrent depression" to one of "hysteria". Treatment was discontinued.

Discussion

It would appear that this method of treatment is an extremely effective way of producing a change in behaviour. How long such changes will last, it is impossible to say, although we have argued elsewhere (Thorpe *et al.*, 1964) that the maintenance of behaviour changes is predominantly due to reinforcers beyond our control.

Our therapeutic results strongly suggest that the use of words rather than actual behaviour will still lead to behavioural change. If this be so, there is no limit to the type of maladaptation that will lend itself to treatment by this method.

The two therapeutic failures are due entirely to the fact that these patients were unable to continue with treatment although symptom changes had already appeared. One is left with the strong suspicion that the reinforcement value of the symptoms of both these patients was considerable, and that they would rather keep their symptoms than lose them. Both patients, as we saw earlier, were later diagnosed as hysterics from which one may suspect that hysterics will not tolerate treatment of this type. These, however, are our only failures so far. It should be added that these two patients were both female. The relevance of this will be studied further.

In regard to neuroticism or anxiety measures before treatment there is no detectable relationship between these and response to treatment. Most of our patients were extremely anxious both clinically and psychometrically, as can be seen from the case details. Not only were they able to tolerate treatment but there was no evidence of exacerbation of symptoms. These observations confirm that aversion therapy can be used in this way without reference to the amount of anxiety present in the patient before treatment.

Eysenck's third assertion that aversion therapy should be combined with therapy by reciprocal inhibition in order to increase its general usefulness requires careful consideration. What he is concerned with is, presumably, avoidance behaviour in which a stimulus evokes anxiety which is reduced by the performance of some act. This act constitutes the maladaptive behaviour and if this behaviour is treated with aversion therapy the anxiety remains. Reciprocal inhibition therapy is then required to eliminate the anxiety response before the patient can be regarded as "cured". Is our technique simply an easy way of applying reciprocal inhibition? If we consider our patient with a cloud phobia, it could be argued that this, in fact, is all that has happened. We have managed to produce a relaxation response to clouds which is incompatible with the previous anxiety response. It should be added, however, that we have also averted him to fear of clouds which may have played a part in successful treatment by breaking into the neurotic paradox of Mowrer (1950). In other words we may have produced in the patient a real fear of his fear of clouds. Further work is clearly required in this connexion but we may conclude that in this example at least, the principle of reciprocal inhibition *may* have been operating.

When we turn to the other examples, the position is apparently different. What we have been attempting is to extinguish a particular pattern and to replace it with another one which is not maladaptive and is socially more acceptable. We have been attempting to replace homosexual behaviour, for instance, with heterosexual behaviour. Insofar as heterosexual behaviour has anxiety evoking properties for the homosexual, then again we may be utilizing the reciprocal inhibition principle. If there is no anxiety, the principle of reciprocal inhibition is not involved and we appear to be dealing simply with new avenues of behaviour which had previously been overlooked. From this analysis we are given positive reinforcement value to objects which previously had comparatively little reinforcement value. Although this analysis is somewhat speculative it is backed by clinical experience in respect of our patients who all report the tremendous affection they develop for the relief stimuli, and follow-ups are consistent in reporting the enhanced stimulus value of these stimuli in real life.

This method therefore lends itself to two main types of problem. First the problem customarily tackled by reciprocal inhibition therapy with the use of electrical aversion more painful than usual in order to increase the intensity of the relief response, and secondly to the problem of the manipulation of motor behaviour. In the latter, new patterns of motor behaviour are substituted for the old.

As one may expect, many problems remain unanswered. The frequency of sessions, the optimal intensity of the shock, the number of shocks, the composition of the list of verbal stimuli etc., all require detailed investigation, and in this connexion further work is under way. The method does, however, appear to carry considerable promise.

Acknowledgements—We would like to express our deep gratitude to Dr. E. P. H. Charlton, Physican Superintendent, Banstead Hospital, without whose co-operation and encouragement this work could never have been carried out. We would also like to thank Drs. E. P. H. Charlton, C. P. Seager, R. P. Kent and C. G. Conway for referring their patients to us and for carrying full clinical responsibility throughout treatments. Finally, thanks are due to Mr. W. M. MacDonald, Mr. W. A. Marriott and Mr. J. H. Syme of the Engineers and Building Departments at the hospital for their assistance in the construction of the apparatus.

References

BANNISTER, D. (1963). The genesis of schizophrenic thought disorder: a serial invalidation hypothesis. *Brit. J. Psychiat.* 109, 680–686.

BEVAN, J. R. (1960) Learning theory applied to the treatment of a patient with obsessional ruminations, in *Behaviour Therapy and the Neuroses* (Ed. H. J. Eysenck). Pergamon Press, London.

BLAKEMORE, C. B., THORPE, J. G., BARKER, J. C., CONWAY, C. G. and LAVIN, N. I. (1963a) The application of faradic aversion conditioning in a case of transvestism. *Behav. Res. Ther.* 1, 29–34.

BLAKEMORE, C. B., THORPE, J. G., BARKER, J. C., CONWAY, C. G. and LAVIN, N. I. (1963b) Follow up note to: Application of faradic aversion conditioning in a case of transvestism. *Behav. Res. Ther.* I, 191.

BROWN, P. T. (1964) On the differentiation of homo- or heteroerotic interest in the male: an operant technique illustrated in a case of a motor-cycle fetishist. *Behav. Res. Ther.* 2, 31–35.

CLARK D. F. (1963) The treatment of monosymptomatic phobia by systematic desensitization. *Behav. Res. Ther.* 1, 63–68.

EYSENCK, H. J. (1959) *Manual of the Maudsley Personality Inventory.* University of London Press, London.

EYSENCK, H. J. (1960) *Behaviour Therapy and the Neuroses.* Pergamon Press, London.

FREUND, K. (1960) Some problems in the treatment of homosexuality, in *Behaviour Therapy and the Neuroses* (Ed. H. J. Eysenck). Pergamon Press, London.

JONES, H. G. (1956) The application of conditioning and learning techniques for the treatment of a psychiatric patient. *J. abnorm. (soc.) Psychol.* 52, 414–420.

JONES, H. G. (1960) Behavioural treatment of enuresis nocturna, in *Behaviour Therapy and the Neuroses* (Ed. H. J. Eysenck). Pergamon Press, London.

LAVIN, N. I., THORPE, J. G., BARKER, J. C., BLAKEMORE, C. B. and CONWAY, C. G. (1961) Behaviour therapy in a case of transvestism. *J. nerv. ment. Dis.* 133, 346–353.

LIVERSEDGE, L. A. and SYLVESTER, J. D. (1955) Conditioning techniques in the treatment of writer's cramp. *Lancet* i, 1147–1149.

McGUIRE, R. J. and VALLANCE, M. (1964) Aversion therapy by electric shock—a simple technique. *Brit. med. J.* 1, 151–153.

MEYER, V. (1957) The treatment of two phobic patients on the basis of learning principles. *J. abnorm. (soc.) Psychol.* 66, 261–266.

MOWRER, O. H. (1950) *Learning Theory and Personality Dynamics.* Ronald Press, New York.

OSGOOD, C. E., SUCI, G. J. and TANNENBAUM, P. H. (1957) *The Measurement of Meaning.* University of Illinois Press, Urbana.

RAYMOND, M. J. (1956) Case of fetishism treated by aversion therapy. *Brit. med. J.* 2, 854–856.

SCHMIDT, E. (1964) A comparative evaluation of verbal conditioning and practical training in an individual case, *Behav. Res. Ther.* 2, 19–26.

TAYLOR, J. (1953) A personality scale of manifest anxiety. *J. abnorm. (soc.) Psychol.* 48, 285–290.

THORPE, J. G. and SCHMIDT, E. (1964) Therapeutic failure in a case of aversion therapy. *Behav. Res. Ther.* 1, 293–296.

THORPE, J. G., SCHMIDT, E. and CASTELL, D. (1964) A comparison of positive and negative (aversion) conditioning in the treatment of homosexuality. *Behav. Res. Ther.* 1, 357–362.

WALTON, D. and BLACK, D. A. (1958) Application of learning theory to the treatment of stammering. *J. psychosom. Res.* 3, 170–179.

WALTON, D. and MATHER, M. D. (1963) The relevance of generalization techniques to the treatment of stammering and phobic symptoms. *Behav. Res. Ther.* 1, 121–125.

WOLPE, J. (1954) Reciprocal inhibition as the main basis of psychotherapeutic effects. *AMA Arch. Neurol. Psychiat.* 72, 205–226.

CHAPTER 9

Cigarette Smoke as a Noxious Stimulus in Self-managed Aversion Therapy for Compulsive Eating: technique and case illustration

KENNETH P. MORGANSTERN[1]

The Pennsylvania State University

Summary– A procedure which uses the inhalation of cigarette smoke as an aversive stimulus is described and illustrated in the successful treatment of an obese compulsive eater. Using a multiple baseline design, three problematic foods were sequentially eliminated by a self-managed aversion procedure in which cigarette smoke served as a noxious stimulus. After dramatic reductions in compulsive eating, the client reported a generalized self-regulatory optimism and initiated substantial changes in her overall diet. Corroborating self-report data on food intake, a weight reduction of 41 lb was observed during 18 weeks of treatment. Additional losses were reported at follow-up. The clinical promise of this aversion procedure and its advantages over alternative treatments are briefly discussed.

Aversion procedures have typically employed either electric shock or nausea-producing chemicals such as emetine and apomorphine. More recently, aversive stimuli have been introduced covertly (Cautela, 1966, 1967). There are times, however, when these standard methods may be inapplicable or impractical. The present report suggests that the inhalation of cigarette smoke may be a potent aversive stimulus for the inexperienced smoker and may be used in a procedure that is simple, efficient, and harmless.

The Technique

Smoking a cigarette usually produces an extremely unpleasant reaction in subjects who have never or rarely smoked before (even for habitual smokers, massed hot smoke can be extremely aversive, cf. Keutzer, 1968; Wilde, 1964). Smoke inhalation elicits an immediate gag response, followed by sensations of dizziness, nausea, and even vomiting. In addition to its demonstrated aversive-

Reprinted with permission from *Behavior Therapy*, 1974, **5**, 255–260, Copyright © 1974 by Academic Press, Inc.

[1] The author acknowledges the many thoughtful comments and helpful suggestions offered by Michael J. Mahoney during the preparation of this manuscript. Requests for reprints should be sent to Kenneth P. Morganstern, Psychology Services, Veterans Administration Hospital, Palo Alto, CA 94304.

ness, there is some evidence to suggest that cigarette smoke may be particularly suited to the treatment of maladaptive eating responses. Several animal studies, for example, have shown that nausea-producing stimuli result in far more effective and generalizeable food avoidance than pain-inducing stimuli such as electric shock (cf. Seligman, 1971). Similar results with human subjects were reported by Stollak (1967) who found that faradic shock had little success in modifying obesity. Moreover, when other aversive procedures are impossible to employ, cigarette smoking may be the most practical physical UCS available.

Case Illustration

BACKGROUND

Miss C. was a 24-year-old, attractive but extremely obese, graduate student when she presented herself for treatment. In addition to eating three regular meals a day, the client reported that she ate candy and "junk" all day long, completely unable to control herself despite countless attempts at dieting and medically prescribed appetite suppressants. Miss C. also stated that she had been in some sort of psychotherapy for 6, nearly continuous, years. This previous treatment had included two instances of hospitalization of very short duration and contact with five separate therapists whose techniques, reportedly, ran the gamut from psychoanalysis to desensitization.

PROCEDURE

Miss C. was seen once a week for a total of 18 treatment sessions. At the start of each week the client was weighed and a record made (starting with Week 2) of her eating behavior. In addition, she was contacted by telephone after Weeks 21 and 24 to report follow-up data on her food consumption and her weight.

A preliminary analysis of Miss C.'s eating habits revealed an enormous consumption of five principal types of food: candy, cookies, doughnuts, ice cream, and pizza. Base-rate data for 3 weeks indicated that the client ate close to 200 pieces of candy, and dozens of cookies and doughnuts per week. In addition, she indulged in pizza and ice cream at least once a day, and often as many as three times in the same day.

At the beginning of the fourth week the rationale for covert sensitization (Cautela, 1966, 1967) was explained and the covert procedure briefly attempted. When it soon became apparent that Miss C. could not consistently maintain a clear image, the intended treatment was abandoned and other possibilities explored. Electric shock was mentioned in passing, only as an example, but the prospect so frightened the client that no serious consideration could be given to its clinical implementation. During previous discussion, Miss C. had reported that a few experiences with smoking had produced extremely unpleasant sensations for her, which included nausea and dizziness; therefore, the possible utilization of smoking as a UCS was suggested to the client. Although skeptical, Miss C. agreed to try the technique. A cigarette was lit and Miss C. was asked to hold it in her hand as she took a bite of candy (the food which showed the highest consumption rate during baseline) and chewed it for a few seconds. Before swallowing the candy she was told to take one long "drag" on the cigarette and then to immediately spit out the food, exclaiming at the same time, "Eating this junk makes me sick." This procedure was repeated 10 times in each session and the client was also asked to practice it on her own twice each day.

During Weeks 5—10, different types of candy were used as target stimuli for aversion treatment. Employing an additive multiple baseline design, cookies were included as target stimuli during Week 11 of treatment and doughnuts were added at Week 15. In this manner, after an initial baseline assessment of these problematic eating behaviors (consumption of candy, cookies, and doughnuts), each response was sequentially targeted in the aversion procedures. In addition to her daily practice assignments at home, Miss C. employed the technique *in vivo* in a variety of problematical situations.

RESULTS

The mean daily number of doughnuts, cookies, and pieces of candy (mostly one-half ounce squares of chocolate or medium bites of candy bars), averaged over weeks, are presented in Fig. 1. The amount of food eaten is quite high and relatively stable over the 3-week baseline period. After aversive contingencies were instituted during Week 4 candy consumption fell to approximately half the base rate level and continued to decline until it was completely eliminated after the ninth weekly treatment session. A similar trend is apparent for the decline of cookie eating during Weeks 11 through 15, although elimination of this behavior is accomplished much more quickly. After Week 15, when the smoking contingencies were applied to the third target food, doughnut consumption fell to zero at this time, Miss C. also began restricting her intake of other problematic foods (e.g., ice cream and pizza) which had shown no noticeable decline during the first 15 weeks. She expressed excited optimism at the possibility of expanding her dietary control and stated, "If I gave up eating all that candy and other stuff, I can do anything!" At this time, the client continued to practice the self-aversion technique twice daily, but no longer found it necessary to use the procedure *in vivo*. When treatment terminated after Week 18, Miss C. was satisfactorily maintaining a low-calorie diet and, because of its success, had terminated the self-aversion procedure. Data obtained by telephone at Weeks 21 and 24 revealed neither the reappearance of compulsive eating nor any subsequent need for the treatment technique. Self-report data revealed no reductions in the subjective aversiveness of cigarette smoke during or

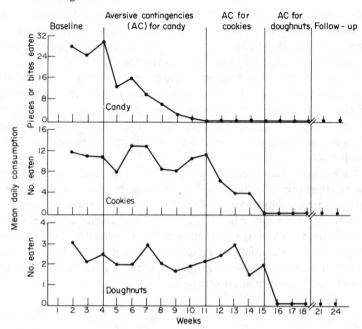

FIG. 1. Mean daily consumption of candy, cookies, and doughnuts
as a function of aversive contingency application.

after treatment. Partially corroborating the self-report data on food consumption, Fig. 2 shows the gradual but consistent weight loss of the client. After 18 weeks of treatment, Miss C. had lost 41 lb. At Weeks 21 and 24, she reported additional weight losses of 9 and 3 lb, respectively, bringing her total reduction to 53 lb. Miss C. left the university after Week 24 and, despite attempts at contact, could not be reached for further follow-up data.

Discussion

The present report offers positive findings and suggests that the use of cigarette smoking may be an effective aversive stimulus in the treatment of compulsive eating behavior. Although there are obvious limitations in the inferences that can be drawn from a single case study, the findings are strengthened by the utilization of a "multiple baseline" design (Baer, Wolf, & Risley, 1968). Thus (Fig. 1), eating rates for cookies and doughnuts show no decline after contingencies were applied to candy consumption (they show, in fact, a brief rise, perhaps a compensation for the reduction of candy). In addition, the dramatic loss of weight appears to be neither a short-lived phenomenon nor the result of a sudden starvation diet. Rather, the reduction is a consistent, steady decline in weight which gradually levels off toward the end

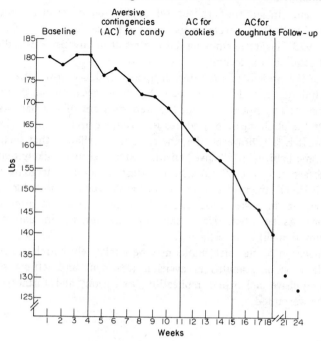

FIG. 2. Weight as a function of aversive contingency
applications to candy, cookies, and doughnuts.

of week 24. Such improvement, considering the long-term intransigence of Miss C.'s eating behavior, offers additional support for the technique. Nevertheless, it is important to recognize the possible role that the implicit demand characteristics inherent in this procedure may have had. Any factor, or interaction of factors, which systematically covaried with the implementation of aversive stimulation (e.g., shifts in attention to one target food at a time, instructions for the client to spit out the food, statements underscoring the inappropriateness of the behavior, or any other placebo effect) is a possible alternative explanation for treatment outcome.

The self-initiated dietary changes after Week 15 highlight the importance of cognitive-symbolic processes in successful self-regulatory maintenance (cf. Kanfer & Phillips, 1970). From the client's statements it may be inferred that she had achieved an important first step in the attainment of self-control skills: the realization that such control is, in fact, possible. That is, she evidenced changes in the perceived "locus of control" of her eating behavior. Previous research has suggested the importance of this variable in the alteration of maladaptive behavior (Lefcourt, 1966).

This consistent self-administration of a potent aversive stimulus also offers encouraging promise to the "contract problem" (Mahoney, 1970) evident in self-punishment. In contrast to the self-application of electric shock, often avoided because of its severe aversiveness (cf. Bandura, 1969; Thoresen & Mahoney, 1973), cigarette smoking did not result in any significant diminution in the application of the technique.

Although the present report offers suggestive evidence of the effectiveness of a new technique, considerable thought has been given to the desirability of teaching clients to smoke when medical reports warn of the dangers of such behavior and a plethora of procedures in recent years have been aimed at its elimination. It is felt, however, that there is little likelihood that such smoking would become habitual for "naive" clients, just as it seems unlikely that subjects would embrace electrical stimulation as a pastime after undergoing treatment with faradic shock (the present case illustration showed no noticeable adaptation to smoking, no increase in its use, and complete cessation after treatment termination). As an alternative to smoking, however, the inhalation of other noxious stimuli might be investigated.

The inhalation of cigarette smoke may be a relatively harmless, economical, and simple noxious stimulus in aversion treatment and self-punishment of certain compulsive behaviors: replication, extension, and further controlled research are warranted.

References

BAER, D. M., WOLF, M. M., & RISLEY, T. R. Some current dimensions of applied behavior analysis. *Journal of Applied Behavior Analysis*, 1968, **1**, 91–97.
BANDURA, A. *Principles of behavior modification.* New York: Holt, Rinehart & Winston, 1969.
CAUTELA, J. R. Treatment of compulsive behavior by covert sensitization. *Psychological Record*, 1966, **16**, 33–41.
CAUTELA, J. R. Covert sensitization. *Psychological Record.* 1967, **20**, 459–468.
KANFER, F. H. & PHILLIPS, J. S. *Learning foundations of behavior therapy.* New York: Wiley, 1970.
KEUTZER, C. S. Behavior modification of smoking: The experimental investigation of diverse techniques. *Behaviour Research and Therapy*, 1968, **6**, 137–157.
LEFCOURT, H. M. Internal versus external control of reinforcement: A review. *Psychological Bulletin*, 1966, **65**, 206–220.
MAHONEY, M. J. Toward an experimental analysis of coverant control. *Behavior Therapy*, 1970, **1**, 510–521.
SELIGMAN, M. E. P. Phobias and preparedness. *Behavior Therapy*, 1971, **2**, 307–320.
STOLLAK, G. E. Weight loss obtained under different experimental procedures. *Psychotherapy: Theory, Research and Practice*, 1967, **4**, 61–64.
THORESEN, C. E., & MAHONEY, M. J. *Behavioral self-control.* New York: Holt, Rinehart & Winston, 1973.
WILDE, G. J. S. Behavior therapy for addicted cigarette smokers. *Behaviour Research and Therapy*, 1964, **2**, 107–110.

CHAPTER 10

Weight Loss Obtained under Different Experimental Procedures[1]

GARY E. STOLLAK[2],[3]

Indiana University

Various techniques have been used in the treatment of obesity (see starred references); the most prevalent have been hypnosis, psychoanalysis, group therapy, and, of course, special foods and diets. In general, the results obtained from the use of these techniques have been less than favorable. Of the people who do lose weight while under treatment, most are found, on follow-ups, to have failed to continue or maintain the weight loss (Consumer Reports, 1963; Kurlander, 1953; Schwartz, 1952; Simmons, 1954). Most of the studies also suffer from lack of control groups, and inadequate specifications of the independent variables, such as the details of the treatment procedures. Replications and definitive statements of the differences between treatments therefore cannot be made. The individual case studies of behavior therapists, although lacking in control groups (as reviewed by Breger and McGaugh, 1965; 1966), at least more clearly specify the details of the therapy procedures. For example, Wolpe (1955) reported the reduction of a food obsession in a woman by pairing electro-shock and fattening food associations.

The present study was designed to evaluate an avoidance conditioning procedure similar to Wolpe's for the treatment of obesity by using large numbers of subjects, a control group and several experimental groups that control for (1) motivation, (2) the subjects attending to their food intake, (3) the experimenter-subject relationship, and (4) the shock-food association contingency.

Reprinted with permission from *Psychotherapy: Theory, Research and Practice*, 1967, **4**, 61–64.

[1] This is an extended version of a paper presented at the 1966 meeting of the Midwestern Psychological Association. The investigation was supported by Public Health Service Research Grant MH-12275 from the National Institute of Mental Health.
[2] The author would like to express his appreciation to Barney Alexander, Larry Clayton, Joan Frankel, Lynn Gottlieb, John Kalivas, Sandra Johnson, and Richard Spear for acting as experimenters and aiding in the collection and analysis of the data.
[3] Now at Michigan State University.

Method

SUBJECTS

The subjects were males and females who were between 20–30% overweight as determined by their weight, height and body build. This range was selected because all individuals more than 20% overweight are required to pay extra premiums on their life insurance policies (Keys, 1955), and over 30% overweight, there is an increased probability of there being a physiological etiology and complication to the obesity (Olson, 1964). Trained personnel estimated the subjects' body builds into small, medium and large.

APPARATUS

A shock apparatus was used with a current range of 0–5 milliamps, and a voltage range of 0–1000 volts. A physician's scale was used to measure the height and weight of the subjects.

PROCEDURE

There were six experimental groups:

Group 1: Control group. This was a control group of twenty male and female subjects who were obtained from the Physical Education Department. At no time during the experiment were they informed that they were participants in a study. After 8 and 10 weeks intervals eighteen of them were weighed again as part of Physical Education "policy."

The subjects in Groups II through VI were volunteers obtained through advertisements in local newspapers. One-hundred and twenty of them who were found to be overweight within specified limits, were randomly assigned to one of the following groups:

Group II: No Contact group. These subjects were asked to return in 8 weeks.

Group III: No Contact–Diary group. These subjects were asked to keep a diary of the kind and approximate amount of food, and the time of each eating occurrence and return with the diary in 8 weeks. They were further told that attending to food intake would result in self-regulation, that they should keep the diary with them at all times, and that they should write down their food intake during or immediately after the occurrence.

Group IV: Contact–Diary group. Along with receiving the same instructions as Group III, these subjects each week for eight weeks, had two fifteen minute discussions of their diaries with a trained experimenter. (The experimenters were one male graduate student, and three male and three female undergraduates.) During each interview, the experimenter commented upon each of the diary items. He gave praise such as "Good" or "You had a well-balanced lunch" etc., for occasions of moderate food intake. When fattening foods such as candy, beer, cake, etc., were consumed, the experimenter obtained through questioning, information as to the details of the situation and the subjects' feelings and thoughts at the time of the occurrence, such as "What was going on when you bought the candy?" "What were you thinking about at the time?" etc. The focus then was on either giving mild praise, or gaining information specific to the diary items. No attempts were made to either explore the past history of the subject, give negative feedback for their over-eating or consumption of fattening foods (although the experimenter's questioning might be interpreted as such), to explore motivations and attitudes, or give interpretations.

Group V: Contact–Diary–Non-specific Shock group. These subjects received the same treatment as Group IV with one exception. These were informed at the beginning of their first interview that "One of the reasons people have difficulty in losing weight is because of lack of physiological motivation" and that "since previous research found that electric shock does increase motivational level, we are interested in studying its effect in this situation." Several who expressed fear at shock, were reassured that the shock was not dangerous and that the experimental procedure would be of benefit to them. The experimenter attached electrodes to the subject's left forearm and gave a progressively stronger shock to determine the level which was very painful to the subject. All subjects found around 1–2 milliamperes to have this effect. The experimenter then set the shock apparatus to deliver 3 milliamperes which was the level used for all subjects. The experimenter then proceeded with the interview and *at predetermined specific times* (unrelated to the subject's discussion) administered shock. Each subject received ten shocks during each interview.

Group VI: Contact–Diary–Shock-Food Association group. These were given the same instructions as Group V with the following additions: "While going through the diary, every once in awhile I will ask you to think about and describe in detail a fattening food you usually eat. During your description I will give you a painful but not dangerous electric shock." The experimenter would administer the shock at that point during the description when he judged the food imagery to be most vivid. Each subject received 10 shocks during each interview, of the same intensity and at the approximately same time intervals as in Group V. While the subjects in Group I were 10 males and 10 females of college age, Groups II through VI each consisted of at least two to three times as many females as males who ranged in age from 18 to 55 with a median age of 20.5.

Follow-up

All subjects in Group III-VI returned for follow-up weighings approximately eight to ten weeks after the end of the eight weeks experimental period. The subjects in Group II were asked to keep a diary during this interval.

E

TABLE 1 Weight Loss Obtained Under Various Experimental Procedures

Groups	No. of premature terminators	No. of Ss remaining through follow-up	Mean weight gain at end of experimental period (lb)	Mean weight gain from end of experimental period to follow-up (lb)	Total mean weight gains during experiment (lb)
I—Control	–	18	+ .8	+ .6	+1.4
II—No contact	8	17	+ .2	+ .4	+ .6
III—No contact–Diary	4	18	−1.1	+5.1	+4.0
IV—Contact–Diary	9	15	−8.5	+4.0	−4.5
V—Contact–Diary–Non-specific shock	10	15	−1.2	+2.2	+1.0
VI—Contact–Diary–Shock–Food association	8	16	−3.8	+ .9	−2.9

Results

An analysis of variance conducted on the weight gain scores at the end of the experimental period yielded an F value significant beyond the .001 level. As can be seen in Table 1, the greatest weight loss was obtained in Groups IV and VI. However, further statistical tests indicated that only Group IV's weight loss was significantly greater than zero and significantly greater than all of the other groups. No other procedure, then, resulted in significant weight loss. But at follow-up, Group IV was found to have gained a sufficient amount of weight so that its total weight loss during the experiment was no longer greater than zero. It was still significantly greater than Group III's but this seems to be due to the overall gain in weight in this latter group.

Discussion

Keeping a diary *and* engaging in a relationship *did* result in significant weight loss. But when another variable such as shock, specific, or non-specific is introduced into this relationship, the positive effect of the relationship disappears.

Although, the simple procedures followed in Group IV and applied by relatively untrained personnel were effective in helping these subjects to lose weight, the termination of these procedures ended the positive effects. Brosin (1953) commenting on similar results in a study using group therapy, stated that "many persons who use food as a means of allaying disquieting feelings can alter their eating patterns effectively when circumstances give the nonfood 'supplies' from other sources." However, he further noted that once the group terminated, these "nonfood supplies" also ended and the individual resorted back to his previous eating habits.

These comments also suggest a possible explanation for the relatively small amount of weight loss in Groups V and VI during the experimental period. It was noted while periodically watching the experimenters through a one-way mirror that there were subtle but observable differences in their behavior when they had to administer shock. They were quieter, seemed less sure of themselves, almost apologetic about having to give shock, sometimes wincing along with the subject. In short, it is possible that they were not supplying the requisite "nonfood supplies" that they were able to give to subjects to whom they had only to relate. Certainly Wolpe would have acted differently with the subjects in the shock groups! Furthermore, subjects in Group V seemed more upset and confused throughout the experimental period about the reasons for the shock (despite our explanation) whereas those in Group VI spontaneously and quickly verbalized the connection between the shock and their food associations.

It is also possible that with the shock level used in this study the expectation of receiving painful shock prevented the occurrence of the "positive" and "satisfying" emotional components during the food description so that no effective avoidance conditioning took place.

One further confounding factor must be noted. Whereas our subjects were selected on the basis of their being overweight, Wolpe treated a food obsession and not obesity. Clearly, specific techniques and procedures which might have value in treating the former problem might not in the latter, and vice versa.

References

BREGER, L. & MCGAUGH, J. L. Critique and reformulation of "learning-theory" approaches to psychotherapy and neurosis. *Psychological Bulletin*, 1965, **63**, 338–358.

BREGER, L. & MCGAUGH, J. L. Learning Theory and Behavior Therapy: A reply to Rachman and Eysenck. *Psychological Bulletin*, 1966, **65**, 170–173.

★BRODIE, B. A. A hypnotherapy approach to obesity. *American Journal of Clinical Hypnosis*, 1964, **6**, 211–215.

BROSIN, H. W. The psychology of overeating. *New England Journal of Medicine*, 1953, 52–69.

★CHAPMAN, A. L. An experiment with group conferences for weight reduction. *Public Health Reports*, 1953, **68**, 439–440.

★Consumer Reports (Eds.) *The Medicine Show*, 1963, Consumer Union, Mount Vernon, N.Y.

★FROMM, ERIKA. Dynamics in a case of obesity. *Journal of Clinical and Experimental Psychopathology*, 1958, **19**, 292–302.

★GRANT, M. Group approach for weight control. *Group Psychotherapy*, 1951, **4**, 156–165.

★HERSHMAN, S. Hypothesis in the treatment of obesity. *Journal of Clinical Experimental Hypnosis*, 1955, **3**, 136–139.

KEYS, A. Weight changes and health of men. E. S. Eppright, P. Swanson and C. Iverson · (Eds.) *Weight Control*, Iowa State College Press, Ames, Iowa, 1955, 108–119.

★KOSOFSKY, S. An attempt at weight control through group psychotherapy. *Journal of Individual Psychology*, 1957, **13**, 58–71.

★KOTKOW, B. Experience in group psychotherapy with the obese. *Psychosomatic Medicine*. 1953, **15**, 243–251.

★KURLANDER, A. Group therapy in reducing. *Journal of American Diet Association*, 1953, **14**, 17–23.

★OACKLEY, RUTH. Hypnosis with a positive approach in the management of "problem" obesity. *Journal of American Society of Psychosomatic Dental Medicine*, 1960, **7**, 28–40.

★OHLSON, M. A., BREWER, W., KERELUK, P., WAGONER A., and CEDARQUIST, D. Weight control through nutritionally adequate diets. E. S. Eppright, P. Swanson and C. Iverson (Eds.) *Weight Control* Iowa State College Press, Ames, Iowa, 1955, 170–188.

OLSON, R. E. Obesity, H. F. Conn (Ed.) *Current Therapy*, W. B. Saunders, Phila, Pa., 1964, 307–312.

★SCHWARTZ, E. Group therapy of obesity in elderly diabetics. *Geriatrics*, 1952, 7, 280–283.

★SIMMONS, W. Group methods in weight reduction in E. S. Eppright, P. Swanson and C. Iverson (Eds.) *Weight Control*, Iowa State College Press, Ames, Iowa, 1955, 219–231.

★SUCZEK, R. Psychological Aspects of weight reduction. E. S. Eppright, P. Swanson and C. Iverson (Eds.) *Weight Control*, Iowa State College Press, Ames, Iowa, 1955, 147–160.

WOLPE, J. Reciprocal inhibition as the main basis of psychotherapeutic effects. *Archives of Neurology and Psychiatry*, 1955, 72, 205–226.

CHAPTER 11

Treatment of Overweight by Aversion Therapy

JOHN PAUL FOREYT and WALLACE A. KENNEDY

Florida State University, Tallahassee, Florida, U.S.A.

Summary– This study describes an aversive conditioning experiment in which favorite foods (CS) were paired with noxious odors (UCS) to help overweight Ss achieve and maintain a weight loss. After the nine-week conditioning period, a significant (obtained $p = 0.002$, significant at $p < 0.05$) average weight loss for the six experimental Ss of 13.33 lb, compared with an average weight loss of 1.00 lb for the six control Ss was reported. After 48 weeks, the experimental Ss had an average weight loss of 9.17 lb, while the control group had a weight gain of 1.33 lb (not significant). The contribution of the aversive conditioning to both the initial weight loss and to the maintenance of the weight loss is discussed.

Hundreds of papers on the treatment of overweight have been published in the last 40 years. Reviews of these studies are in general accord; the results of treatment with this population are remarkably poor. Although many articles report initial weight losses, few report follow-up results where subjects have managed to maintain their weight loss. Of the many treatments for overweight, none has been shown to have more than even a modest success.

The use of aversive conditioning with human subjects, used formerly almost exclusively on alcoholics, has more recently been extended to other behavioral disorders and several authors (Wolpe, 1954; Meyer and Crisp, 1964; Thorpe, *et al.*, 1964) have reported the use of electric shock (UCS) with overweight subjects. Wolpe (1969) reported the treatment of two overweight subjects using a solution of asafetida (UCS) and Kennedy and Foreyt (1968) described a technique using butyric acid (UCS) to help subjects lose weight.

This paper describes the application of a classical aversive conditioning procedure using a variety of noxious odors (UCS) to help overweight subjects achieve an initial weight loss and, with the development of conditioned avoidance responses, help them maintain the weight loss over an extended time period.

Reprinted with permission from *Behaviour Research and Therapy*, 1971, 9, 29–34.

Method

SUBJECTS

The experimental group (Group E) consisted of six volunteer women: three undergraduate students and three members of a local Take-Off-Pounds-Sensibly (TOPS) weight reduction club. The control group (Group C) consisted of six volunteer women from the TOPS club. All 12 Ss had been defined as "over-weight" according to the New Weight Standards for men·and women (Statistical Bulletin, November–December, 1959), i.e. at least 10 per cent above their best weight, and also by their physicians.

Average age for the six Ss in Group E was 31.00 years, with the range being 18–53 years; average age for the six Ss in Group C was 48.17 years, with the range being 34–60 years. Average initial weight for Group E was 190.83 lb with the range being 152–233 lb. Average weight for Group C was 172.50 lb, with the range being 155–237 lb.

APPARATUS

The apparatus consisted of an oxygen mask connected to a short piece of glass tubing. This glass tubing connected with a turret holding six test tubes, each containing a different noxious odor, the unconditioned stimuli (UCS). The turret could be rotated so as to allow any one of the six test tubes to connect with the glass tubing and oxygen mask. A small fan connected to the tubing blew the UCS odor to the mask. Seven odors were used (six at a time): butyric acid, pure skunk oil, trimethylamine, pyridine, diisopropylamine, benzylamine and methyl sulfide, each mixed with water in various proportions.

The Ss' favorite high-caloric foods, the conditioned stimuli (CS), were warmed, when appropriate, on a small heating coil.

PROCEDURE

Before conditioning began, the Ss in Group E were told briefly that the study was an attempt to help them achieve an initial weight loss through the use of noxious smells which when paired with favorite foods would eventually make the favorite foods less desirable.

The only contact with Group C was a general talk about the importance of weight loss and a request by the TOPS club president for volunteers to allow us to use their monthly weight data. Since all Ss in Group C were members of this weight loss club and all six attended their weekly meetings quite regularly, it was assumed that weight loss was an important goal in their life.

A hierarchy of desirable craved-for-foods was collected from each S in Group E before any conditioning began. Foods high in calories, fat or carbohydrates were the ones designated to be eliminated. These foods, for example, consisted of pies, cakes, sweet rolls, candy, french fries, potato chips, doughnuts, roasted peanuts, etc.

An aversive conditioning paradigm was used for the *S*s in Group E. A favorite food, such as a doughnut (CS), was heated in front of the *S*. The *S* was told by *E*, who was seated next to her, to smell the doughnut, to take it in her hands and feel it, to think about putting it to her lips, chewing it, rolling it around her mouth, swallowing it, etc. When *S* signalled by nodding her head that she was smelling it, and was thinking about it, she immediately was told to put her nose up to the oxygen mask and one of the six noxious odors (UCS) was blown up to her. The time from leaving the smell of the CS to receiving the smell of the UCS was about one second.

The *S* would determine whether the UCS was strong enough for her on that particular day. If not strong enough, other UCS were tried until a sufficiently noxious one was found. The CS–UCS pairings were repeated approximately 15 times throughout each session, depending on the individual *S*. An average of two different foods was run at each session. A food was run generally on consecutive sessions until the *S* reported that she was experiencing no desire for it and her food lists indicated that she was apparently not eating it.

A random intermittent reinforcement schedule was used, i.e. approximately 3–4 of the 15 CS–UCS pairings consisted of the food smell (CS) paired with air. Each session lasted about 30 min. Approximately three sessions a week were run for the first 4 weeks, then two sessions a week for the next 5 weeks.

*S*s were weighed at the beginning of the experiment and at the beginning of each session. Weight data from Group C for this same time period were obtained from the official club weight taker. *S*s in Group E were also given food data sheets on which they recorded the time, nature, quantity and circumstance of all food and drink intake and they also converted all food and drink into calories. These food data sheets were reviewed with the *S* at each experimental session. Attempts were made by the *S*s to limit their intake to 1000–1300 calories per day.

Monthly follow-up data were obtained for three TOPS Group E *S*s and the six Group C *S*s from the official TOPS weight-taker. Monthly follow-up data were obtained for the three Group E students by having them mail their monthly weights signed by their physician to *E*. At the end of 48 weeks, a questionnaire regarding their participation in the project was mailed to the *S*s in Group E.

Results

The average weight for *S*s in Group E at the start of the study was 190.83 lb with the range being 152–233 lb, that for Group C was 172.50 lb with the range being 155–237 lb. An analysis of variance on these initial weights was not significant ($F = 0.87$, $df = 1.10$).

The average number of conditioning sessions for Group E was 21.67, with the range being 15–24 sessions. Average weight loss for Ss in Group E at the end of the 9-week conditioning period was −13.33 lb, the range being −19 to −5 lb, that for Group C at the end of the same nine-week period was −1.00 lb, the range being −6 to +3 lb. A Mann–Whitney U test (Siegel, 1956) on this weight data was significant (obtained $p = 0.002$, significant at $p < 0.05$). A median test (Siegel, 1956) was also significant (obtained $p = 0.039$, significant at $p < 0.05$).

Average weight loss for Group E at the end of 48 weeks was −9.17 lb, the range being −23 to +14 lb. For Group C, the average weight change after the same 48-week period was +1.33 lb, the range being −15 to +9 lb. A Mann–Whitney U test on these results was not significant (obtained $p = 0.090$). A median test was significant (obtained $p = 0.039$, significant at $p < 0.05$).

Table 1 presents each Group E S's age, total number of conditioning sessions, initial weight change after conditioning and weight change after 48 weeks. Comparable data are also included for Group C.

Figure 1 presents the cumulative weight change in pounds for both groups during the conditioning period and the follow-up period.

Discussion

As expected, the six Group E Ss lost weight during the conditioning period. After 48 weeks, five of the six Ss still showed some weight loss, although not as much as right after the conditioning. Responding to a questionnaire at the end of 48 weeks, five of the six Ss reported that they felt they had been "conditioned", i.e. feelings of uneasiness, lessened desire for certain foods, etc., during the actual conditioning period. It was apparent from most of the Ss that they were indeed experiencing considerable discomfort during the experimental sessions and from their food data reports, reports from their husbands, and anecdotal stories they related, there was a high probability that some conditioning did occur with each of these five Ss.

The one S, E5, who did not feel that she had been "conditioned" had insisted through-out the conditioning sessions that the odors were not having any effect on her but she continued coming because she felt that the food checking done each session was helping.

The Ss frequently related stories about how they had been offered certain conditioned foods and subsequently had become quite ill. E6, for example, told how she had been at a drive-in restaurant with friends and some of her friends had bought french-fries. One smell was enough; she had to open the windows or, she reported, she would have vomited. French-fries had at that time not been run at all with her although other greasy foods had been worked with. Apparently some generalization was working. Incidentally, the S was not "psychologically-minded" and seemed quite genuinely perplexed about why this had happened since she had never worked with french-fries.

TABLE 1. Weight change of Ss after condition and 48-weeks

S	Age (yr)	Number of sessions	Initial weight (lb)	Weight change after conditioning (lb)	Weight change after 48 weeks (lb)
E1	37	21	233	−18	−21
E2	36	24	162	−11	−6
E3	53	21	217	−5	−23
E4	23	23	152	−10	−7
E5	19	15	168	−17	+14
E6	18	24	213	−19	−12
T	186	128	1,145	−80	−55
$\bar{X}$	31.0	21.3	190.8	−13.3	−9.2
C1	59	−	157	+3	+9
C2	51	−	162	+1	+9
C3	41	−	155	−6	−15
C4	44	−	237	−1	+3
C5	34	−	181	−4	−1
C6	60	−	143	+1	+3
T	289	−	1,035	−6	+8
$\bar{X}$	48.2	−	172.5	−1.0	+1.3

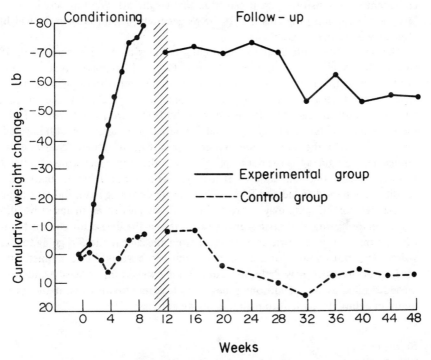

FIG. 1. Cumulative weight change in lbs for both groups during the conditioning period and the follow-up period.

Even though the conditioning may have been successful to some degree with each of the Ss except perhaps E5, it certainly was not the only factor involved in the weight loss. Without question, the experimenter—patient relationship was vital in achieving the initial weight loss. E formed positive relationships with each of the six Ss. He talked with them at length, was quite interested in them and listened to their daily problems, their troubles with their children, husbands and schoolwork. He insisted that they lose weight; he checked their food lists thoroughly during each session and told them repeatedly that they were to stop eating certain foods. This relationship cannot be overemphasized as being crucial in the initial period.

The experiment would not have to have been run this way. If one were interested only in the effects of the aversive procedure, the sessions could have been run with little or no interaction at all. This, however, was not our goal. Our purpose was to help these Ss achieve an initial weight loss by whatever means possible including the conditioning. It was therefore not surprising to see that at the end of the nine-week conditioning period there was a significant difference between the two groups. The research generally indicates that with almost any technique the S is going to lose weight. However, no technique has been able to consistently demonstrate that it can keep the weight off. What usually happens in weight reduction programs is that the Ss generally begin to regain the weight after they leave the program.

The apparent length of the conditioning effect was asked at the end of 48 weeks. One S (E1) who at 48 weeks had lost 21 lb reported that the conditioning was still in effect with all chocolate foods and with doughnuts. These were the foods that were most regularly worked with and she was the one that appeared most strongly conditioned during the first 9 weeks. E4 reported that the full effects of the conditioning lasted 3 months, although traces still lingered; E6 reported that the conditioning lasted 2 months, but added "Sweets don't bother me, so I guess the gas did help". E3 wrote that the effect wore off after 1 month; E2 said that she thought it lost its effect about a month before the conditioning period ended and E5 said that the conditioning never did take hold.

Aversive conditioning may prove to be useful as part of an inclusive weight-reduction program, in that it seems to help lessen the desire for certain foods which have to be cut down or eliminated from the diet if the S is going to lose weight. It is not enough for a patient who must lose weight but combined with other procedures it may help the patient lose weight more easily and with reconditioning as the conditioning begins to lose its effectiveness, it should be useful in aiding the patient to maintain his weight loss.

References

KENNEDY, W. A. and FOREYT, J. P. (1968) Control of eating behavior in an obese patient by avoidance conditioning. *Psychol. Rep.* 22, 571–576.
MEYER, V. and CRISP, A. H. (1964) Aversion therapy in two cases of obesity. *Behav. Res.*

& *Therapy* **2**, 143–147.

SIEGEL, S. (1956) *Nonparametric Statistics: for the Behavioral Sciences.* McGraw-Hill, New York.

STATISTICAL BULLETIN (1959) New weight standards for men and women. *Metropolitan Life Insurance Statistical Bulletin,* November–December **40**, 4–7.

THORPE, J. G., SCHMIDT, E., BROWN, P. T. and CASTELL, D. (1964) Aversion-relief therapy: A new method for general application. *Behav. Res. & Therapy* **2**, 71–82.

WOLPE, J. (1954) Reciprocal inhibition as the main basis of psychotherapeutic effects. *Am. Med. Assoc. Archs Neurol. Psychiat.* **72**, 205–226.

WOLPE, J. (1969) *The Practice of Behavior Therapy.* Pergamon Press, New York.

PART III

COVERT SENSITIZATION

Introduction[1]

RICHARD L. HAGEN
Florida State University

Just a little over a decade ago, Miller and his colleagues called themselves "subjective behaviorists" (Miller, Galanter and Pribram, 1960), observing uncomfortably that the term seemed as paradoxical as "round squareness" or "black whiteness". Indeed, their discomfort was appropriate, for at that time in our history, few behaviorists openly embraced a psychology which elevated cognitive or subjective events to a position of theoretical prominence. By contrast, a new breed of learning theorists now include and theorize broadly about the importance of cognitive behaviors (e.g. Irwin, 1971; Segal and Lachman, 1972) and behavior therapists speak freely of modifying such unobservables through conditioning principles.

Wolpe (1958) might well receive a lion's share of the credit for blending the cognitive with the behavioral in clinical treatment, but the movement has no doubt gained impetus from the unprecedented revival of general psychological interest in "the image" during the 1960s (Richardson, 1969).

The topic considered here, covert sensitization (along with coverant conditioning, Part IV), appears to represent the cognitive ultimate in behaviorism. Whereas Wolpe and his followers instruct the individual to produce relaxation responses which, with the proper instrumentation, are measurable, in covert sensitization, all events necessary for treatment change are produced "in the mind's eye" of the client.

In the first article of this Part (Cautela, 1972), Joseph Cautela, who developed the procedure, outlines its theoretical basis, application to obesity, and advantages over other similar treatments. The theoretical rationale derives from its parent, aversive conditioning (Part II) and is based upon an "escape-avoidance" paradigm. Theoretically, by pairing a highly aversive event (nausea) with a stimulus which formerly elicited approach responses (a food, for example), the stimulus assumes properties which cause discomfort to the individual. When this occurs, the individual will "escape" from the stimulus (the food) and will eventually learn to avoid that stimulus (Cautela, 1966, 1967).

The procedure is "covert" because neither the conditioned (undesirable)

[1] This introduction was written especially for this book.

stimulus nor the unconditioned stimulus is actually presented, and it is called "sensitization" because its goal is to build up avoidance responses to the undesirable stimulus (Cautela, 1967).

Cautela suggests that the procedure is applicable to a wide variety of behaviors, including, in addition to obesity, alcoholic problems, homosexuality and juvenile delinquency — indeed, to any of the problems which the overt aversion therapies have been applied. Suggested advantages of this procedure over other aversion therapies are: greater control of the CS and UCS pairing; reduced attrition from treatment (those who find electric shock or vomiting too painful or uncomfortable); the danger of physical harm to the client is removed; and the treatment can be taken home with the client via homework assignments. Furthermore, Cautela claims that the effects of covert sensitization are very specific. That is, if one food is treated, there will be little generalization to other foods.

The next two articles in this Part (Murray and Harrington, 1972; Maletzky, 1973) report single case studies involving the use of covert sensitization in the treatment of obesity. Although such case studies, these included, inevitably involve a host of additional treatment techniques which render the reports only "suggestive" of evidence for the techniques in question (Paul, 1969), case studies are an appropriate place to begin clinical research in that their tentative data can generate efforts of greater control.

It is difficult to give any meaningful interpretation to the results presented by Murray and Harrington (1972) because their subjects were presumably attending TOPS (Take-Off-Pounds-Sensibly) club meetings throughout the duration of the study. Hence, one does not know whether the effects observed were related to the covert sensitization treatment or if they were the result of procedures utilized at the TOPS meetings. If a stable baseline had been presented, the study would have been strengthened considerably. Murray and Harrington suggest that they did take baseline measures and that the weight change during treatment was significantly greater than that observed during baseline; however, inspection of their data reveals that the mean weight loss during 3 to 5 weeks of baseline was 2.9 lb while that during 10 weeks of treatment was 5.9 lb. The authors do not point out that average weekly loss was actually *greater* during baseline (0.72 lb) than it was during the treatment period (0.59 lb). Maintenance at 3 and 6 months was good, but again, it appears that the subjects continued to attend TOPS meetings throughout follow-up. The study provides promising data for either TOPS or covert sensitization; one cannot be sure which.

Maletzky's (1973) report of two case studies indicates that the introduction of a nauseous odor (valeric acid) along with suggestions of nausea and vomiting may enhance the covert sensitization treatment technique.

The last five articles in this Part (Janda and Rimm, 1972; Manno and Marston, 1972; Sachs and Ingram, 1972; Foreyt and Hagen, 1973; Diament and Wilson, 1975) represent designs which allow for a higher level of product (Paul,

1969). All investigators randomly assigned subjects to two or more treatment groups and attempted to hold certain variables constant. The studies differ, of course, in both independent and dependent variables since they are directed toward somewhat different questions.

The Janda and Rimm (1972) study represents the strongest demonstration to date that the procedural manipulations of covert sensitization are themselves effective in the treatment of obesity. The authors point out that uncontrolled variables such as credibility of the treatment, suggestion, or the relative emphasis placed on specific foods may have contributed to the success of the covert sensitization group; nevertheless, they did include an attention placebo group and a no-treatment control group. Although the number of subjects was small (only six subjects in each group), results at the end of a 6-week follow-up were quite impressive in that the covert sensitization group showed a mean loss of 11.7 lb, significantly different from the control subjects (−0.9 lb) and the attention-placebo group, which showed a gain in weight of 2.3 lb.

The study by Manno and Marston (1972) also represents an attempt to parcel out the effect of therapist attention by the use of a "minimal treatment control". A second treatment group involved covert sensitization and a third, positive covert reinforcement, a technique Cautela recommends to be used along with covert sensitization.

Manno and Marston found no difference between the two treatment groups, but both groups lost more weight than the minimal treatment control, again providing evidence for the effectiveness of the techniques involved in Cautela's treatment package. The only serious question to be raised about the study has to do with just what the minimal treatment control did not involve which the treatment groups did. It appears, for example, that the minimal treatment control subjects were not weighed weekly and that the treatment subjects were, but not enough information is given for a clear evaluation.

The last three studies in this Part focus not on the question of the effectiveness of covert sensitization as a technique, but on the theoretical model upon which the procedure is based.

Sachs and Ingram (1972) compared covert sensitization as it is normally used (UCS following the image of food) with a treatment in which the UCS preceded the food. Their results suggest that subjects equally decreased their food intake under either forward or backward conditioning, thus, as the authors point out, violating the principles of learning used to explain the effects of covert sensitization. However, these results must be considered in the light of a number of procedural weaknesses. The reader should note, for example, that each treatment was administered during only one 20-minute session, and the dependent measures were the subjects' reported consumption of certain foods. No direct measures were taken.

Foreyt and Hagen (1973) also attempted to shed some light on the claimed "conditioning principles" involved in covert sensitization by developing a placebo group, which if conditioned, would find the target food even more desirable than before treatment. Cautela (1969) appeals to Mowrer's (1947) two-factor theory of avoidance learning in explaining the avoidance behavior observed after covert sensitization. Foreyt and Hagen point out that just as Mowrer's theory would predict that stimuli associated with unpleasant events would be avoided so also stimuli associated with pleasant events should be even more actively sought or approached. As Mowrer states, "If a ... stimulus is paired with a rewarding state of affairs, that stimulus acquires the capacity to ... attract the subject toward it" (Mowrer, 1960, p. 9). Upon this basis, these investigators included a placebo treatment which was identical in all respects to the covert sensitization treatment except that pleasant scenes were substituted for the scenes of nausea and vomiting. The same foods and situations comprised the "conditioned stimuli" in both treatments.

Thus the two groups were presumably being conditioned in opposite directions although all subjects were told they would come to dislike the foods and would lose weight. Conditioning then was pitted against suggestion. The investigators argue that suggestion appears to be the strong winner since all subjects reported significant decreases in the palatibility of the target foods, and weight loss did not significantly differ for the two groups.

Diament and Wilson (1975) did a follow-up on the Foreyt—Hagen study but strengthened the procedure considerably by using in addition to weight loss and subjective ratings of palatability, measures involving (1) amount of target foods consumed during a laboratory analogue test and (2) amount of salivation while the subject imagined eating a target food. Their findings replicated those of Foreyt and Hagen: that both CS and CS Placebo subjects reported decreases in palatability to the target foods but none of the behavioral measures reflected such a decrease. I must agree with the authors in their statement that the study "represents perhaps the most relevant and appropriate experimental test of the aversion conditioning rationale of CS to date" (Diament and Wilson, 1975). The only serious challenge which could be made to this study by those who continue to hold a "conditioning" model of covert sensitization involves the small number of treatment sessions (six in all).

How does one summarize the status of research on the treatment of obesity by covert sensitization at the present time? The theoretical rationale upon which it was based by Cautela has been seriously challenged by two carefully done studies; nevertheless, as a treatment technique with a great deal of placebo going for it, one must say that it appears to be as effective as any technique. Furthermore, as an adjunct to other treatment procedures it should certainly be considered. Covert sensitization is easy to use and in some respects is more enjoyable for the therapist than some other methods.

To the researcher, encouragement must be given for more carefully planned and controlled research in this area. Indeed, the subject population abounds, the dependent measure is both reliable and valid, and the questions surrounding both "technique" and "theory" are plentiful. Several specific suggestions for the researcher follow.

Very little attention has been given to control of the expectations of the subjects. The rationale for placebo groups must be as believeable as that presented for covert sensitization, which by the way, sounds very convincing to the layman, and this rationale should be clearly reported so that the reader can judge how believeable it is. In addition, subjective reports from the subjects should be obtained indicating the degree of their own belief in the procedure and satisfaction with it.

A somewhat more difficult variable to control, but just as important, is that of therapist expectations. A step in this direction was made by Foreyt and Hagen (1973) by inviting observers into the groups to make subjective appraisals of the therapist's enthusiasm, encouragement, reinforcement, etc., but this method leaves much to be desired. A far superior remedy is to use therapists who have as much faith in the placebo treatment or alternate treatment as they do in the treatment under scrutiny. Paul's (1966) monumental work on systematic desensitization is the only therapy outcome study to this writer's knowledge in which each therapist conducted all treatments and the therapy actually practiced and believed in by the therapists came out second best. Therein lies its strongest argument. An alternative research strategy is to use different therapists for each treatment, in each case using therapists who are comfortable with and believe in the particular therapy to which they are assigned (e.g. Penick, *et al.*, 1971, see Part VI). Although the design does not control for confoundings within the therapist domain, it is certainly preferable to using all therapists who are "true believers" in the main treatment under scrutiny. There are many, even among behavior therapists, who have doubts about covert sensitization. It should not be too difficult for the serious investigator to strengthen his study by soliciting therapists from unbelieving ranks.

In addition, researchers will have to be willing to use minimal interpersonal pressure and thereby run the risk of getting minimal weight loss if they are to give the technique itself a chance to demonstrate whether or not it is effective. This writer has talked to a broad cross-section of investigators in obesity, and has found that all report the temptation to "throw in the kitchen sink" in order to produce weight loss. At our present stage of knowledge, the "kitchen sink" method is appropriate for treatment, but certainly not for research if we are to learn anything from our efforts. No doubt, the reticence of journal editors to publish negative results adds to the pressure to "produce weight loss regardless". Hopefully, their attitudes will change as they become more aware of the needs of this area of research.

References

Cautela, J. R. Treatment of compulsive behavior by covert sensitization. *The Psychological Record*, 1966, 16, 33–41.

Cautela, J. R. Covert sensitization. *Psychological Reports*, 1967, **20**, 459–468.

Cautela, J. R. Behavior therapy and self-control: Techniques and implications. In C. M. Franks (Ed.), *Behavior therapy: Appraisal and status*. New York: McGraw-Hill, 1969.

Cautela, J. R. The treatment of over-eating by covert conditioning. *Psychotherapy: Theory, Research and Practice*, 1972, **9**, 211–216.

Diament, C. and Wilson, G. T. An experimental investigation of the effects of covert sensitization in an analogue eating situation. *Behavior Therapy*, 1975, 499–509.

Foreyt, J. P. and Hagen, R. L. Covert sensitization: Conditioning or suggestion? *Journal of Abnormal Psychology*, 1973, **82**, 17–23.

Irwin, F. W. *Intentional behavior and motivation: A cognitive theory*. New York: Lippencott, 1971.

Janda, L. H. and Rimm, D. C. Covert sensitization in the treatment of obesity. *Journal of Abnormal Psychology*, 1972, **80**, 37–42.

Maletzky, B. M. "Assisted" covert sensitization: a preliminary report. *Behavior Therapy*, 1973, **4**, 117–119.

Manno, B. and Marston, A. R. Weight reduction as a function of negative covert reinforcement (sensitization) versus positive covert reinforcement. *Behavior Research and Therapy*, 1972, **10**, 201–207.

Miller, G. A., Galanter, E., and Pribram, K. H. *Plans and the structure of behavior*. New York: Holt, 1960.

Mowrer, O. H. On the dual nature of learning – a reinterpretation of "conditioning" and "problem solving". *Harvard Educational Review*, 1947, **17**, 102–148.

Mowrer, O. H. *Learning theory and the symbolic processes*. New York: Wiley, 1960.

Murray, D. C. and Harrington, L. G. Covert aversive sensitization in the treatment of obesity. *Psychological Reports*, 1972, **30**, 560.

Paul, G. L. *Insight vs. desensitization in psychotherapy: An experiment in anxiety reduction*. Stanford, California: Stanford University Press, 1966.

Paul, G. L. Behavior modification research: Design and tactics. In C. M. Franks (Ed.), *Behavior therapy: Appraisal and status*. New York: McGraw-Hill, 1969.

Penick, S. B., Filion, R., Fox, S., and Stunkard, A. J. Behavior modification in the treatment of obesity. *Psychosomatic Medicine*, 1971, **33**, 49–55.

Richardson, A. *Mental imagery*. New York: Springer Publishing Co., Inc., 1969.

Sachs, L. B. and Ingram, G. L. Covert sensitization as a treatment for weight control. *Psychological Reports*, 1972, **30**, 971–974.

Segal, E. M. and Lackman, R. Complex behavior or higher mental process: Is there a paradigm shift? *American Psychologist*, 1972, **27**, 46–55.

Wolpe, J. *Psychotherapy by reciprocal inhibition*. Johannesburg: Witwatersrand University Press, 1958.

CHAPTER 12

The Treatment of Over-eating by Covert Conditioning

JOSEPH R. CAUTELA

Boston College, Chestnut Hill, Massachusetts 02167

A major assumption of behavior theory is that behavior is influenced by the consequences that follow the behavior. Evidence (Skinner, 1969) indicates that if the frequency of a particular behavior is to be decreased, a combination of punishment for the behavior and reinforcement for antagonistic behavior is most effective.

It is the purpose of this paper to present a treatment procedure for the modification of eating behavior which punishes particular eating responses and reinforces responses antagonistic to eating. A number of studies (Ferster *et al.*, 1962; Meyer & Crisp, 1964; Hermatz & Lapuc, 1968; Moore & Crum, 1969; Upper & Newton, 1971) indicate that the manipulation of the consequences of eating can be successfully employed to reduce over-eating.

In the procedure to be described both the punishing stimulus and reinforcing stimulus are presented in imagination *via* instructions. The method presenting a punishing stimulus in imagination to decrease behavior is labeled covert sensitization (Cautela, 1966, 1967). The presentation of a reinforcing stimulus in imagination is designated as covert reinforcement (Cautela, 1970). A major assumption of this paper is that an aversive stimulus and a reinforcing stimulus presented in imagination *via* instructions have the same functional relationship to covert and overt behavior as externally presented aversive and reinforcing stimuli. The assumption that covert events obey the same laws as overt events has been held by learning theorists such as Pavlov (1955, p. 285), Skinner (1969, p. 242), Kimble (1961), and Franks (1967). There is ample experimental evidence that both covert sensitization (Ashem & Donner, 1968; Barlow *et al.*, 1969; Stuart, 1967; Viernstein, 1968; Wagner & Bragg, in press) and covert reinforcement (Cautela *et al.*, in press; Cautela *et al.*, 1971; Flannery, in press; Krop *et al.*, 1971) are effective in the modification of behavior.

Reprinted with permission from *Psychotherapy: Theory, Research and Practice*, 1972, 9, 211–216.

Description of Procedure

After the usual assessment procedure (Cautela, 1968), the client is given a weight questionnaire which is used to determine weight history and eating habits. The patient is also asked to write down everything he eats including the time and place and exact amount. He is also asked to indicate the amount of calories and grams of carbohydrates for each food item. Sometimes just recording eating behavior results in a loss of weight but in the author's experience the loss is only temporary and the client will usually gain weight unless covert sensitization is used.

Data are accumulated for 2 weeks. Meanwhile during the two sessions (the client is usually seen once a week), the client is tested for clarity of imagery, and the Fear Survey Schedule (Wolpe & Lang, 1964) and the Reinforcement Survey Schedule (Cautela & Kastenbaum, 1967) are administered to determine possible aversive and reinforcing situations that may be presented in imagination.

The client is told that over-eating is a habit which gives him pleasure. The habit consists of eating too much food and food containing more fuel than is necessary to maintain his normal activity. He is told that one way to reduce his food intake is to have him associate particular eating behaviors with something unpleasant and to reward him for not engaging in the maladaptive eating behavior. He is also told that this will be done by asking him to imagine certain unpleasant and pleasant scenes. The client is reassured that he will not develop a dislike for food in general but only for over-eating and eating particular kinds of foods. The client and therapist then agree on the desired loss of weight and keep charts on the progress of weight loss.

After the client turns in his eating habits data on the second week, the therapist circles with a pencil the eating behavior that has to be eliminated. This behavior includes:

(1)   eating between meals
(2)   eating foods with high caloric content
(3)   eating too much food at one sitting (e.g. eating two 4-ounce steaks or five lamb chops or too much bread).

The client is simply told that he is to stop engaging in these behaviors and to continue to accumulate the eating data. The client is also asked to weigh himself every day.

At the beginning of the fourth session, the therapist indicates to the patient where he has failed to eliminate the undesirable behavior. At this time, covert sensitization and covert reinforcement are applied to those situations in which he did not eliminate the maladaptive eating behavior.

THE APPLICATION OF COVERT SENSITIZATION

The following instructions concern the general applications of covert sensitization given to the client.:

> I am going to ask you to imagine this scene as vividly as you can. I do not want you to imagine that you are seeing yourself in these situations. I want you to imagine that you are actually in these situations. Do not only try to visualize the scenes, but try to feel, for example, the fork full of food in your hand, or the chair on which you are sitting. Actually smell the warm apple pie on the plate before you. Try to use all of your senses as if you were really there. The scenes I will pick are concerned with situations in which you are about to eat. It is very important that you try to visualize the scenes as clearly as possible and try to actually feel yourself in the situation.

If the client has eaten between meals he is presented with a scene similar to the following:

> I want you to imagine that you are walking along the street and as you pass a candy counter, you stop and pick up a few candy bars. As you begin to open the wrapper of the first bar you get a very queasy feeling in the pit of your stomach. You start to feel weak, nauseous, and sick all over. As you raise the candy bar to your mouth, you feel a bitter liquid come up into your throat. You try to swallow it down and put the candy in your mouth. As soon as the candy reaches your lips, you puke. The vomit rushes out all over your hands, the candy, and down the front of your dress. The sidewalk is a mess and people stop to stare at you. Your eyes are burning, and slimy mucous continues to run down your chin and your neck. The sight of all the vomit makes you vomit even more until you can not vomit any more than a little trickle of watery substance. You feel so horrible and so sick, and so embarrassed. You turn and run away from all that mess and feel much better.

A typical covert sensitization scene for eating highly caloric foods is as follows:

> I want you to imagine that you are at your dinner table and have just finished your first serving of steak. You reach across the table to get yourself another piece, and just as your hand reaches the plate, you feel a queasy, churning feeling in your stomach. You transfer the steak to your plate and just as you do a bitter spit comes up into your throat and mouth. You swallow it down and raise a piece of meat on your fork. Just as the fork reaches your lips, you puke all over your hand, all over the plate in front of you. The vomit goes all over the table and splashes on the people eating with you. They look at you horrified. You feel miserable, slimy and the sight of the vomit mixed with food particles spread all over the table makes you vomit even more and more. You hurry and get up from the table and rush out of the room and you feel better.

After presentation of each scene which applies to the client, he is questioned concerning the clarity of the scene and how much discomfort he felt. If the client reports that the scene was not clear or he could not get any discomfort from the scene, the scene is presented again in more detail. After the client reports that the scene is clear, he is asked to carefully imagine the scene by himself. Again he is questioned concerning the clarity and degree of discomfort. He is asked to keep practicing the scene until it is clear and discomfort is experienced.

In each session, the scenes are presented to the subject in which he gives in to the temptation to eat and vomits. Then the client presents the same scenes to himself.

Besides the above scenes in which the client gives in to temptation, ten escape (or self-control) scenes are presented in which the client is tempted to eat, feels nauseous, and then decides not to eat. A typical escape scene is:

> I want you to imagine that you have just finished eating your meal and you decide to have some dessert. As soon as you make that decision you start to get a funny feeling in the pit of your stomach. You say, "Oh, no. I will not eat dessert." Then you immediately feel calm and comfortable.

As in the other scenes the client is asked to repeat the scene to himself. At the end of the session, the client is told to practice each scene performed in the office at least twice a day at his home. He is cautioned to make the scenes as clear as possible and to include a self-control scene with each failure scene.

The client is also instructed to say, "Stop!" to himself and to imagine he is vomiting on food whenever he is tempted to eat maladaptively in real life situations.

At each subsequent session, the client is weighed, and asked if he did all his homework. The therapist then goes over all the eating data from the previous week and covert sensitization is applied where necessary. At this time, daily calorie and carbohydrate maximums are determined and the client is told not to exceed the limit set.

THE APPLICATION OF COVERT REINFORCEMENT

Covert reinforcement is employed to increase the probability of behaviors antagonistic to over-eating.

Reinforcers are chosen from the Reinforcement Survey Schedule (RSS) and from questioning the client. The items are then tested for their reinforcing properties. The client is asked to close his eyes and imagine that he is receiving the stimulus, e.g. if the item selected is rock and roll music, the patient is instructed in the following manner:

> Choose your favorite rock and roll song – one that you know quite well – and try to imagine that you really hear it. As soon as you feel that you can really hear it, signal me by raising your right index finger.

The client is then questioned about the clarity of the image. Practice receiving the reinforcer is continued until he can imagine it clearly and without any delay.

After a number of reinforcers have been chosen and tested by the client, it is explained to him that these certain items or activities that give him pleasure will be paired in imagination with the behaviors that he finds difficult to do (e.g. walking away from the table after a meal). He is then instructed as follows:

> In a minute I am going to ask you to try to relax and close your eyes. Then I will describe a scene to you. When you can imagine the scene as clearly as possible, raise

your right index finger. I will then say the word, "reinforcement." As soon as I say the word, "reinforcement," try to imagine the reinforcing scene we practiced before – the one about your swimming on a hot day, the feeling of the refreshing water, and feeling wonderful. As soon as the reinforcing scene is clear, raise your right index finger. Do you understand the instructions? Remember to try to imagine everything as vividly as possible, as if you were really there. All right, now close your eyes and try to relax.

After the patient has closed his eyes and appears comfortable, the therapist presents a scene such as this one:

> You are sitting at home watching TV . . . you say to yourself, "I think I'll have a piece of pie." You get up to go to the pantry. Then you say, "This is stupid. I don't want to be a fat pig." (Reinforcement)

Other examples of covert reinforcement scenes are:

> You are at home eating steak. You are just about to reach for your second piece and you stop and say to yourself, "Who needs it, anyway?" (Reinforcement)
> I want you to imagine that as you eat a dish of your favorite ice cream, you see it turn to fat on your arm. (Reinforcement)
> Imagine that you have lost 50 pounds and you are standing naked in front of a mirror. You congratulate yourself for getting rid of all the flab. (Reinforcement)

As with the covert sensitization procedure, the client is asked to practice each scene twice a day at home. Sometimes covert reinforcement is combined with covert sensitization in the following ways:

(1) After the client has imagined himself vomiting, he tells himself that doing that (i.e. giving in to temptation) was stupid and that he will not do it again and administers reinforcement to himself.

(2) The client imagines he is tempted to eat and feels a little nauseous but decides not to eat and feels better and administers a reinforcement to himself.

OTHER PROCEDURES COMBINED WITH COVERT SENSITIZATION AND COVERT REINFORCEMENT RELAXATION

If anxiety appears to be an antecedent condition to eating, the client is taught to relax using a modified Jacobson (1938) procedure. He is taught to use relaxation as a self-control procedure (Cautela, 1969). He is taught to relax before he enters into what he feels will be an anxiety-provoking situation and after he has just experienced anxiety which may still persist in part. He is also instructed to relax and covertly reinforce himself for not eating if he feels anxious and is about to eat.

DESENSITIZATION

If it is clear that specific anxiety-provoking situations are antecedent to maladaptive eating, the client is desensitized (Wolpe, 1958) to the situation.

Covert reinforcement can also be used to reduce anxiety in specific situations by reinforcing antagonistic responses.

STIMULUS CONTROL

The client is instructed to try to eat only in proper eating situations such as the kitchen or dining room. He is told not to eat in such situations as while watching TV or while reading since these situations may act as stimuli for eating. In Hullian terms, they may pick up secondary drive properties (Hull, 1952); or in operant terms, they may become discriminative stimuli (SD) for eating.

COVERT CONDITIONING AS A SELF-CONTROL PROCEDURE

It is clear from the description of the home-work assignments that the client learns to make responses that are antagonistic to eating. Also, before the client is discharged he is given a weight range (e.g. 160–165 lbs.). The client is instructed to weigh himself once a week and to apply the covert conditioning procedure whenever the maximum weight is reached. The procedure is again carefully explained for possible future use.

LENGTH OF TREATMENT

The length of treatment, of course, depends on the desired amount of weight loss. The client is usually seen once per week for a period of 3 months and then once every 2 weeks until the desired weight is reached. The average goal for weekly pound loss is 2 or 3 pounds.

Results

Though the author has found the procedure outlined above quite effective, anecdotal results such as these are not sufficient evidence for the acceptance of the treatment procedure. The procedure outlined above is confounded by a number of interacting variables such as the behavior of the therapist which is not specified in the procedure. Also, a combination of procedures has been used. Questions arise such as — would desensitization or covert sensitization alone be sufficient to modify maladaptive eating behavior? Of course, the questions can be properly answered by experimental analysis. Although no experimentation has been completed investigating the efficacy of combining covert sensitization and covert reinforcement to the modification of eating behavior, the author is of the opinion that the procedures outlined deserve serious consideration for further investigation for the following reasons:

(1) Experimental studies indicate that covert sensitization is effective in modifying other approach behaviors such as alcoholism (Ashem & Donner,

1968), sexual deviation (Barlow *et al.*, 1969), smoking (Wagner & Bragg, in press).

(2) Studies employing covert reinforcement (Cautela *et al.*, in press; Cautela *et al.*, 1971; Flannery, in press; Krop *et al.*, 1971) indicate that it is a powerful procedure for the modification of behavior.

(3) In one study (Sachs *et al.*, 1970) in which covert sensitization was compared to an operant self-control procedure in eliminating smoking behavior, covert sensitization appeared more effective.

The few studies investigating the efficacy of covert sensitization in the treatment of weight control generally report positive results. Stuart (1967) presented additional anecdotal evidence of the successful combination of covert sensitization with other operant self-control procedures in the elimination of over-eating.

Ashem *et al.* (1970) compared covert sensitization with an overt aversive stimulus in the treatment of over-eating. They concluded that:

> Results using covert sensitization with obesity appear good. There seems to be no need to use overt stimuli as adjuncts. Undoubtedly, results could be enhanced by conditioning a response incompatible with the compulsive eating response, once the covert sensitization has taken effect.

Sachs & Ingram (1972) found covert sensitization effective in reducing intake of selective foods.

An important question that needs experimental testing is whether the combination of covert sensitization and covert reinforcement is superfluous because maybe either of the procedures alone would be sufficient to eliminate a certain behavior. In the author's experience, the combination of both covert sensitization and covert reinforcement seems to hasten treatment and decrease the probability of relapse.

Problems Encountered in the use of Covert Conditioning

A number of factors have been found to hinder the successful application of covert conditioning. These factors do not preclude the use of covert conditioning since modification in procedure can usually eliminate or reduce the detrimental effects.

Poor Imagery. The inability to obtain clear imagery is reported by a few (about five per cent) of the clients. They claim they cannot get sufficiently clear imagery whenever a scene is described. Usually poor imagery can be overcome by: describing scenes in more detail; emphasizing the sense modality that enables the client to get the clearest imagery; and having the client observe certain real life situations and then try to imagine them immediately after.

Ineffective aversive stimuli. Rarely a client will claim that even after very vivid and detailed description of the vomiting scenes, he never can feel nauseous or get any discomfort. For such clients, other possible aversive stimuli are chosen from the Fear Survey Schedule (FSS) or from the interview situation. One client was asked to imagine that the food was covered with worms just as she was about to eat. Another client was asked to imagine that the food turned to blubber as it was entering her body.

Incomplete homework. Some clients report that they forget or are too busy to do the homework. It is again emphasized that homework will make treatment more effective thereby saving them time or money. Covert reinforcement is applied by having them imagine they are practicing the procedures at home and then a reinforcement is presented.

Health problems. Contrary to what some colleagues have expected would occur, the clients treated by covert conditioning do not lose their taste for all food. They only lose the "urge" to eat in a maladaptive manner. The author also insists that every patient have a thorough physical examination before treatment is begun. This rarely has to be done, however, since by the time clients come to the author for treatment, they have made many attempts to lose weight and have had physical examinations in the process.

Summary

In summary, the covert conditioning procedure combines punishment in imagination for eating and reinforcement in imagination for responses antagonistic to eating. Often it is necessary to eliminate the drive component (anxiety) of the eating behavior. In such cases, procedures such as desensitization and relaxation are also employed.

Thus far, there have been no reported adverse effects such as *anorexia nervosa* or physical complaints. The data supporting the general effectiveness of covert sensitization and covert reinforcement as applied to other maladaptive behaviors, the author's experience with the techniques, and all the reports of colleagues warrant serious consideration of the procedures described in this paper. However, hardcore experimental investigations are still needed.

References

ASHEM, B. & DONNER, L. Covert sensitization with alcoholics: A controlled replication. *Behavior Research and Therapy*, 1968, 6, 7–12.

ASHEM, B., POSER, E., & TRUDELL, P. The use of covert sensitization in the treatment of over-eating. Paper presented at the Association for the Advancement of Behavior Therapy, Miami, September, 1970.

BARLOW, D. H., LEITENBERG, H., & AGRAS, W. S. Experimental control of sexual deviation through manipulation of the noxious scene in covert sensitization. *Journal of Abnormal Psychology*, 1969, 5, 596–601.

CAUTELA, J. R. The treatment of compulsive behavior by covert sensitization. *Psychological Record*, 1966, 16, 33–41.

CAUTELA, J. R. Covert sensitization. *Psychological Record*, 1967, 20, 459–468.

CAUTELA, J. R. Behavior therapy and need for behavioral assessment. *Psychotherapy: Theory, Research and Practice*, 1968, 5,(3) 175–179.

CAUTELA, J. R. Behavior therapy and self-control: Techniques and implications. In C. Franks (Ed.), *Behavior Therapy: Appraisal and Status.* New York: McGraw-Hill, 1969, 323–340.

CAUTELA, J. R. Covert reinforcement. *Behavior Therapy*, 1970, 1, 33–50.

CAUTELA, J. R. & KASTENBAUM, R. A reinforcement survey schedule for use in therapy and research. *Psychological Reports*, 1967, 20, 115–130.

CAUTELA, J. R., WALSH, K., & WISH, P. The use of covert reinforcement to modify attitudes toward the mentally retarded. *Journal of Psychology*, 1971, 77, 257–260.

CAUTELA, J. R., STEFFAN, J., & WISH, P. An experimental test or covert reinforcement. *Journal of Clinical and Consulting Psychology*, in press.

FERSTER, C. B., NURNBERGER, J. I., & LEVITT, E. E. The control of eating. *Journal of Mathetics*, 1962, 1, 87–109.

FLANNERY, R. An investigation of differential effectiveness of office vs. *in vivo* therapy of a simple phobia: an outcome study. *Behavior Therapy and Experimental Psychiatry*, in press.

FRANKS, C. Reflections upon the treatment of sexual disorders by the behavioral clinicians: an historical comparison with the treatment of the alcoholic. *Journal of Sex Research*, 1967, 3, 212–222.

HERMATZ, M. G. & LAPUC, P. Behavior modification of over-eating in a psychiatric population. *Journal of Consulting and Clinical Psychology*, 1968, 32, 583–587.

HULL, C. *A behavior system.* New Haven: Yale University Press, 1952.

JACOBSON, E. *Progressive relaxation.* Chicago: University of Chicago Press, 1938.

KIMBLE, G. A. *Hilgard & Marquis' Conditioning and Learning.* New York: Appleton-Century-Crofts, 1961.

KROP, H., CALHOON, B., & VERRIER, R. Modification of the "self-concept" of emotionally disturbed children by covert reinforcement. *Behavior Therapy*, 1971, 2, 201–204.

MEYER, V. & CRISP, A. H. Aversion therapy in two cases of obesity. *Behavior Research and Therapy*, 1964, 2, 143–147.

MOORE, C. H. & CRUM, B. C. Weight reduction in chronic schizophrenia by means of operant conditioning procedures: a core study. *Behavior Research and Therapy*, 1969, 7, 129–131.

PAVLOV, I. P. *Selected works.* Translated by S. Belsky. J. Gibbons (Ed.). Moscow: Foreign Languages Publishing House, 1955.

SACHS, L. B., BEAN, H., & MORROW, J. E. Comparison of smoking treatments. *Behavior Therapy*, 1970, 1, 465–472.

SACHS, L. B. & INGRAM, G. L. Covert sensitization as a treatment for weight control. *Psychological Reports*, 1972, 30, 971–974.

SKINNER, B. F. *Contingencies of reinforcement.* New York: Appleton–Century-Crofts, 1969.

STUART, R. Behavioral control of over-eating. *Behavior Research and Therapy*, 1967, 5, 357–365.

UPPER, D. & NEWTON, J. G. A weight reduction program for schizophrenic patients on a token economy unit: Two case studies. *Journal of Behavior Therapy and Experimental Psychiatry*, 1971, 2, 113–115.

VIERNSTEIN, L. Evaluation of therapeutic techniques of covert sensitization. Unpublished data, Queens College, Charlottesville, North Carolina, 1968.

WAGNER, M. K. & BRAGG, R. A. Comparing behavior modification methods for habit decrement – smoking. *Journal of Consulting and Clinical Psychology*, in press.

WOLPE, J. *Psychotherapy by reciprocal inhibition.* Stanford: Stanford University Press, 1958.

WOLPE, J. & LANG, P. J. A fear survey schedule for use in behavior therapy. *Behavior Research and Therapy*, 1964, 2, 27–30.

CHAPTER 13

Covert Aversive Sensitization in the Treatment of Obesity

DAVID C. MURRAY and L. GARTH HARRINGTON

Veterans Administration Hospital, Syracuse, New York

Cautela (1966) described a case of obesity in which covert aversive sensitization (pairing a noxious stimulus or scene with food in a patient's imagination) led to marked weight reduction. Harris (1969) reported that, for Ss who had already had 2½ mo. of self-control training, 3 wk. of covert aversive sensitization was not superior to 3 additional wk. of self-control training.

To test the effects of a longer term covert aversive sensitization, 16 adult female volunteers, all members of TOPS (Take Off Pounds Sensibly) clubs, were seen individually once weekly by one of 4 therapists, 2 male Ph.D. psychologists and 2 female psychology trainees. Missed sessions were made up either the same week or by extending treatment a week. Six Ss terminated between the second and the eighth sessions (average 3.8). The others received 2 to 4 sessions of either relaxation training (4 Ss) or free-associating about food (6 Ss), 1 session practicing imagining both eating and experiencing unpleasant sensations and nausea, and 10 sessions in which they were treated with covert aversive sensitization as described by Cautela (1966, 1967). Those free-associating about food lost slightly, nonsignificantly more weight than those receiving relaxation training, so the 2 groups were combined for statistical analysis.

Average weights of the 10 Ss completing treatment and the 6 prematurely terminating Ss at their local TOPS clubs 14 wk. before treatment began were 244.8 and 224.4 lb. respectively, compared to 251.0 and 223.5 lb. at the time preliminary training began. Those completing treatment lost 2.9 lb. during the preliminary sessions (probably due to attention) and an additional 5.9 lb. during the 10 wk. of covert aversive sensitization. A comparison of the baseline change with the change during covert aversive sensitization for 10 Ss completing treatment, taken from a single factor analysis of variance for repeated measures, was significant ($F = 6.31$, $df = 1/27$, $p < .05$). Of 10 Ss 8 gained weight during the 14 wk. prior to treatment, 9 of 10 lost weight during treatment ($p < .01$ by exact test from 2×2 contingency table). Although average change was quite modest in relation to total body weight, it was maintained relatively well during

Reprinted with permission from *Psychological Reports*, 1972, **30**, 560.

follow-up (+1.5 and +0.4 lb. after 3 and 6 mo.). Most of those terminating did so before receiving much actual covert aversive sensitization, and on average gained 4.5 lb. before dropping out, with an additional 3.8 lb. gain on 3-mo. follow-up, but during the following 3 mo. they lost 2.3 lb.

Of 6 Ss terminating treatment, all but one were seen by a very young, small female psychology trainee. The 6 women seen by the experienced male therapists all completed treatment. Because of small N, high drop-out rate, differences between therapists, lack of a control group, and the variations in pre-training sessions, results cannot be considered a conclusive test of covert aversive sensitization but do suggest the technique may have potential for weight reduction.

References

CAUTELA, J. R. Treatment of compulsive behavior by covert sensitization. *Psychological Record*, 1966, **16**, 33-41.
CAUTELA, J. R. Covert sensitization. *Psychological Reports*, 1967, **20**, 459-468.
HARRIS, M. B. Self-directed program for weight control: pilot study. *Journal of Abnormal Psychology*, 1969, **74**, 263-270.

CHAPTER 14

"Assisted" Covert Sensitization: a preliminary report

BARRY M. MALETZKY[1]

Department of Neuropsychiatry, U.S. Army Lyster Hospital, Fort Rucker, Alabama

Summary— Because covert sensitization alone had proven ineffective with several patients, a modification of the standard technique was attempted by the introduction of a malodorous substance at critical points during scene presentations. The technique is described as applied to the treatment of homosexuality and compulsive eating. The substance used, valeric acid, is safe, inexpensive, readily available, and may considerably strengthen the technique of covert sensitization in selected cases.

Despite early acclaim, several critical reports of covert sensitization demonstrating only marginal effect have now been published (Ashem & Donner, 1968; Sachs, Bean, & Morrow, 1970). This has also been our experience. To bolster the strength of conditioning in such cases, an odiferous substance, valeric acid,[2] was introduced at points during scene presentations coincident with verbal suggestions of nausea and vomiting. The following examples demonstrate the use of this technique:

Case Report 1

A 52-year-old house painter complained of a long-standing compulsion to commit fellatio five to seven times monthly. For the past 35 years he had "given in" and solicited men in public toilets for this purpose. He came to our clinic because, as he grew older, religion became important to him and, in addition, he feared apprehension. He denied other forms of homosexual behavior, and he and his wife described adequate heterosexual adjustment.

Failing to diminish soliciting thoughts or behaviors to any significant degree with routine covert sensitization, the following modification was attempted:

Reprinted with permission from *Behavior Therapy*, 1973, 4, 117-119. Copyright © 1973 by Academic Press. Inc.

[1] Requests for reprints should be sent to Barry M. Maletzky, Chief, Department of Neuropsychiatry; U.S. Army Lyster Hospital, Fort Rucker, Ala. 36360.

[2] I am indebted to Dr. Donald Molde for first experimenting with the use of valeric acid in conditioning therapies. Valeric acid is an inexpensive, relatively noncorrosive substance easily purchased from many chemical supply firms. Its odor is powerful, yet it can be used repeatedly without loss of potency.

F

when the therapist introduced verbal suggestions of nausea and vomiting coincident with the act of fellatio, he also introduced an offensive odor by uncapping a bottle of valeric acid and holding it under the patient's nose. He also practiced with tape recordings of scenes and by smelling this acid in the rest rooms he used to frequent. This technique induced rapid sensitization with brief extreme feelings of nausea and several episodes of actual vomiting.

    * After 15 sessions of sensitization using valeric acid, neither acts of fellatio nor bothersome urges to perform the act were reported. Verification was obtained from his wife and associates. "Booster" sessions were held at 3-month intervals for 1 year. A 12-month follow-up indicated sensitization had been sustained.

    Eight additional homosexual patients have now been sensitized using this "assisted" technique and a 12-month follow-up indicates a total absence of homosexual urges, dreams, and overt behavior. A tenth patient has achieved only a partial remission. The technique has been applied to other types of maladaptive approach behaviors as well.

Case Report 2

    A 27-year-old married woman was progressing slowly in a weight-control group. She had difficulty not eating anything made of chocolate. After relaxation training she was presented with scenes of chocolate goodies she had just tasted infested with lice and maggots. At the appropriate moment, the smell of valeric acid was introduced, incuding nausea and gagging. After 10 such sessions, she has refrained from eating chocolate on most occasions and a 7-month follow-up revealed a continued weight loss.

    There is ample precedent for the use of foul-smelling substances to sensitize behavior (e.g. Kennedy & Foreyt, 1968; Wolpe, 1969). Valeric acid seemed remarkably suitable in these cases, however, as the protocols called for imagining fecal and putrid odors and tastes in various scenes. This substance not only assaults the olfactory senses with an odor benignly termed foul, but adds a certain human decaying quality as well, which seemed appropriate in helping these subjects more vividly experience a noxious visceral response. Moreover, as Bandura (1969) has recently reported, stimuli producing nauseous reactions may yield "more natural and symbolically reproducible aversions" than the more commonly used electroshock techniques.

    The purist may well assert that the procedure employed with these subjects is hardly covert sensitization inasmuch as a physical stimulus was utilized. This is indisputably correct; nonetheless, the procedure originally derived from covert sensitization which, when proving too tenuous for these particular patients, was modified accordingly.

References

ASHEM, B., & DONNER, L. Covert sensitization with alcoholics: A controlled replication. *Behaviour Research and Therapy,* 1968, 6, 7–12.

BANDURA, A. *Principles of behavior modification.* New York: Holt, Rinehart and Winston, Inc., 1969, pp. 507–508.

KENNEDY, W. A., & FOREYT, J. Control of eating behavior in an obese patient by avoidance and conditioning. *Psychological Reports,* 1968, 23, 571–573.

SACHS, L. B., BEAN, H., & MORROW, J. E. Comparison of smoking treatments. *Behavior Therapy,* 1970, 1, 465–472.

WOLPE, J. *The practice of behavior therapy.* New York: Pergamon Press, 1969.

CHAPTER 15

Covert Sensitization in the Treatment of Obesity[1]

LOUIS H. JANDA[2] and DAVID C. RIMM[3]

Arizona State University

Summary– One group of overweight *S*s received six sessions of covert sensitization. A second group received six sessions of a realistic attention–control condition, while a third group served as nontreated controls. At the end of treatment, covert sensitization *S*s reporting the greatest reaction to the imagined scene showed greater weight loss than the attention–control and control groups. At a 6-wk. follow-up, the treatment effect including all covert sensitization *S*s was highly significant. Self-report measures indicated that covert sensitization *S*s perceived their treatment positively and were highly motivated. Anxiety reduction and weight loss were found to be uncorrelated. These results offer considerable support for the efficacy of covert sensitization in the treatment of obesity.

The literature concerning attempts to modify maladaptive overeating suggests that this behavior is quite resistant to change. A rather wide variety of treatments has been employed including dietary instruction and nutrition clinics (Young, *et al.*, 1955; Yule, Martin & Young, 1957), the use of appetite depressants (Silverstone & Solomon, 1965), various types of group therapies (Holt & Winick, 1961; McCann & Trulson, 1955), hypnosis (Erickson, 1960), a combination of self-control procedures (Stuart, 1967), aversion therapy (Meyer & Crisp, 1964), aversion-relief therapy (Thorpe *et al.*, 1964), and operant techniques (Bernard, 1968).

Positive results, when they are reported, are often difficult to evaluate because of the lack of adequate controls. For example, Stuart (1967) reported marked weight reduction in each of his eight *S*s, following presentation of several self-control procedures (e.g., meal interruption, pairing eating with no other activity, use of the Premack principle). While such results would seem to be impressive, the role of factors such as attention and spontaneous improvement cannot be evaluated because of the absence of controls. Harris (1969), employing similar self-control procedures, did include a nontreated control group. The group undergoing treatment showed considerably greater weight loss

Reprinted with permission from *Journal of Abnormal Psychology*, 1972, 80, 37-42.

[1] This paper is based on an MA carried out by the first author under supervision of the second author.

[2] Requests for reprints should be sent to Louis H. Janda, Department of Psychology, Arizona State University, Tempe, Arizona 85281.

[3] Now at the Department of Psychology, Southern Illinois University.

than the controls. These results are also impressive although the absence of an attention–control group precludes the possibility of assessing the role of this important variable. Foreyt and Kennedy (1971) reported significantly greater weight loss for obese Ss receiving 9 wk. of aversion therapy (employing noxious odors as the UCS) than for nontreated controls. Failure to include an attention–control group coupled with the fact that at a 48-wk. follow-up most of the experimental Ss had regained a portion of the lost weight weakens these findings somewhat. Nevertheless, these results strongly suggest that aversion therapy using noxious odors may hold considerable promise. Wollersheim (1970) conducted a study with the necessary attention and nontreated control groups and a follow-up. She obtained significant results with a group therapy utilizing learning principles (e.g., stimulus control, self-rewards, development of incompatible behaviors, etc.).

In recent years considerable interest has been shown in the use of covert sensitization (Cautela, 1966) in the treatment of maladaptive appetitive responses. Case studies suggest that this technique may be useful in the treatment of obesity (Cautela, 1966; Stuart, 1967), alcoholism (Anant, 1968), sexual deviance (Kolvin, 1967), and cigarette smoking (Tooley & Pratt, 1967). Barlow, Leitenberg, and Agras (1969) were able to modify subjective reports of sexual arousal in one homosexual and one pedophile using covert sensitization. The acquisition–extinction–reacquisition design employed provides evidence that the covert sensitization procedures *per se* was responsible for the reported changes. However, the absence of objective measures as well as a follow-up weakens any firm conclusions one might draw from this study.

Ashem and Donner (1966) in their application of covert sensitization to alcoholics included a "pseudoconditioning" (backward conditioning) control group. Both the experimental (forward conditioning) and control groups showed similar improvement, and the authors argued that the control condition was not a pseudotreatment after all. However, in view of the considerable literature indicating the general failure to obtain backward conditioning (e.g., Kamin, 1963; Spooner & Kellogg, 1947), it is at least possible that the positive findings for both groups resulted from non-specific factors such as attention. Harris (1969), in her aforementioned study, presented covert sensitization along with the other self-control procedures, but she reported no additional increment in weight loss. Wagner and Bragg (1970) used covert sensitization as one of their treatment conditions with cigarette smokers. At the time of the follow-up, only those Ss receiving both covert sensitization and systematic desensitization remained significantly different from the controls.

Results of the aforementioned studies and case histories taken together are strongly suggestive of the efficacy of covert sensitization. Nevertheless, as a consequence of factors such as the lack of adequate controls, presentation of other techniques, etc., no single study has yet provided evidence that covert sensitization used alone is an effective treatment procedure. The present investigation represents an attempt to overcome some of the limitations of prior research. It examines the effect of covert sensitization, used by itself, on overeating, with the necessary attention-control group and no-contact controls included.

Method

SUBJECTS

The *S*s were recruited from among Arizona State University undergraduates who had contacted the Student Health Service for assistance in losing weight. Nineteen *S*s were referred to the *E*, and 1 was eliminated in the initial interview because she was 2 lb. underweight according to the *Mayo Clinic Manual* (The Committee on Dietetics, 1955). The remaining 18 *S*s (15 females and 3 males) ranged from 2 to 149 lb. overweight with a mean of 41.4 lb. All *S*s received a medical examination prior to participation in the study, and each was instructed to check into the Health Service weekly to be weighed. The dietician also provided calorie charts and recommended diets for all *S*s. At the weekly weigh-in at the Student Health Service, the dietician discussed the problems that *S*s were having with their diet and answered any questions that they had about dieting in general.

During the initial interview with *E*, *S*'s height and weight were taken. The *S* was then told that two relatively new methods for helping overweight people were to be tested. One method involved reducing anxiety so that the individual would find it easier to control his eating. The second method involved helping *S* develop self-control so as to eliminate fattening foods from his diet. Each *S* was told that *E* would not be able to see all of the volunteers, so there was a possibility he might not be included in either group.

THERAPIST

All interviews and therapy sessions were conducted by the first author, a second-year clinical psychology graduate student. He was not firmly committed to any specific orientation, but his expectations in this case were that both the attention—control and the covert sensitization groups would lose weight during the treatment period, and only the covert sensitization group would maintain their weight losses during the follow-up period.

PROCEDURE

Following the initial interview, *S*s were divided into triplets based on their percentage of excess weight, with members of each triplet randomly assigned to one of three groups: the control group, the attention—control group, and the covert sensitization group. The *S*s in the attention—control and covert sensitization groups were seen individually for six 40-min. weekly sessions. Prior to the first treatment session, *S*s in both groups were given the Taylor Manifest Anxiety Scale (Taylor, 1953).

Control group. The *S*s in this group were informed that as a result of a random selection procedure they were to be excluded from participation in the study. However, they were to continue to come once a week to the Health Service in order to be weighed.

Attention—control group. The *S*s were weighed at the beginning of each treatment session. The *E* was careful not to offer praise or punishment for weight losses or gains, but responded in a neutral manner. During the first treatment session, *S* received training in deep muscle relaxation (Wolpe & Lazarus, 1966), with *E* informing *S* of the benefits associated with relaxing in situations that typically gave rise to anxiety. The *S* was then asked to prepare a list of such anxiety-producing situations prior to the next treatment session. Throughout the remaining five 40-min. treatment sessions, *E* and *S* discussed these situations, with *E* responding in a nondirective, reflective manner. The *E* continued to discuss the benefits to be derived from relaxing, specifically encouraging *S* to practice on his own. In Sessions 2—6, *S*s did from one to three specific exercises from the deep muscle relaxation procedure if they reported feeling tense or anxious. Comments by *S* relative to dieting were not encouraged by *E*, but they were not discouraged when they did occur; *E* simply responded in the usual nonevaluative and reflective manner. The *S*s in the attention—control group, as well as *S*s in the covert sensitization group, who had specific questions about their diets, were referred to the dietician at the Student Health Service.

Covert sensitization group. All *S*s were weighed at the beginning of each treatment session. Again, the *E* did not offer praise or punishment for weight losses or gains. The *S*s were also given relaxation training during the first treatment session (Cautela, 1966). Following this, *S* was required to imagine vividly approaching a food to be eliminated from the diet, feeling increasingly ill, and, finally, vomiting just as he is about to place the forbidden food in his mouth. A typical scene is as follows:

> Imagine yourself sitting in your room late in the evening studying. All of a sudden you notice a craving to have something sweet to eat. You decide to go to the snack room (in the dormitory) and buy a candy bar. As you walk into the room and toward the candy machine, you notice kind of a sick feeling in the pit of your stomach. You walk over to the machine anyway, and as you are standing in front of it, you are *really* starting to feel sick! You have that unpleasant, queasy feeling in your stomach. But you decide you want the candy anyway so you drop your money into the machine. As you pick up the candy, you are really feeling sick! You can now feel the vomit start to come up your throat but you manage to choke it back down. You then unwrap the candy and lift it toward your mouth. Just as you're ready to put it in your mouth your stomach *violently* rebels. You can feel the vomit in your throat. You try to choke it back down but you can't! You finally vomit all over yourself, all over the candy bar, and all over the person standing next to you. The taste of the vomit in your mouth and the smell of it make you so sick you vomit *again* and *again*.

Finally you decide to leave, and as soon as you start to walk away from the candy bar and candy machine, you begin to feel better. You go to your room, take a shower, put on clean clothes, and now you feel much better. Your stomach now feels completely calm, and you feel good about yourself for not eating that candy bar [Adapted from Cautela, 1967].

For the second of the series of three situations, *S* was asked to imagine vividly eating a meal consistent with *S*'s reducing diet, enjoying it thoroughly, and feeling very proud of sticking to the diet. The *E* did not suggest what types of foods *S*s should imagine eating in this type of scene; they were only told "to imagine yourself eating a meal which is consistent with your diet." Such scenes were introduced in order to sharpen *S*'s ability to discriminate between forbidden and acceptable foods. For the third situation, *S* was to imagine approaching a forbidden food, feeling increasingly ill, then turning away from the food and feeling better. He was asked to imagine feeling considerable pride at being able to resist temptation.

For each of the remaining five sessions, *S* was presented with 15 scenes: 5 each of the vomiting or punishment scenes, the discrimination scenes, and the avoidance scenes. At the end of each weekly session, *S* was asked to make note of any fattening foods (or eating habit) he was having particular difficulty with. During the following session, the two or three foods or habits causing the most difficulty were incorporated in the sensitization scenes (e.g., ice cream, second helpings).

For two of the six *S*s, the scenes were modified slightly because the above was observed to have little apparent negative effect. For one *S*, the vomiting was replaced with "dry heaves" with emphasis on the spitum caught in his throat, and for the second *S*, more emphasis was placed on friends observing his vomiting and evidencing disgust with him. After three sessions, one *S* requested not to continue because she had lost about 50% of her excess weight and was fearful lest she never be able to eat fattening foods again.

The week following completion of the treatment, *S*s in all three groups were again weighed and those in the covert sensitization and attention—control groups were readministered the Manifest Anxiety Scale. In addition, they were given a seven-item questionnaire relating to possible side effects; their perception of the therapist in relation to warmth, interest, and ability; and self-ratings dealing with motivation, visualization ability, and physiological reaction (subjective distress) to the scenes (the last two items were presented to the covert sensitization group only). Six weeks later, a follow-up weight check was conducted.

Results

WEIGHT LOSS

Prior to treatment, the mean weight in pounds for the control, attention—control, and covert sensitization groups, respectively, was 164.7, 182.0, and

178.5 ($F < 1$, $df = 2/15$). Following treatment, the controls showed a mean decrement of 4.5 lb., the attention—control Ss showed a mean increase of .7 lb., and the covert sensitization Ss showed a mean decrement of 9.5 lb. (with five of six Ss showing a decrease). Although these results are in the predicted direction for the covert sensitization group, an analysis of variance indicated that they are not statistically significant ($F = 2.64$, $df = 2/15$). However, an analysis of Ss' self-rated reactions to the scenes revealed a relatively high correlation ($r = .53$) between rated subjective discomfort and weight loss. With this in mind, the difference scores were reanalyzed, including in the covert sensitization group only those three Ss reporting the highest degree of arousal when presented with the scenes (mean weight loss = 17.3 lb). This analysis revealed a highly significant treatment effect ($F = 7.80$, $df = 2/12$, $p < .01$). The proportion of variance in weight loss attributable to treatment effects was quite sizable ($w^2 = .48$; Hayes, 1963). An individual means comparison (Scheffé, 1959) revealed clearly significant differences between the covert sensitization and attention—control groups ($p < .01$) and between the covert sensitization and the two control groups combined ($p < .025$). The difference between the covert sensitization and control groups was marginally significant ($p < .10$). Contrary to E's expectation, the attention—control group did not differ significantly from the control group.

At the 6-wk. follow-up, control Ss ($n = 5$, one S could not be located) showed a mean weight loss of $-.9$ lb. (relative to their pre-experimental weight); the attention—control Ss showed a mean gain of 2.3 lb.; the covert sensitization group showed a mean loss of 11.7 lb., with five Ss showing a decrease. With all six covert sensitization Ss included, the treatment effect was now highly significant ($F = 9.19$, $df = 2/14$, $p < .005$; $w^2 = .49$). The Scheffé analysis revealed the covert sensitization group to be significantly different from the attention—control group ($p < .025$), and significantly different from the attention—control and control groups combined ($p < .05$). With only those three covert sensitization Ss showing the highest self-ratings to the scenes included (mean weight loss = 21.0 lb.), the treatment effect is again highly significant ($F = 8.88$, $df = 2/11$, $p < .01$; $w^2 = .53$), with covert sensitization differing significantly from the controls ($p < .05$) and from the attention—control Ss ($p < .01$). Again, there was no significant difference between the control and the attention—control groups.

MANIFEST ANXIETY SCALE

Prior to treatment, the Manifest Anxiety Scale means for the attention—control and covert sensitization groups were 25.00 and 19.83. A t test indicated that this difference was not significant ($t = 1.09$, $df = 10$). Following treatment, both groups showed a slight but nonsignificant decrease in anxiety (mean decrease of 3.17 for the attention—control group and a mean decrease of 3.67

for covert sensitization *S*s). The correlation for the 12 *S*s in both groups between anxiety reduction and weight loss does not approach significance ($r = -.10$).

POSTTREATMENT QUESTIONNAIRE

The questionnaire consisted of one unstructured question pertaining to side effects and six 7-point rating scales. The responses to the question in no case indicated adverse side effects or anything remotely resembling "symptom substitution." The mean ratings for the six rating scales for the attention—control and covert sensitization groups were as follows: warmth of *E* (7 indicates maximum warmth), 5.33 versus 5.50; interest of *E* (7 indicates maximum interest), 5.83 versus 6.33; *E*'s competency (7 indicates maximum competence), 5.17 versus 5.00; *S*'s motivation (7 indicates maximum motivation), 3.17 versus 5.67 ($t = 3.33$, $df = 10$, $p < .01$). Aside from motivation, none of the other comparisons approached significance. For the covert sensitization *S*s the mean physiological (subjective) reaction to the scenes (maximum reaction of 7) was 5.00, with the mean rating of image clarity of 6.17 on a 7-point scale.

Discussion

In the present investigation, covert sensitization was shown to be an effective and an extremely rapid means of dealing with maladaptive overeating. In contrast to prior studies (Harris, 1969; Stuart, 1967) which employed this technique adjunctively, or in concert with other methods, in the present study, covert sensitization was presented by itself. This, coupled with the inclusion of an attention—control group, strongly suggests that the covert sensitization package accounted for the observed weight loss. Additionally, in contrast to most previously reported results (McCann & Trulson, 1955; Yule *et al.*, 1957), *S*s in the present study (five out of six) continued to lose weight during the 6-wk. follow-up period. While 6 wk. is hardly sufficient to establish the permanency of the treatment effects, these results are nevertheless quite encouraging.

One surprising result of the study was that the attention—control group did not lose weight, but showed a slight increase of .7 lb. at the end of the treatment period. This suggests that nonspecific factors such as lower credibility of the rationale and less expectation for relief could have negated the extra attention that these *S*s received. Because there were no significant differences between the attention—control and the control groups at the end of treatment, or at the end of the follow-up, it is possible that nonspecific variables which may have a positive effect on weight loss were not controlled for. It is, of course, also possible that such variables are not effective in dealing with overeating.

It must be pointed out that this study was not intended to deal with the question of whether covert sensitization is effective because of the aversive conditioning aspect of the procedure. It is possible that nonspecific factors such as credibility of the treatment, suggestion, or the relative emphasis placed on specific foods contributed to the success of the covert sensitization group. This study did control for the important variable of therapist attention, but it is possible that one or more of the above factors were responsible for the results. However, the difference in weight loss between the three Ss with reported high arousal and the three Ss with reported low arousal (21.0 versus 2.3 lb.) is at least suggestive that aversive conditioning was the important variable.

The results of the questionnaire are instructive in that they provide an indication of S's general reaction to this particular type of aversion therapy. It is possible that a negative sensation such as nausea, having been paired with E, the experimental room, etc., would in some manner negatively valence Ss perception of E or decrease S's motivation to return. The present results are very much to the contrary. The E was perceived as being just as warm, interested, and competent following covert sensitization as following the highly permissive attention—control treatment; additionally, Ss receiving covert sensitization missed fewer appointments (6% in contrast to over 30% for the attention—control Ss; all missed appointments were rescheduled). The significantly higher level of reported motivation obtained for the covert sensitization Ss at the end of the study in all likelihood does not reflect an initially higher level of motivation (all Ss were sufficiently concerned about their weight problem to seek professional help). Instead, it seems reasonable to conclude that S's interest in covert sensitization was maintained as a consequence of some degree of immediate success. For example, one S reported being able to eliminate soft drinks after only one presentation of an associated scene.

One finding of the present study that may have considerable diagnostic significance was the positive relationship between rated subjective distress and weight loss. At the time of follow-up, the three Ss reporting the most intense reactions to the imagined scenes showed a mean weight loss of 21.0 lb. in contrast to only 2.3 lb. for the three reporting the least intense response. This suggests that covert sensitization might be rendered more efficient, if prior to treatment patients were given some sort of standardized test measuring subjective distress while imagining a pertinent scene. Those individuals reporting little distress might be given additional training in visualization, or perhaps an attempt might be made to elicit negative emotions other than nausea. For example, in the present investigation, one S who reported experiencing only minimal distress to the scenes nevertheless indicated that the scenes were at least somewhat effective because they made her feel guilty about eating.

The failure to find a relationship between weight loss and anxiety reduction provides little support for the rather widely held view (Cauffman & Pauley, 1961) that obese people frequently overeat because they are anxious. However, it should be pointed out that the present investigation was primarily concerned with the manipulation of weight, not anxiety, and a fairer test of the relationship between these variables would involve a treatment specifically aimed at the modification of anxiety as well.

References

ANANT, S. S. The use of verbal aversion (negative conditioning) with an alcoholic: A case report. *Behaviour Research and Therapy*, 1968, 6, 695–696.

ASHEM, B. & DONNER, L. Covert sensitization with alcoholics: A controlled replication. *Behaviour Research and Therapy*, 1966, 6, 7–12.

BARLOW, D. H., LEITENBERG, H., & AGRAS, W. S. Experimental control of sexual deviation through manipulation of the noxious scene in covert sensitization. *Journal of Abnormal Psychology*, 1969, 74, 596–601.

BERNARD, J. L. Rapid treatment of gross obesity by operant techniques. *Psychological Report*, 1968, 23, 663–666.

CAUFFMAN, W. J. & PAULEY, W. G. Obesity and emotional status. *Pennsylvania Medical Journal*, 1961, 64, 505–507.

CAUTELA, J. R. Treatment of compulsive behavior by covert sensitization. *Psychological Record*, 1966, 16, 33–41.

CAUTELA, J. R. Covert sensitization. *Psychological Reports*, 1967, 74, 459–468.

ERICKSON, M. A. The utilization of patient behavior in the hypnotherapy of obesity: Three case reports. *American Journal of Clinical Hypnosis*, 1960, 3, 112–116.

FOREYT, J. P. & KENNEDY, W. A. Treatment of over-weight by aversion therapy. *Behaviour Research and Therapy*, 1971, 9, 29–34.

HARRIS, M. B. Self-directed program for weight control: A pilot study. *Journal of Abnormal Psychology*, 1969, 74, 263–270.

HAYES, W. L. *Statistics for psychologists*. New York: Holt, Rinehart & Winston, 1963.

HOLT, H. & WINICK, C. Group psychotherapy with obese women. *Archives of General Psychiatry*, 1961, 5, 156–168.

KAMIN, L. J. Backward conditioning and the conditioned emotional response. *Journal of Experimental Psychology*, 1963, 56, 517–519.

KOLVIN, I. "Aversive imagery" treatment in adolescents. *Behaviour Research and Therapy*, 1967, 5, 506–515.

McCANN, M. & TRULSON, M. F. Long-term effect of weight-reducing programs. *Journal of the American Dietetic Association*, 1955, 31, 1108–1110.

MEYER, V. & CRISP, A. H. Aversion therapy in two cases of obesity. *Behaviour Research and Therapy*, 1964, 2, 143–147.

SCHEFFE, H. *The analysis of variance*. New York: Wiley, 1959.

SILVERSTONE, J. T. & SOLOMON, T. The long-term management of obesity in general practice. *British Journal of Clinical Practice*, 1965, 19, 395–398.

SPOONER, A. & KELLOGG, W. N. The backward conditioning curve. *American Journal of Psychology*, 1947, 60, 321–334.

STUART, R. B. Behavioral control of overeating. *Behaviour Research and Therapy*, 1967, 5, 357–365.

TAYLOR, J. A. A personality scale of manifest anxiety. *Journal of Abnormal and Social Psychology*, 1953, 48, 285–290.

THE COMMITTEE ON DIETETICS. *Mayo Clinic Diet Manual*. Philadelphia: Saunders, 1955.

THORPE, J. G., SCHMIDT, E., BROWN, P. T., & CASTELL, D. Aversion relief therapy: A new method for general application. *Behaviour Research and Therapy*, 1964, 2, 71–82.

TOOLEY, J. T. & PRATT, S. An experimental procedure for the extinction of smoking behavior. *Psychological Record*, 1967, 17, 209–218.

WAGNER, M. K. & BRAGG, R. A. Comparing behavior modification approaches to habit decrements – Smoking. *Journal of Consulting and Clinical Psychology*, 1970, 34, 258–263.

WOLLERSHEIM, J. P. Effectiveness of group therapy based upon learning principles in the treatment of overweight women. *Journal of Abnormal Psychology*, 1970, 76, 462–474.

WOLPE, J. & LAZARUS, A. A. *Behavior therapy techniques*. New York: Pergamon Press, 1966.

YOUNG, C. M., MORE, N. S., BERRESFORD, K., EINSET, B. M., & WALDNER, G. The problem of the obese patient. *Journal of the American Dietetic Association*, 1955, 31, 1111–1115.

YULE, J. B., MARTH, E. L., & YOUNG, C. M. Weight control: A community program. *Journal of the American Dietetic Association*, 1957, 33, 47–52.

CHAPTER 16

Weight Reduction as a Function of Negative Covert Reinforcement (sensitization) versus Positive Covert Reinforcement

BEATRICE MANNO and ALBERT R. MARSTON

University of Southern California, Los Angeles, California 90007, U.S.A.

Summary— The use of covert or imaginal procedures for weight reduction was evaluated using both positive covert reinforcement and negative (covert sensitization) in group treatment. The results indicate that both of these groups had significantly greater weight losses than a minimal treatment control group. Although the covert, positive reinforcement group did not significantly differ from the negative, its mean weight loss (in lb) was greater at the end of the four week program. Both groups showed a further weight loss at a 3-month follow-up, although the changes in mean loss were not statistically significant. The control group, on the other hand, lost a significant amount of weight between the end of treatment and follow-up. However, at follow-up both positive and negative groups still had significantly greater weight losses than the control.

The renewed interest in cognitive factors in desensitization is to some extent related to the assertion that covert operants are indeed responses. Skinner went so far as to state, "We need not suppose that events which take place within an organism's skin have special properties for that reason" (Skinner, 1953, p. 237). Cautela (1966) reports success in modifying maladaptive approach behavior through what he labels a covert sensitization procedure. Similar results were reported by Barlow *et al.* (1969) and Anant (1967). Cautela describes the method whereby the subject (*S*) visualizes a pleasurable but undesirable stimulus followed by imagining noxious sensations such as vomiting. This would appear to be essentially an escape learning procedure since the *S* is told that turning away from the stimulus image will relieve the discomfort. After repeated trials the *S* reports the absence of temptation for the object. Ashem and Donner (1968) attempted a systematic investigation of covert sensitization with alcoholic *S*s using forward and backward conditioning and a no-contact control. They found a significant difference between the combined treatment and the control groups. The fact that the backward conditioning group showed improvement raises doubts about an aversive conditioning explanation of the covert sensitization results.

The need, however, for more adequately controlled studies seems apparent in

Reprinted with permission from *Behaviour Research and Therapy*, 1972, **10**, 201–207.

light of certain obvious advantages in the covert techniques in which many of the problems involved in chemical and electrical stimulation are circumvented. In addition, *S*s are given a procedure which they can take with them and apply under their own control whenever temptation occurs. In this way, more frequent conditioning trials can occur, although with less control over the programming and strength of the stimuli. Finally, aversive stimuli can be made more relevant and appropriate to the response in question, the importance of which has been demonstrated by Garcia and Koelling (1966).

As with treatment of addictions via overt responses, the prominent treatments using covert responses have focused on aversive or negatively reinforcing stimuli. Aversive conditioning, whether it be overt or covert, runs into a special set of problems in the case of obesity. Harris (1969) reviews the extent of attempts to deal with this problem and indicates that, in part, the difficulty stems from the peculiar nature of this type of addictive behavior. While immediate positive reinforcement seems to be provided by eating, positive reinforcement for refraining from eating is usually delayed, presenting a problem for any aversive therapy procedure. Moreover, as Ferster, Nurnberger and Levitt (1962) noted, because eating behaviors occur in many different situations, they are under the control of various stimuli apart from those physiological cues which accompany hunger. The problem is further compounded by the fact that one *must* eat. Therefore, we cannot deal exclusively with avoidance response acquisition, as in the case of smoking or alcoholism, but rather, must attend to the establishment of limiting cues which in themselves have reinforcing properties.

Selective positive reinforcement might serve a function more efficiently than negative reinforcement (as used by Cautela) because of the probable greater likelihood of avoidance of such negative stimuli when away from the control of a therapy group.

The present study then deals with two issues: (1) experimentally testing the efficacy of aversive covert sensitization (replicated from Cautela, 1966) as a treatment procedure in weight reduction, relative to a minimal treatment control; and (2) evaluating aversive covert sensitization against a selected, covert positive reinforcement treatment.

Method

SUBJECTS

The *S*s for this study were 41 students and staff personnel from the University of Southern California who responded to an advertisement in the college paper for a weight-reduction clinic (36 women, 5 men). All *S*s had a desired weight loss of a minimum of 15 lb and none were under medical care at the time of the study. All agreed to make a $15.00 deposit prior to the beginning of the first session. The deposit was refunded at the end of the treatment, contingent only on attendance.

MATERIALS

A Detecto bathroom scale was used. The *S* were also required to fill out several forms. (1) A history sheet contained chronological data. (2) Rating scales were designed to determine eating habit strength, general food approach tendency and preferred foods. These rating scales included items designed to assess the *S*'s responses to eating. Two scores were obtained. One score, the habit score, measured the tendency of the *S* to reach for food "automatically", that is without sub-vocal intentions such as "I'm hungry" or "That food really looks good, I think I'll eat it". The other score, the total food approach score, measured the degree to which the *S* reports pleasure in handling food, such as food preparation, the degree of relaxation he feels food affords him, the extent of his craving for food, etc. In addition, this score includes, as one of its items, the habit score. (3) A rating scale was designed to determine *S*'s attitude about being overweight and weight reduction. (4) The *S*s completed a body image form on which they were required to make an outline drawing of the ideal body and their own bodies (Real body). (5) A food data sheet was used to record all food intake. (6) Rotter's I-E Scale (Rotter, 1966) was completed. (7) A scale of vividness of visual imagery scale (Sheehan, 1967) was filled out.

PROCEDURE

All *S*s were assigned on a random basis to one of three groups: Group 1, covert reinforcement (sensitization); Group 2, positive covert reinforcement; Group 3, minimal treatment control. The five men were distributed relatively evenly among the three groups (one to negative, three to positive, and one to control). Each group was seen as a group for eight sessions, two per week. The first session was the same for all groups, followed by six differential treatment sessions. The final session was devoted to filling out the various forms and discussion of previous sessions. Each session was approximately 1 hour in length. The first author, a third-year graduate student, served as experimenter–therapist (*E*) for all groups.

Session 1: This introductory session was the same for all groups. The *E* introduced herself and explained that the research program combined treatment and the collection of information about weight reduction. The *S*s were told that the program was oriented around the idea that eating was a habit, and that they would concentrate on reducing the frequency of that habit. They were then weighed and asked to fill out the history sheet, the two rating scales and the body image form. They were given food data sheets and asked to record the day, time, amount and surrounding circumstances of all food and drink intake throughout each day. Finally, the Ss were then given Rotter's I-E Scale. The remainder of the hour was spent answering questions and discussing some of the responses given on the rating scales. There was no mention of the actual treatment group procedures. The Ss were told that time would be allotted during each meeting to discuss problems related to weight reduction and any questions they might have about the program. They were asked to get a calorie guide and maintain the caloric intake necessary for weight reduction at their weights. They were initially asked to select their own diets which they felt were sensible and which they could maintain, although E later provided each group with a nutritionist's standard diet at their request.

Sessions 2–7: Negative covert sensitization group. The Ss were weighed at the beginning of each session. Simple aversive conditioning was explained to the group. They were told that the inappropriate eating habits would become less frequent through this procedure. The Ss were then given simple relaxation instructions, in which they were asked to close their eyes, get as comfortable as possible and think of neutral, non-arousing images, and asked to raise their hand if they felt they were not experiencing the instructions as directed. They were then asked to keep their eyes closed and imagine one specific class of food (E enumerated several high frequency foods that had appeared on the rating scales). When the S could imagine the food item, he was asked to imagine picking it up, being tempted by it, bringing it to his lips. This was followed by an adaptation of Cautela's procedure in which a feeling of nausea is vividly elicited. The Ss were asked to imagine the scene three more times, using different classes of foods from the high-frequency items on the hierarchy. The session was ended following collection and discussion of the food data sheets. Sessions 3–7 followed essentially the same procedure with several exceptions. (Session 3): S was asked to see a food item, pick it up (but not bring it to his mouth), feel tempted to eat it and then get ill. Putting the food down makes him stop vomiting and he feels better. (Session 4): S was asked to see the food, reach for it, just as he becomes nauseous and is about to vomit, pull his hand away, prevent vomiting and feel better. (Session 5): S was asked to imagine seeing the food, begin to feel ill as soon as he is tempted to eat it, turn away from the food and feel better. (Sessions 6 and 7): S was asked to think about food and start to feel slightly ill. He then was to say to himself, "I don't want it", imagine not wanting it and feel wonderful. Each session, then, consisted of weighing, four trials of the covert stimulus complex, review of food data sheets and discussion.

Sessions 2–7: Covert positive reinforcement group. (Session 2): Simple conditioning procedures were explained to the group and Ss were told about the positive covert procedure, and given simple relaxation instructions. The Ss were asked to imagine that they saw a high frequency food, reach for it, pick it up and bring it to their mouth. Just as they are tempted to eat it, they say "I don't want it", they put it down and imagine feeling wonderful that they were able to resist. They are thrilled with themselves. A friend, whom they want to impress was imagined seated beside the S and she (he) is pleased with the S's self-control. This was repeated for three more trials using different specific foods on the hierarchy. The S was also asked to imagine how wonderful he will look in new clothes. The last part of the hour was devoted to discussion of the food data sheets and any questions that arose. Sessions 3—7 were essentially the same with several exceptions. (Session 3): S was asked to see the food item, pick it up (but not bring it to his mouth), say "I don't want it" and put it down. He then feels wonderful and is praised by his friends who notice his self-control. (Session 4): S imagined reaching for the food, imagined not really wanting it, imagined himself with the ideal body and other advantages of losing weight (E enumerates several of the reasons for weight reduction gathered from the scales). (Session 5): S imagines seeing the food item and being thrilled that he doesn't want it; imagines himself with the ideal body, in a bathing suit and feels wonderful. (Sessions 6 and 7): S imagined the food, has no desire for it, imagined the dial on a scale showing a 5 lb weight loss, then a 10 lb weight loss, feeling marvelous.

Sessions 2—7: Contact control group. The control group was a minimal treatment group. Each session was devoted to a review of the food data sheets, discussion of problems arising from dieting and eating habits, with emphasis upon the notion of the learning and habit aspects to food intake.

Followup. Three months after the end of the treatment all Ss were telephoned by E who simply asked for a report of current weight. Telephone followup was used because of the intervening summer school vacation, and the dispersal of many of the Ss away from the treatment locale. Even by telephone, it was not possible to reach 10 of the Ss; fortunately this attrition was relatively even across treatment groups.

Results

An analysis of variance was done on pre-treatment weights (Session 1) for all three groups; $F = 0.1609$, df $= 2, 58, p > 0.05$. The mean weight loss at the end of treatment for the Positive group was 5.1 lb ($n = 15$); for the Negative group, 4.13 lb ($n = 13$); and for the Control group, 0.83 lb ($n = 13$). The mean total weight loss at followup (relative to pretreatment) for the Positive group was 8.9 lbs ($n = 10$); for the Negative group 8.9 lb ($n = 11$); and for the Control group, 5.2 lb ($n = 10$). An analysis of variance (Treatment X Trials repeated measured) performed on the arc sines of percentage weight loss at the end of treatment and followup yielded a Treatment main effect F of 7.3 (df $= 2, 28$), $p < 0.01$. The Trials main effect F (Session 8 end of treatment vs. Followup) was 7.4 (df $= 1, 28$), $p < 0.01$; across all groups there was a continued loss of weight during the followup period. The interaction of trials by treatment (F $= 0.74$; df $= 2, 28$) was not significant.

A Newman—Kuels analysis on treatment means yielded a significant value of

8.454 (Qr, df = 3, 28) for the Negative vs. Control conditions, $p < 0.01$. For the Positive conditions vs. Control condition, the value was 7.218 (Qr, df = 2, 28), $p < 0.01$. The difference between the positive and aversive conditions was not significant.

A Newman–Kuels analysis showed a significant weight loss between the end of treatment and followup for the control condition (difference = 2.522, Qr, df = 2, 28, $p < 0.05$) while changes in weight loss from end of treatment to followup for the Negative and Positive conditions were not significant. Differences between Positive and Control groups at end of treatment were significant at the 0.01 level (difference = 4.529, Qr, df = 3, 28). The difference between the negative and control conditions at end of treatment was also significant (difference = 4.988, Qr, df = 4, 28, $p < 0.01$). The difference between the Positive and Negative groups at end of treatment was not significant. At followup, the Positive group again significantly differed from the Control (difference = 2.689, Qr, df = 4, 28, $p < 0.05$). Similarly, the Negative group significantly differed from the Control (difference = 3.486, Qr, df = 5, 28, $p < 0.05$). The Negative and Positive groups were not significantly different.

T-tests were used to assess the differences between Session 1 and Session 8 (post-treatment) on the food habit scores, the total food approach scores, and the body image discrepancy scores (Ideal minus Real). Body image scores were derived from each drawing by combining girth scores measured at three points on the body. The Positive covert reinforcement treatment was the only group to yield significant changes in any of these measures; for the Food Habit score t (df 14) = 3.54, $p < 0.01$; for the Total Food Approach score t (df 14) = 3.23, $p < 0.01$. Both of these changes were in the direction of reports of weaker inappropriate eating habits and lower attraction to food at post-treatment.

A number of variables were correlated with post-treatment and followup weight loss. Few of these correlations were statistically significant, and fewer still evidenced a meaningful pattern across treatment groups; only the latter are summarized in what follows. In the period of time during which initial significant weight loss occurred (post-treatment for the treatment groups and at followup for the control group), there were several measures which correlated with the weight loss: (1) Discrepancy between Real and Ideal body image in pre-treatment drawings showed a significant correlation with post-treatment weight loss ($r = -0.47$, $p < 0.05$) in the positive reinforcement group and similar, but non-significant r's in the negative covert sensitization group ($r = -0.13$) and in the control group (at followup $r = -0.45$). A negative correlation indicates that larger discrepancies relate to smaller weight losses. (2) Eating habit scores taken at the final treatment session showed a significant correlation with post-treatment weight loss ($r = -0.64$), $p < 0.01$) in the negative covert sensitization group and similar, but non-significant r's in the positive reinforcement group ($r = -0.37$) and in the control group (at followup $r = -0.18$). The negative correlation indicates that a verbal report of excessive eating relates to smaller actual weight loss. Similarly, a report of strong attraction to undesirable foods relates to smaller actual weight loss (r for negative covert sensitization group = -0.61, $p < 0.05$; r for positive reinforcement group = -0.24, for control at followup $r = -0.07$). A measure of reduction in this food attraction score from pre- to post-treatment correlated positively with weight loss in the two treatment groups (r for positive = 0.43, $p < 0.05$; r for negative = 0.26), but negatively in the control group (r at followup = -0.46). In the control group there was a tendency for improvement in food perception during treatment to relate to a poorer response during the followup period when control Ss tended to show their weight loss. The other correlation of note in the control group was an r of -0.57 ($p < 0.05$) between I-E scale scores and weight loss at followup (greater weight loss is associated with an internal control orientation). The I-E scores correlate negatively (-0.39) with pre-treatment weight in the control group. However, pre-treatment weight correlates positively (0.49) with weight loss at followup in this group. Thus, while heavier Ss generally lost more, externally oriented Ss weighed more at pre-treatment, yet, lost less at followup. Of 28 correlations with followup weight loss in the two treatment groups, only one was significant ($r = -0.60, p < 0.05$); verbal reports of strong eating habits pre-treatment were associated with smaller weight loss in the Positive group.

Discussion

Compared with a group form of Cautela's covert sensitization procedure, a similar method employing only positive covert reinforcement achieved comparable results. Both treatments showed continued weight loss at a 3-month followup, with continued superiority over a minimal treatment control (despite significant weight loss in the control group during the followup period). Self-reports of changed habits *vis-à-vis* eating, correlated with actual weight loss. However, only the positive covert reinforcement group showed a significant change in the verbal measures. Predictor measures for success in treatment were generally unsuccessful. Large discrepancies between real and ideal body image prior to treatment were associated with lower weight loss. Scores on Rotter's I-E scale correlated with loss at followup. While Ss who weighed more generally lost *more* weight, externals (person's attributing little control over reinforcements to themselves) tended to weigh more at the outset and lose *less*.

The success of the control group Ss *after* treatment indicates the importance of *commitment* in the effort to achieve behavior change (Marston and Feldman, 1970). Unless one posits a delayed effect of minimal treatment, it would appear that self-directed efforts proved effective. One might conclude that all Ss came into treatment with such a commitment; that the experimental treatments facilitated carrying out the commitment, while minimal treatment inhibited behavior change. At any rate, it is clear that the treatment (or facilitation) effect is as well achieved with positive as negative covert reinforcement. Further, only positive reinforcement achieved changes in verbal behavior which may prove useful to the S in the long term effects of the program. Given some of the problems of aversive stimulation discussed in the introduction, the present findings seem to indicate that at least in the use of covert processes, aversive stimuli can be avoided.

The correlational findings, while generally disappointing, hold out some possibilities of understanding cognitive or attitudinal variables which relate to successful behavioral change. The pre-treatment body-image discrepancy seemed to account for a significant part of weight loss variance (correlation of discrepancy with pre-treatment weights were not significant). Apparently, some overweight individuals experience a body-image that is sufficiently discrepant from ideal so as to inhibit behavioral change. It will be important to determine whether this discrepancy is a function of obesity history and whether systematic intervention can modify the discrepancy, thereby facilitating weight loss. Similarly, the tendency for Externals to weigh more and lose less reflects a possible cognitive variable which could be manipulated in order to mediate change. Training in environmental (particularly reinforcement) control may be helpful. Alternatively, training in self-reinforcement and freedom from dependence on external evaluation (e.g. Rehm and Marston, 1968) may provide an important therapeutic strategy.

References

ANANT, S. S. (1967) A note on the treatment of alcoholics by a verbal aversion technique. *Can. Psychol.* **8a** (1), 19–22.

ASHEM, B. and DONNER, L. (1968) Covert sensitization with alcoholics: A controlled replication. *Behav. Res. & Therapy* **6**, 7–12.

BARLOW, D. H., LEITENBERG, H. and ARGAS, W. S. (1969) Experimental control of sexual deviation through manipulation of the noxious scene in covert sensitization. *J. abnorm. Psychol*, **74**, 597–601.

CAUTELA, J. R. (1966) Treatment of compulsive behavior by covert sensitization. *Psychol. Rec.* **16**, 33–41.

FERSTER, C. B., NURNBERGER, J. I. and LEVITT, E. E. (1962) The control of eating. *J. Mathetics* **1**, 87–109.

GARCIA, J. and KOELLING, R. A. (1966) Relation of cue to consequence in avoidance learning. *Psychon. Sci.* **4**, 123–124.

HARRIS, M. B. (1969) Self-directed program for weight control: A pilot study. *J. abnorm. Psychol.* **74**, 263–270.

MARSTON, A. R. and FELDMAN, S. E. (1970) Toward the use of will in behavior modification. Paper presented at the meeting of the American Psychological Association, Miami Beach. *J. consult. clin. Psychol.* (in press).

REHM, L. and MARSTON, A. R. (1968) Reduction of social anxiety through modification of self-reinforcement: An instigation therapy technique. *J. consult. clin. Psychol.* **32**, 565–574.

ROTTER, J. B. (1966) Generalized expectancies for internal versus external control of reinforcement. *Psychol. Monographs* **80**, 1–28.

SHEEHAN, P. W. (1967) A shortened form of the Betts' questionnaire upon mental imagery. *J. clin. Psychol.* **23**, 386–389.
SKINNER, B. F. (1953) *Science and Human Behavior.* MacMillan, New York.

CHAPTER 17

Covert Sensitization as a Treatment for Weight Control

LEWIS B. SACHS

Veterans Administration Hospital, San Francisco, California

and

GILBERT L. INGRAM

Robert F. Kennedy Youth Center, Morgantown, West Virginia

Summary.– Factors responsible for the success of covert sensitization were investigated with regard to effectiveness in initiating an aversion toward selected foods. 5 volunteers first were given forward-conditioning, then backward-conditioning trials using Cautela's covert sensitization procedures, and 5 Ss were given the opposite sequence. Conditions were then reversed allowing each S to serve as his own control. Significant reductions were found for all Ss in the intake of selected foods but no differential effect was found for the two conditioning procedures. This study supported the efficacy of using the rehearsal of an aversive scene to reduce food intake but suggests that motivational rather than learning factors may account for the results.

Since the first descriptions of covert sensitization by Cautela (1966, 1967), several investigators have applied the technique across a variety of clinical problems. Research by Ashem and Donner (1968) with alcoholism, Barlow, Leitenberg, and Agras (1969) with sexual deviation, Wagner and Bragg (1968) and Sachs, Bean, and Morrow (1970) with smoking have all provided support for the effectiveness of covert sensitization. Further data on effectiveness have been summarized by Cautela (1971).

The purpose of this study was to investigate some of the factors responsible for the success of covert sensitization. In particular, the study focused on the effectiveness of covert sensitization in initiating an aversion toward foods selected in a weight-control program. In an effort to analyze separately the components of the covert sensitization procedure, the escape or self-control scene was eliminated so the effect of presenting the aversive scene alone could be determined. In a further attempt to investigate the mechanisms involved in covert sensitization the effect of altering the temporal contingency between the

Reprinted with permission from *Psychological Reports*, 1972, **30**, 971–974. © Psychological Reports 1972.

conditioned stimulus (CS) and the unconditioned stimulus (UCS) of the aversive scene was assessed.

Method

Seventeen volunteers from Robert F. Kennedy Youth Center[1] residents and West Virginia University students served as *S*s. The data were based on the 10 volunteers who completed the experiment.

Each *S* was seen individually for three 20-min. sessions over a period of 3 wk. Advanced graduate students conducted the treatment sessions after *S*s were cleared by the medical staff.

In the first session, *S*s were given the following instructions. "You have volunteered to take part in this study because you want to lose weight. In order to work with you, we need information on your usual eating habits. That is why we want you to keep daily records of the foods you eat so that we will know where to begin in your case."

*S*s were given daily charts for recording all food eaten during the next 3 wk. The charts included: a description of the intensity of desire to eat the food (rated on a 7-point scale; 1 = weak, 7 = strong); a description of the event, thought, or feeling that led to eating; a list of all food eaten; the amount of food; the caloric value; the intensity of pleasure (rated on a 7-point scale); and, a description of the pleasurable attributes of eating. After an explanation of how to use the charts, *S*s were instructed not to allow their daily recording to interfere with their normal eating patterns. They were told to start using the charts immediately and to return the next week.

*S*s were introduced to treatment during the second session. The treatment condition was described as a very effective technique but not yet perfected for every individual. Therefore, in keeping with the still needed research on these techniques, *S*s were asked not to confound evaluation by exerting willpower or by attempting any of their own treatment techniques.

In the second session, each *S* selected two problem foods based on the frequency and caloric value as recorded during the previous week. *S*s then received conditioning trials in which the aversive scene was paired with the food they selected first. *S*s were randomly assigned to either a forward conditioning or a backward conditioning treatment.

The conditioning sessions were carried out subsequent to minimal relaxation training, which involved alternate tensing and releasing of major muscle groups (Jacobson, 1938). In forward conditioning *S*s followed termination of the pleasurable sensations of the selected food with the visualizations of the aversive scene (vomit, mucus, etc.). In backward conditioning *S*s followed termination of

[1] This study would not have been possible without the cooperation of Roy E. Gerard, Director of the Robert F. Kennedy Youth Center, and the Federal Bureau of Prisons. The Bureau assumes no responsibility for the material contained herein.

the visualizations of the aversive scene with the pleasurable sensations of the selected food. In both treatments Ss were told to discontinue the visualizations of one scene before presentation of the next scene. Three such pairings occurred during each treatment session, and Ss were instructed to practice the same procedure on their own 10 times each day.

In the third session Ss received conditioning trials in which the aversive scene was paired with the food they selected second. For this session the conditions were also reversed in that Ss previously assigned to forward conditioning were changed to backward conditioning and vice versa for the other half. Thus, each S selected two foods from his first week of daily recording and then received forward and backward conditioning during his second and third week. In this way each S was allowed to serve as his own control.

Results

Reduction of selected food intake occurred so quickly that frequency data were the only dependent measure providing information adequate for statistical analysis.

Table 1 indicates the frequency of the two foods selected by each S during the week of their basic-rate assessment and during the week following their forward and backward conditioning. The analysis of data for forward conditioning, regardless of whether initiated for the first or second week of treatment,

TABLE 1. Frequency of two foods selected by Ss measured during base-rate assessment, forward-conditioning, treatment, and backward-conditioning treatment

	FC-BC Sequence ($N = 5$)		BC-FC Sequence ($N = 5$)	
Food 1	BR 9	FC 2	BR 24	BC 0
Food 2	BR 5	BC 1	BR 20	FC 0
Food 1	BR 3	FC 0	BR 12	BC 1
Food 2	BR 5	BC 0	BR 9	FC 0
Food 1	BR 13	FC 9	BR 7	BC 1
Food 2	BR 7	BC 0	BR 13	FC 10
Food 1	BR 17	FC 2	BR 16	BC 0
Food 2	BR 13	BC 0	BR 14	FC 7
Food 1	BR 23	FC 0	BR 20	BC 4
Food 2	BR 34	BC 9	BR 25	FC 3

Code.– BR = base rate, FC = forward conditioning, BC = backward conditioning.

indicated a significant reduction ($t = 4.47$, $df = 9$, $p < .01$, one-tailed) for Ss' selected food. Also the data for backward conditioning, regardless of whether initiated for the first or second week of treatment, indicated a significant reduction ($t = 5.09$, $df = 9$, $p < .01$, one-tailed) in Ss' selected food. There were no statistically significant differences between the conditioning treatments at either the beginning or end of treatment. Thus, the analysis indicated that both treatments produced significant reductions and that there was no differential effectiveness.

On the assumption that reversing the order of the conditioned and unconditioned stimulus presentation would negate the effectiveness of treatment, Ashem and Donner (1968) attempted to use backward conditioning as a pseudo-conditioning control group. Their results indicated both forward and backward conditioning were significantly better in eliminating subsequent drinking in alcoholics than the no-contact control Ss. However, the Ashem and Donner (1968) comparison was confounded as the CS and UCS were simultaneously present during presentations in both backward and forward conditioning.

The results of the present study, even after controlling for the separation between CS and UCS indicated both treatments were equally effective in significantly reducing the consumption of the target foods. Thus, there was no support for differential classical conditioning; however, it is possible that any differences were masked by the powerful effects of Ss' set and expectations. Also, Cautela's duration of pain hypothesis (1965) needs to be examined. This hypothesis asserts that the perception of pain caused by the external unconditioned stimulus may serve as an internal stimulus after the noxious stimulus is removed. Occurring simultaneously with the conditioned stimulus, Ss respond to the perception of pain thus accounting for the observed backward-conditioning phenomenon. A crucial test of the effectiveness of backward conditioning would necessitate an interval of several minutes between the CS and UCS. In the present study, Ss were told to discontinue visualization on one scene before presentation of the next scene. However, they were not questioned about how well they were able to perform this instruction. If they perseverated on an aversive scene, a possible source of error was introduced.

Further assessment of the reversal of the CS-UCS contingency and the CS-UCS interval is of importance for determination of the variables responsible for the effectiveness of covert sensitization. For instance, if either backward conditioning or long CS-UCS intervals are as effective as either forward conditioning or short intervals, then the phenomena violate learning parameters. Motivational variables (for example, Ss' desire to lose weight) which have affected results in other experimental situations rather than learning factors appear responsible for the effectiveness of presentation of the aversive scenes in the technique of covert sensitization.

References

ASHEM, B. & DONNER, I. Cover sensitization with alcoholics: a controlled replication. *Behavior Research and Therapy*, 1968, 6, 7-12.
BARLOW, D., LEITENBERG, H., & AGRAS, W. S. Experimental control of sexual

deviation through manipulation of the noxious scene in covert sensitization. *Journal of Abnormal Psychology*, 1969, 5, 596-601.

CAUTELA, J. R. The problem of backward conditioning. *Journal of Psychology*, 1965, 60, 135-144.

CAUTELA, J. R. Treatment of compulsive behavior by covert sensitization. *Psychological Record*, 1966, 16, 33-41.

CAUTELA, J. R. Covert sensitization. *Psychological Record*, 1967, 20, 459-468.

CAUTELA, J. R. Covert conditioning. In A. Jacobs & L. B. Sachs (Eds.), *The psychology of private events*. New York: Academic Press, 1971. Pp. 109-130.

JACOBSON, E. *Progressive relaxation*. Chicago: University of Chicago Press, 1938.

SACHS, L. B., BEAN, H., & MORROW, J. E. Comparison of smoking treatments. *Behavior Therapy*, 1970, 1, 465-472.

WAGNER, M. K. & BRAGG, R. A. Comparing behavior modification methods for habit decrement-smoking. *Journal of Consulting and Clinical Psychology* (in press).

CHAPTER 18

Covert Sensitization: Conditioning or Suggestion?

JOHN PAUL FOREYT and RICHARD L. HAGEN[1]

Florida State University

Summary— Using thirty-nine female college students, this investigation attempted to assess the strength of the underlying theoretical basis of covert sensitization by comparing a covert sensitization group of overweight subjects with a placebo control (suggestion) group and a no-treatment control group. Results showed no differential weight change among groups; however, while the control group reported no change in the palatability of any foods, both the covert sensitization and the placebo suggestion group reported significant decreases in their "liking" for favorite foods after treatment, while their liking for other foods did not change. The data imply that the results obtained by covert sensitization may be interpreted as being the result of factors such as suggestion and attention.

The practicing clinician is being deluged with new techniques and approaches to psychotherapy (Bandura, 1969; Franks, 1969; Levis, 1970; Ullmann & Krasner, 1969). While case studies suggest that some of these may be effective for certain types of clinical problems, very few of these new techniques have been subjected to evaluation under conditions designed to control for the influence of confounding factors, such as attention, demand characteristics, and other nonspecific variables involved in the treatment process (Hagen, 1974). Consequently, clinicians often find dissonance created between their "scientific conscience" which requires rigorously tested procedures and the demands of service which seem unwilling to wait for the slow process of scientific investigation.

Covert sensitization (Cautela, 1966) is one of these new techniques which has become increasingly popular over the last few years in the treatment of alcoholism, sexual deviancy, smoking and other maladaptive behaviors. This technique involves the construction of visualized scenes depicting events leading to some particular deviant behavior. An example would be an overweight individual visualizing himself buying and eating a chocolate pie. These visualized events are then interspersed with visualized aversive scenes such as images of himself becoming nauseous and vomiting.

Reprinted with permission from *Journal of Abnormal Psychology*, 1973, 82, 17–23.

[1] Order of authorship is arbitrary since both authors participated equally in the research.

Requests for reprints should be sent to Richard L. Hagen, Department of Psychology, Florida State University, Tallahassee, Florida, 32306.

As an aversive conditioning technique, covert sensitization is a fairly simple one to learn and administer to an individual, and it gives the clinician all the advantages of aversive conditioning without the elaborate equipment and the difficulties involved in having to administer electric shocks or nauseous chemicals.

Covert sensitization claims conditioning as its theoretical rationale. Presumably, the stimuli previously associated with the performance of some deviant act take on aversive properties by virtue of their association, during treatment, with aversive events. The person then seeks to avoid these stimuli in his daily environment.

Although many published reports have appeared purporting to show covert sensitization as an effective procedure, the theoretical underpinnings of the technique have received little attention. It is possible that the reported effectiveness of covert sensitization is a function of the clients' expectations rather than a result of a conditioning process.

The purpose of this investigation was to assess the strength of the underlying theoretical basis of covert sensitization by comparing a covert sensitization group of overweight individuals with a placebo control (suggestion) group and a no-treatment control group.

Method

SUBJECTS

A total of 45 female subjects were selected to participate in the program. The program was advertised in the university newspaper, and selection of the subjects was made on the basis of percent overweight. All subjects were students at Florida State University, varying in age from 18 years to 24 years. Using the same procedure as Wollersheim (1970), the weight criteria were based on the 1959 Metropolitan Life Insurance Company norms for desirable weight for women (U.S. Department of Health, Education, and Welfare, 1967). A subject was included in the program only if her weight was at least 10% above her desirable weight at the time of initial contact.

All subjects were required to deposit $5.00 with the therapists at the beginning of the program, with the stipulation that it would be returned to them at the end of the follow-up period if they: (a) attended at least 80% of the sessions, (b) weighed themselves in the therapist's presence at the end of the nine-week conditioning period, and (c) weighed themselves again at the end of a nine-week follow-up period. Data were used only from the 39 of the 45 subjects who completed these requirements.

ASSESSMENT INSTRUMENTS

The pretreatment assessment battery administered included height (to the nearest inch without shoes) and weight (to the nearest pound in indoor clothing without shoes) obtained on a standard physician's balance scale; an Eating Patterns Questionnaire (Wollersheim, 1970); a modification of Schifferes' (1966) Physical Activity Scale; and a Food Palatability Scale devised by the investigators. The Food Palatability Scale was developed by asking the subjects at the initial meeting to list the 10 foods which caused them the most problem in overeating. These lists were tabulated by frequency, and the 8 foods which appeared with the greatest frequency were included in the scale. Eight fruits and eight vegetables were also included in the scale. The 24 foods were then rated by all subjects on a 5-point scale, ranging from 1 — "can't stand" to 5 — "wild about . . . would eat very often if I could afford it and wouldn't gain weight".

Assessment instruments at posttreatment included weight, the Food Palatability Scale, and a 5-point scale rating the program on (a) "How well did you like the program?" and (b) "How helpful was the program?" Assessment at follow-up included only weight.

THERAPISTS

The two investigators served as therapists. Both hold PhD degrees in clinical psychology and are licensed in the State of Florida. Both have conducted major investigations in the treatment of obesity. Their orientation may be described in general as cognitive-behavioral.

TREATMENT

Subjects were stratified on the basis of percentage overweight and were randomly assigned from blocks of three to one of three experimental conditions: (a) covert sensitization, (b) covert sensitization placebo, (c) no-treatment control.

One week before treatment began, letters were sent informing treatment subjects of the time and place for their first meeting and control subjects that they would not receive treatment until 18 weeks later.

For the covert sensitization and covert sensitization placebo conditions, subjects were told that they were assigned to a particular group because their scores on the initial assessment instruments indicated that they would benefit most from that particular treatment. Subjects were treated in groups of six or seven, with each of the therapists conducting one group under each condition. Treatment groups met twice weekly for 9 weeks (18 sessions total), each session lasting approximately 50 minutes with 15 scenes being covered each session. In both treatment conditions, subjects were told that the basic cause of their overweight was that more calories were coming into their system than were being burned up in energy. Subjects were encouraged to eat less in general. Furthermore, they were told that their treatment program would enable them to exercise better control over those foods which were particularly tempting and high in calories. The rationale used was specific to the type of treatment administered.

COVERT SENSITIZATION GROUP

During the first session, the standard treatment rationale was presented (Cautela, 1966) and the subjects were given relaxation training as outlined by Wolpe (Wolpe & Lazarus, 1966), with instructions to practice the relaxation at home two times daily. In addition, information was collected concerning favorite foods and the conditions in which the subjects found themselves most likely to overeat. From this information, the investigators prepared twenty scenes involving six different situations and the eight foods most frequently mentioned by the subjects. Ten of these scenes involved acts up to and including bringing the food to the lips and then vomiting all over it (Cautela, 1966). The other ten scenes involved "turning away from eating" and feeling much better (Cautela, 1966). In addition, time was given for subjects to imagine scenes and foods that they each found particularly applicable to their own problems in eating. The following is an example of the type of scenes used:

> Imagine yourself approaching your favorite restaurant. You and your friends enter and sit down and get very comfortable. Look around you. Be very aware of all the details surrounding you . . . look at the furniture, people, colors . . . odors. Take your time and get as clear a picture as possible (time allowed for the subject to conjure up the images). Now, you decide that you'd like to order a pizza.
>
> As you decide to order the pizza, you begin to have a funny feeling in the pit of your stomach. Your stomach feels all queasy and nauseous. As the waiter comes up to take your order, you feel very sick but you go ahead and order your favorite pizza. You begin to feel sicker and sicker. As the waiter brings your pizza and places it in front of you, notice its color . . . notice its texture . . . take a deep breath and be very aware of its odor. Look carefully at the pizza and study it.
>
> As you do this, your stomach feels more and more nauseous. Some liquid comes up in your throat, and it is very sour. You manage to swallow it back down. You are feeling sweaty and a little bit dizzy. Now, reach forward to pick up a piece of the pizza. As you are touching the pizza, puke comes up into your mouth. You feel and taste the bitter liquid and the food particles coming up your throat into your mouth. You are feeling dizzy and weak all over. You are sweating . . . trying to hold back the vomit. You manage to swallow it back, but you have this horrible, sick, bitter taste in your mouth and stomach. Now picture yourself bringing the pizza up to your mouth. As it gets nearer and nearer to your mouth, you become sicker and sicker. You can clearly see the color of the pizza, you can smell it, and the sight and smell of the pizza makes you overwhelmed with sickness. You can't hold the vomit down any longer. You try to hold your mouth closed, but the vomit rushes forward into your throat. You feel it going up into your nose and running out of your nose. You feel the particles of food in your mouth and nose. You finally open your mouth and out gushes the vomit all over the pizza . . . all over your hand . . . all over your clothes and the floor. You feel terribly sick. Again and again you vomit. You are dizzy. The room seems to sway. Your hands, your clothes, and the pizza are covered with slimy, putrid, stinking vomit. You have dry heaves now, with a terrible feeling in your

stomach. Snot and mucous are running out of your nose. Look now at the pizza. Putrid pieces of yellow vomit are running all over it. It is slimy and sticky. See the color of the pizza . . . and notice the vomit covering it . . . dripping off it onto your clothes and onto the floor. You want to get rid of the pizza and get yourself cleaned up. You immediately start to feel better. You go and clean yourself up. You get washed and you change your clothes. Then you go outside and into the clean fresh air. You feel much better now. It feels so good to get away from the pizza.

Some subjects reported that they could not capture strong feelings of nausea; therefore, the investigators also added some scenes which involved a pairing of favorite foods with other kinds of aversive situations (Deitchman, 1972).

After the sixth session, relaxation training was shortened, and most of the treatment session was devoted to the presentation of the scenes. Therapists stressed the importance of daily practice of the scenes (each scene twice daily) as an instrument toward long-range weight control rather than stressing weight loss *per se*; nevertheless, subjects were congratulated and praised as success was noted.

COVERT SENSITIZATION PLACEBO GROUP

The placebo treatment was designed to follow as closely as possible the covert sensitization treatment with one exception — pleasant scenes were substituted for the scenes of nausea and vomiting. The same foods and situations were used for both treatments.

The supposed rationale for this treatment was presented during the first treatment sessions. The investigators endeavoured to make it as convincing as possible to control for the expectations on the success of treatment. It included a lengthy discussion of classical and operant conditioning principles (using diagrams on-board, etc.) to explain how the pairing of thoughts of eating with thoughts of pleasant scenes would make the thoughts of eating tension reducing, thus weakening the chain of events which normally leads to eating behaviors.

Pleasant scenes were identified by asking subjects at the initial session to describe situations in which they found themselves to be relaxed and happy. These scenes included taking a walk in the country, lying on a blanket in a beautiful field of flowers looking up at a clear blue summer sky, lying on a raft in the water, canoeing on a slow-moving river, etc. In addition, time was given for subjects to imagine scenes and foods that they each found particularly applicable to their own problems in eating. The following is one example of the type of specific situation used:

Imagine yourself approaching your favorite restaurant. You and your friends enter and sit down and get very comfortable. Look around you. Be aware of all the details surrounding you . . . look at the furniture, people, colors . . . odors. Take your time and get as clear a picture as possible (time allowed for the subject to conjure up the images). Now you decide that you'd like to order a pizza.

As you decide to order the pizza, you find yourself switching to a scene in which you are walking through a field of beautiful flowers (spoken in a slow, relaxed voice).

It is a warm summer day, and you feel very relaxed and happy. You look up at the sky . . . it is a beautiful clear blue . . . little puffy clouds form all sorts of pictures. There is a warm breeze on your face. You feel as if you could stay here forever. Now, put yourself back in the restaurant. As the waiter comes up to take your order, you feel very good and you go ahead and order your favorite pizza. You are feeling very relaxed and comfortable. As the waiter brings your pizza and places it in front of you, notice its color . . . notice its texture . . . take a deep breath and be very aware of its odor. Look carefully at the pizza and study it.

As you do, picture yourself once again out in the field of flowers. You are barefoot, and you feel the cool soft grass beneath your feet. You have a blanket under your arm, and you decide to spread the blanket and stretch out in this beautiful peaceful field. The breeze is soft . . . the smell of the flowers is delightful . . . you feel completely relaxed and very happy . . . relaxed and very happy. Once again you are in the restaurant. Now reach forward to pick up a piece of the pizza. As you are touching the pizza, quickly switch once again to the beautiful field of flowers. You are lying on your back on the blanket. Around you, you can see lovely flowers. The odor is fresh and sweet. Above you, the blue sky looks peaceful. You have a wonderful sense of deep relaxation and happiness. You feel completely satisfied. You would like to lie there forever. Now put yourself back into the restaurant. You are now bringing the pizza up to your mouth. As it gets nearer and nearer to your mouth, you can clearly see the color, you can smell it very well. Once again, quickly change scenes and put yourself back into the field. Notice the deep sense of peace and relaxation which you feel. Look around and notice the colors, the sweet odors. You are in an open field, lying among colorful flowers. It is a warm day and you are feeling very drowsy and warm and wonderful. The sun and the flowers make you feel very relaxed and happy. Nothing else matters . . . you have no worries . . . you feel only the warmth of the sun and the beautiful flowers.

As with the covert sensitization subjects, the importance of daily practice of the scenes was emphasized, and subjects were congratulated on weight loss and encouraged to restrict their calorie intake. The therapists were very much aware that their own expectations and hopes concerning the efficacy of the various treatments might well affect the enthusiasm with which they conducted their programs. Accordingly, they made a conscious effort to display the same enthusiasm in both treatments. Graduate student assistants who sat in on the therapy sessions as observers reported that indeed differences among groups did not seem to exist.

NO-TREATMENT–WAIT–CONTROL GROUP

Subjects in this group received letters informing them that they had been accepted into the program, but because of the constraints of research and other considerations it was impossible for them to receive a treatment program until 18 weeks later. They were told that a treatment manual was still being developed and revised and that they would receive this self-help manual at that time. The only contact with the subjects during the following 18 weeks involved getting their weight at the ninth (posttreatment) and eighteenth (follow-up) weeks and giving them the self-help manual.

Results

Of the 45 subjects who began the program, 39 met the criterion of 80% attendance. Attrition was distributed as follows: no-treatment control, 1 subject; covert sensitization placebo, 2 subjects; covert sensitization, 3 subjects. A chi-square analysis revealed no differential attrition rate across groups. In addition, attrition did not affect group equivalence on age, percentage overweight, and body weight. One-way analyses on these variables indicated that all groups were well equated (all *ps* > .20). Correlations were also performed to test for relationships between attrition and subject characteristics (age, percentage overweight, and actual weight). None of these correlations were significant. Means and standard deviations of age, percentage overweight, and initial weight appear in Table 1.

TABLE 1. Descriptive statistics for treatment groups

Treatment group	N	Age (in yr.)		Percent overweight		Pretreatment weight (in lb.)		Posttreatment weight (in lb.)		Follow-up weight (in lb.)	
		X	SD	X	SD	X	SD	X	SD	X	SD
Covert sensitization	12	20.8	1.59	31.1	21.33	161.7	26.05	157.6	25.50	160.5	24.02
Covert sensitization placebo	13	20.2	1.71	29.5	19.62	159.5	24.72	151.0	24.60	152.4	25.19
No-treatment control	14	20.1	1.82	28.1	21.27	158.3	29.77	154.6	30.22	152.2	28.02

COMPARATIVE TREATMENT EFFECTS: WEIGHT

Mean weights at pretreatment, posttreatment, and nine-week follow-up also appear in Table 1. Mean weight loss (in pounds) for each of the groups at posttreatment were: covert sensitization, 4.1; covert sensitization placebo, 8.5; no-treatment control, 3.7. Mean weight losses from pretreatment to follow-up were: covert sensitization, 1.2; covert sensitization placebo, 7.1; no-treatment control, 6.1.

In order to determine treatment effects, the major analyses were done with residual gain scores (DuBois, 1957), which are derived by expressing the posttest score as a deviation from the posttest-on-pretest regression line. Thus, one is able to partial out the part of the posttest score which is predictable from pretest information (Cronbach & Furby, 1970). Analyses of variance are then used on the residual gain scores to determine differential gain across groups. For other studies using body weight as the major dependent variable in residual gain score analyses, the reader is referred to Wollersheim (1970) and Hagen (1974).

Results from analyses of variance on residual gain scores were not significant (pretreatment to posttreatment: $F = 2.10, p > .05$; pretreatment to follow-up: $F = 1.90, p > .05$).

In order to test for differences in therapist effectiveness, a supplementary analysis for therapist effects were performed using the covert sensitization and covert sensitization placebo subjects only and subjecting posttreatment and follow-up residual gain scores to two-way analyses of variance (Treatments X

Therapists). Therapist and Treatments X Therapists effects were not significant on either set of scores ($p > .05$, $p > .05$, respectively).

COMPARATIVE TREATMENT EFFECTS: PALATABILITY OF FOODS

Using pretreatment and posttreatment ratings, residual gain scores were computed for changes in reported palatability of three classes of foods: target foods (those favorite foods visualized during the treatment sessions), fruits (foods not visualized), and vegetables (foods not visualized), and one-way analyses of variance were performed on each of these foods.

The analysis on the target foods revealed a significant effect ($F = 5.62$, $p < .01$), indicating that changes in palatability differed across treatment groups. Figure 1 shows the change in the reported palatability for the three classes of

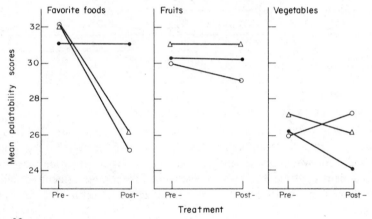

△ CS group
○ CSP group
● NTC group

FIG. 1. Mean palatability scores at pretreatment and posttreatment for three types of foods.

food at pretreatment and posttreatment. A multiple comparison among means using Duncan's multiple-range test revealed that both treatment groups (covert sensitization and covert sensitization placebo) differed significantly from the control group (both $ps < .05$), but that the two treatment groups did not differ significantly from each other.

Analyses on the nontarget foods (fruit and vegetables) revealed no significant effects, indicating that the subjects who received treatment did not report increases or decreases in palatability for either of these groups of foods.

EVALUATION OF TREATMENT BY SUBJECTS

At the time of the posttreatment assessment, each subject who had received treatment (covert sensitization and covert sensitization placebo groups) was asked to rate on a five-point scale: (a) "How well did you like the program?" and (b) "How helpful was the program?" In each case, the higher score indicated the more positive rating.

Analyses of these data for the two treatment groups revealed no significant differences on either of the two scales ($t = 1.28$, $p > .20$; $t = .96$, $p > .20$, respectively). In both instances, the programs were rated as likable (covert sensitization $X = 3.83$; covert sensitization placebo $X = 4.38$), and helpful (covert sensitization $X = 3.42$; covert sensitization placebo $X = 3.85$). The mean ratings for both groups combined on likability and helpfulness were 4.12 and 3.62, respectively.

Discussion

Cautela (1969) appeals to the two-factor theory of avoidance learning first proposed by Mowrer (1947) and elaborated upon by Solomon and Wynn (1954) and Turner and Solomon (1962), in explaining the avoidance behavior observed after covert sensitization. Within such a framework, one would presume that the unpleasant sensations produced by the unpleasant imagery (e.g., vomiting) become respondently conditioned to other stimuli embedded within the imagined scene (e.g., the food, the behaviors involved in getting the food from the refrigerator, etc.). In the absence of the unconditioned stimulus (vomiting imagery), the image or presence of the food itself then produces an unpleasant state in the individual.

The second factor involves operant conditioning. In order to reduce or eliminate the unpleasant state, the organism avoids the conditioned stimuli which produced this state. For Cautela's subjects, the sight and smell of certain foods were conditioned to arouse unpleasant emotional states because of their association with vomiting. After treatment, the subjects then avoided these foods in order to reduce the unpleasant emotional experience that the foods produced.

Dependent measures for the two types of conditioning represented by Mowrer's two factors were included in the present study. For the covert sensitization groups, the first factor, the respondent conditioning phase, should have produced a decrease in the attractiveness or palatability of the foods paired with the aversive stimuli. Such a decrease in palatability was noted in the data. It is possible, however, that this decrease in palatability ratings was the result of suggestion or demand characteristics (Orne, 1962) of the treatment setting. To investigate the question of whether conditioning or suggestion was responsible for this decrease, the covert sensitization placebo group was used.

Subjects in the covert sensitization placebo group also gave strong testimony to the effectiveness of that technique in reducing their desire for target foods. For example, one subject in a placebo group reported that she had gone to a restaurant with friends and when she saw a pizza that her friends had ordered she had no desire at all for the food and could not bring herself to even look at it or taste it. Another placebo group subject reported during the seventh week of treatment that she went to a doughnut store to test the treatment and found that she had lost all desire for doughnuts. She reported that she drank a cup of coffee there and left. Another placebo group subject volunteered that she had no more desire for fudge cake (which had been a big favorite of hers). A fourth placebo group subject reported that she went to a restaurant for spaghetti but found that she couldn't eat it when brought to her. She was so pleased with the program that she taught the procedure to a friend who wanted to quit smoking. Sure enough, she reported that it worked well with cigarettes. Subjects in the covert sensitization groups reported similar types of experiences except that they generally reported feelings of nausea when seeing favorite foods like pizza. One subject, for example, reported that when she had forced herself to eat a hamburger, she became sick to her stomach after eating it. Others reported the mere sight of target foods made them ill.

If, as the data indicate, suggestion rather than conditioning was operating for the covert sensitization placebo group, it is reasonable to assume that suggestion was also a critical independent variable for the covert sensitization group.

The second factor of Mowrer's theory, the operant component of the design, is also used to account for the behavior of avoiding foods after treatment. One measure of avoiding food is the number of pounds lost. In the present study, neither placebo nor covert sensitization subjects showed a significant weight loss when compared to the control subjects. The number of subjects in each group was too small for any definitive conclusions, but it is worth noting that the trend of the data favors the covert sensitization placebo treatment over the covert sensitization treatment.

In an effort to keep therapist pressure from obscuring the results, the therapists used only as much pressure as was necessary to maintain morale of the groups. This involved mild reprimands, mild encouragement, and weighing in before the entire group. By holding therapist pressure to a minimum, avoidance of foods and accompanying weight loss should have been primarily a result of either (a) conditioning according to Mowrer's theory or (b) suggestion that the foods would become aversive. Both groups showed a mean weight loss, though not significant. One would expect a weight loss from the covert sensitization group based upon either conditioning or suggestion since both were designed to produce decreased attractiveness of the foods. However, the placebo group also lost weight, and the mean loss in weight was even greater than for the covert sensitization subjects.

In summary, the data imply that the results obtained by covert sensitization may just as easily be interpreted as being the result of factors such as suggestion and attention rather than any actual conditioning.

References

BANDURA, A. *Principles of behavior modification.* New York: Holt, Rinehart & Winston, 1969.

CAUTELA, J. R. Treatment of compulsive behavior by covert sensitization. *Psychological Record,* 1966, **16**, 33–41.

CAUTELA, J. R. Behavior therapy and self-control: Techniques and implications. In C. M. Franks (Ed.), *Behavior therapy: Appraisal and status.* New York: McGraw-Hill, 1969.

CRONBACH, L. J. & FURBY, L. How we should measure "change" – or should we? *Psychological Bulletin,* 1970, **74**, 68–80.

DEITCHMAN, P. The use of covert sensitization in the treatment of obesity. Unpublished doctoral dissertation, Florida State University, 1972.

DUBOIS, P. H. *Multivariant correlation analysis.* New York: Harper, 1957.

FRANKS, C. M. (Ed.) *Behavior therapy: Appraisal and status.* New York: McGraw-Hill, 1969.

HAGEN, R. L. Group therapy versus bibliotherapy in weight reduction. *Behavior Therapy,* 1974, in press.

LEVIS, D. J. (Ed.), *Learning approaches to therapeutic behavior change.* Chicago: Aldine, 1970.

MOWRER, O. H. On the dual nature of learning–a reinterpretation of "conditioning" and "problem solving". *Harvard Educational Review,* 1947, **17**, 102–148.

MOWRER, O. H. *Learning theory and the symbolic processes.* New York: Wiley, 1960.

ORNE, M. T. On the social psychology of the psychological experiment with particular reference to demand characteristics and their implications. *American Psychologist,* 1962, **17**, 776–783.

SCHIFFERES, J. J. *What's your caloric number?* New York: Macmillan, 1966.

SOLOMON, R. L. & WYNNE, L. C. Traumatic avoidance learning: The principles of anxiety conservation and partial irreversibility. *Psychological Review,* 1954, **61**, 353–385.

TURNER, L. H. & SOLOMON, R. L. Human traumatic avoidance learning: Theory and experiments on the operant-respondent distinction and failures to learn. *Psychological Monographs,* 1962, **76** (40, Whole No. 559).

ULLMANN, L. P. & KRASNER, L. *A psychological approach to abnormal behavior.* Englewood Cliffs, N. J.: Prentice-Hall, 1969.

UNITED STATES DEPARTMENT OF HEALTH, EDUCATION, AND WELFARE. *Obesity and health: A sourcebook of current information for professional health personnel.* Arlington, Va.: Author, 1967.

WOLLERSHEIM, J. P. Effectiveness of group therapy based upon learning principles in the treatment of overweight women. *Journal of Abnormal Psychology,* 1970, **76**, 462–474.

WOLPE, J. & LAZARUS, A. A. *Behavior therapy techniques: A guide to the treatment of neuroses.* New York: Pergamon Press, 1966.

CHAPTER 19

An Experimental Investigation of the Effects of Covert Sensitization in an Analogue Eating Situation[1]

CHARLES DIAMENT[2] and G. TERENCE WILSON[3]

Rutgers University

Summary— Covert sensitization (CS) was compared to an attention—placebo group and a no-treatment control group in a controlled outcome study with obese college students as subjects. In addition to weight loss, the dependent measures included quantity of food consumed in an analogue eating situation, and a salivary response measure of the palatability of the target food. The results showed no differential effect among the three treatment groups on any of these three objective behavioral measures. However, both CS and attention—placebo groups reported significantly greater treatment-produced negative subjective reactions to the taste and odor of the target food than the no treatment control group. These findings seriously call into question the purported efficacy of CS as an aversive conditioning technique.

Covert sensitization (CS) is described as an aversion conditioning technique in which imaginal representations of undesirable behaviors are repeatedly paired with noxious images of nausea and vomiting as aversive stimuli. This technique has been widely applied to such diverse disorders as obesity, alcoholism, drug addiction, and sexual deviance, and presented as a tried and tested behavior modification technique (Cautela, 1973). Several potential therapeutic advantages recommend the experimental investigation of this procedure. Firstly, nausea appears to be a more biologically appropriate stimulus for establishing conditioned aversive reactions than a relatively artificial event like electric shock (Wilson and Davison, 1969). Secondly, CS is a self-control procedure which the client can use to regulate his behavior in the extratherapeutic environment (Thoresen and Mahoney, 1974). And finally, both practical and ethical con-

Reprinted with permission from *Behavior Therapy*, 1975, 6, 499–509.

[1] This research was supported by a grant from the Busch Foundation Endowment Fund, Rutgers University, to G. Terence Wilson. We are indebted to Russell Leaf for his constructive criticism in designing the study, Cherie Diament for her help in conducting the experiment, and Elaine Wilson for assistance with the data analysis.

[2] This paper is based on the senior author's Master thesis completed under the direction of G. Terence Wilson.

[3] Requests for reprints should be addressed to G. Terence Wilson, The Psychological Clinic, Rutgers University, New Brunswick, New Jersey 08903.

siderations favor its use over other forms of aversive stimulation such as electric shock.

However, the enthusiastic advocacy of CS as an effective therapeutic technique is based more upon uncontrolled clinical studies and case reports than acceptable scientific research. Cautela (1972) has claimed that CS is an effective treatment of over-eating. Yet the available experimental evidence seems to contradict this contention. Janda and Rimm (1972) compared CS, attention—placebo and no-treatment conditions, and found no significant difference at the end of treatment. By excluding half of the CS group who did not report very high subjective discomfort during the six treatment sessions from the data analysis, there was a statistically significant difference between the restructured covert sensitization group and the attention—placebo group. The difference between CS and the no-treatment control group was still insignificant. At a 6-week follow-up, CS subjects showed significantly greater weight loss even with all subjects included, although it is not clear whether the CS and the no-treatment control groups differed. The small number of subjects ($n = 6$) and the presentation of the data in terms of raw pounds rather than percentage of overweight lost renders this study suggestive at best.

In a well-controlled outcome study Foreyt and Hagen (1973) compared CS to attention—placebo and no-treatment control conditions. Using larger numbers of subjects in the treatment groups, with many more treatment sessions than in the Janda and Rimm 1972 study (18 as opposed to 6), Foreyt and Hagen found no difference between groups in terms of weight loss. Both CS and placebo groups reported that their liking for the target foods focused upon during the treatment sessions had diminished. Foreyt and Hagen (1973) concluded that CS is no more effective than a placebo treatment and that its effects are probably due to the role of suggestion and demand characteristics as opposed to any conditioning process. Romanczyk et al. (1973) showed that CS did not facilitate weight loss over and above the effects of self-monitoring of daily caloric intake. Moreover, the finding that self-monitoring of eating habits and caloric intake can result in successful weight loss (cf. Romanczyk, 1974; Romanczyk et al. 1973) suggests another plausible alternative explanation of the effects of CS. Cautela (1972) emphasizes the fact that the administration of CS procedure entails instructing the patient "to write down everything he eats including the time and place and exact amount. He is also asked to indicate the amount of calories and grams of carbohydrates for each food item" (p. 211). Given the possible reactivity of self-monitoring it is impossible to unequivocally attribute weight loss to the imagery. Both Harris (1969) and Lick and Bootzin (1971) have also reported negative findings on the treatment of obesity with CS.

Manno and Marston (1972) found that CS produced greater weight loss than a minimal treatment control group following treatment. Unfortunately, their follow-up data are suspect in so far as they were based on self-reported weight estimates obtained from subjects over the phone. Sachs and Ingram (1972) reportedly demonstrated that CS was effective in reducing intake of selective foods. However, their results are uninterpretable since they not only failed to include a placebo control group but also found no difference between forward and backward conditioning conditions.

In sum, not only are the empirical findings on CS applied to obesity negative, but any effects which might be obtained are attributable to a number of potential confounding social influence processes, including placebo effects, demand characteristics, and self-monitoring of caloric intake. The conditioning rationale of CS posits that pairing noxious symbolic scenes with imagined participation in undesirable behaviors (e.g. eating high caloric food) directly endows those behaviors with conditioned aversive properties. The client then avoids those foods which have been aversively conditioned in the natural environment. Accordingly, this conditioning hypothesis would be best tested by assessing the hypothesized suppressant effects of CS on the consumption of specific foods or on decreasing eating in specific situations (Abramson, 1973). Weight loss is too molar a dependent measure since it is a function of several complex variables which are not specifically affected by CS. For example, Lick and Bootzin (1971) reported that while CS appeared to modify the food preferences of some subjects, they did not lose weight because of their increased consumption of foods which has not been included in the treatment sessions.

Consistent with this strategy, Foreyt and Hagen (1973) measured the effects of CS on the palatability of specific target and non-target foods. However, their procedure relied upon subjects' subjective self-reports of palatability which are particularly vulnerable to placebo influences. Both their CS and placebo groups reported changes in the expected direction on palatability ratings. The present study is an attempt to improve upon the conceptual and methodological problems of previous research by using objective measures of eating behavior under counter-therapeutic demand instructions to assess unambiguously the effects of covert sensitization on specific target foods.

Method

SUBJECTS

Four males and thirty-two females were selected from respondents to an advertisement of a weight-control program in the university newspapers. All met the following criteria: university students; aged 18–25 years; a minimum of 5% overweight based upon the 1959 Metropolitan Life Insurance Company norms. (U.S. Department of Health, Education and Welfare, 1967); the absence of medical problems; not currently involved in any other weight reduction program; and an expressed willingness to attend all sessions and deposit $10 at the beginning of the program, refundable contingent on their attendance at all sessions.

THERAPIST

The senior author acted as therapist. He was experienced in the application of behavior modification principles in the treatment of obesity and specifically trained in the use of CS.

DEPENDENT MEASURES AND ASSESSMENT PROCEDURES

Pretreatment assessment included height and weight (without shoes and in indoor clothing) obtained on a standard physician's balance scale; an Eating Patterns Questionnaire (Wollersheim, 1970); an analogue eating or "taste-rating" task adapted from Schachter, Goldman, and Gordon (1968); and the Strongin-Hinsie-Peck (SHP) salivary response measure as used by Wooley and Wooley (1973).

Taste-rating Task. This task, based on Schachter *et al.*'s (1968) original procedure for studying the eating behavior of volunteer subjects, provides subjects with a legitimate rationale for eating in the laboratory situation. Subjects were asked to sample and compare the tastes of four different foods on ten different dimensions (e.g., "saltyness", "taste", "freshness", "odor", etc.). The foods consisted of pretzels, potato chips, crackers, and popcorn, and were individually presented to subjects in sealed, plastic baggies, the weights of which had been prerecorded. To encourage *ad lib.* eating, each subject was instructed to consume as much of the various foods as was necessary to make as accurate a judgement as possible about their respective tastes. Subjects were unaware of the duration of the test period which was terminated 15 minutes after the beginning of the task. Unknown to each subject, each bag of food was then reweighed to determine the quantity which had been eaten.

It is important to emphasize that subjects were deliberately kept unaware of the fact that food intake was being measured so as to keep the task free from experimental demand effects or expectancy factors. To minimize the confounding influence of demand characteristics subjects were given counter-therapeutic demand instructions. The study was presented as an experiment designed to assess the effects of weight loss on taste. Subjects were then informed that: "We will take several measures of your subjective liking of certain foods three times during the course of the program. Two baseline measures will be taken before you begin to lose weight and one measure will be taken in 8 to 12 weeks after you lose some weight. In this way we can assess how weight loss affects your subjective taste rating of certain foods."

Subjects were clearly led to expect changes in taste-rating task and weight loss only after the baseline, pretreatment period. In fact, the "two baseline" taste-rating tasks served as the dependent measure of amount of food eaten before and after the administration of the experimental treatment conditions. The third taste-rating task was never administered.

Salivary response measure. Following Wooley and Wooley's (1973) procedure, three 1½ in. dental rolls were placed in the mouth of each subject (one sublingually, two bucally bilaterally) and left in place for three 2-minute intervals. Subjects were instructed to avoid any mouth movements during the measurement procedure. While the dental rolls were in the subjects' mouths, they were shown a potato chip and asked to imagine a scene involving eating potato chips. To facilitate vivid imagery, the therapist presented a detailed description of just such a scene. After each 2-minute collection period subjects removed the dental rolls and rested for a minute. The dental rolls were packaged in plastic baggies with locking covers which had been weighed before, and were weighed a second time within an hour, after the measurement procedure. The average amount of saliva obtained in the three collections constituted the salivation measure. The rationale given subjects was the same as for the taste-rating task, viz. that these were baseline measures in a study of the influence of weight loss on salivation.

Wooley and Wooley (1973) have shown that this salivary response measure is significantly and positively correlated with palatability of food. Accordingly, if covert sensitization acts to decrease the palatability of specific target foods by endowing them with conditioned aversive properties, this effect might be reflected in significantly reduced salivary response levels following covert sensitization treatment.

Questionnaire measures. Throughout the study, subjects in the CS and placebo conditions completed a Therapy Session Assessment Questionnaire at the end of each session. Subjects rated the clarity of their imagery and the intensity of their affect during aversive scenes on seven-point rating scales. The same subjects also completed a between-session Progress Assessment Questionnaire at the beginning of each treatment session. This questionnaire yielded information on the frequency with which subjects practiced the technique between sessions; how much time they devoted to practice; how clear their imagery had been; how helpful the technique had proved to be; and whether there were any difficulties associated with its use.

Posttreatment assessment, conducted at the sixth session, included weight and readministration of both the taste-rating task and the salivary response measure. In addition all subjects completed a Therapist and Program Assessment Questionnaire designed to provide data about the subjects' perceptions of their treatment experience. The taste-rating task was carried out by an assistant who was unaware of which treatment condition subjects had been in.

TREATMENTS

Subjects were stratified on the basis of percentage overweight and then randomly assigned from each of three blocks to one of the following treatment conditions: (a) CS (n = 14); (b) CS placebo (n = 12); and (c) no-treatment control (n = 10). Scheduling difficulties resulted in an unequal number of subjects across groups. Subjects in the no-treatment control condition were told that they would not receive treatment until 3 weeks later. The CS and CS placebo groups were told that for the next 3 weeks they would be practising procedures which would eventually facilitate their losing weight. They were informed that two baseline assessments of the taste-rating task and salivary response measures were to be made before the actual weight-reduction treatment program would begin. The clear implication was that they would not lose weight and that the baseline measures would thus remain relatively unchanged until the "real" treatment program began. Subjects were treated in small groups of four of five by the same therapist. Treatment groups met twice weekly for 3 weeks (six sessions in all), with sessions lasting approximately 60 minutes, and with six imaginary scenes, each of about 5—8 minutes' duration, being covered in every session.

Covert sensitization condition. At the first treatment session, Cautela's (1966) therapy rationale was presented and the subjects trained in the relaxation procedures of Wolpe and Lazarus (1966), with instructions to practice at home at least twice before the next session. Potato chips were designated as the target food and included in each of three aversive scenes which were then repeated. The nature of the scenes was taken from Foreyt and Hagen (1973). Half of the six imaginal scenes presented subjects were punishment trials in which the subject began to eat and then vomited all over the chips. The other half were avoidance trials in which the subject turned away from the chips without either eating or vomiting. Each presentation was deliberately presented so as to give subjects sufficient time to rehearse the full details of the scene. The following is an example of a punishment scene:

> Imagine the following scene as clearly as you can. You and your friends are approaching your favorite restaurant. You enter and sit down and get very comfortable. Look around you. Look at the furniture, colors, people and odors. Take your time and get as clear a picture as possible. While you are waiting for your meal, the waitress brings some potato chips to the table. Your stomach begins to feel all queasy and nauseous. As you look at the potato chips you begin to feel sicker and sicker. Notice their texture and become very aware of what they look and smell like. Some liquid begins to come up in your throat and it is very sour. You manage to swallow it back down. You are feeling sweaty and a little bit dizzy. Now, reach forward to pick up one potato chip. As you touch the chip, puke comes up into your mouth. You are feeling dizzy and weak all over. You are sweating trying to hold back the vomit. You manage to swallow it back but you have this sick horrible taste in your mouth and in your stomach. Now picture yourself bringing the potato chip to your mouth. As it gets nearer and nearer to your mouth you get sicker and sicker. You can't hold the vomit down any longer. You try to hold your mouth closed but the vomit rushes forward into your throat. You feel it going up into your mouth and in your nose. You finally open up your mouth and out gushes the vomit all over the potato chips . . . all over your hand . . . all over your clothes and the floor. You feel terribly sick. Again and again you vomit. You are dizzy. The room seems to sway. Your

hands, your clothes, and the potato chips are covered with slimy, putrid, stinking vomit. You have dry heaves now with a terrible feeling in the pit of your stomach. Snot and mucous are running out of your nose. Look now at the potato chips. Putrid pieces of yellow vomit are running all over them. They are slimy and sticky. Look at their color and notice the vomit dripping off them onto the floor and onto your clothes. You want to get rid of the potato chips and get yourself cleaned up. You get washed and, you change your clothes. Then you feel much better now. It feels so good to get away from those potato chips.

All subsequent sessions followed the same format as the first session except that the initial relaxation instructions were shortened to about 10 minutes and subjects completed the Progress Assessment and Therapy Session Assessment Questionnaires. At all sessions, the therapist stressed the importance of rehearsing the aversive scenes at home.

Covert sensitization placebo condition. Modeled after Foreyt and Hagen's (1973) placebo group, this condition was identical to the CS treatment, with the single difference that pleasant scenes were substituted for the aversive scenes of nausea and vomiting. The foods and situations used were the same in both conditions. The rationale given subjects at the first session emphasized how the technique was based on the powerful principles of "social learning theory". An explanation stated that pairing pleasant thoughts with eating would counter-condition the eating urges elicited by the food-related thoughts and thereby interfere with the behavioral sequence which previously led to eating. Further-more, subjects were informed that, according to the principle of *covert catharsis*, the act of imagining eating certain foods would symbolically satisfy their need to eat. The following is an excerpt of one of the scenes used:

> Imagine yourself approaching your favorite restaurant. You and your friends enter and sit down and get very comfortable. Look around you. Be aware of all the details surrounding you. Look at the furniture, colors, people and odors. Take your time and get as clear a picture as possible. While you are waiting for your meal the waitress brings some potato chips to your table. As you look at the potato chips you find yourself switching to a scene in which you are walking through a field of beautiful flowers. It is a warm summer day and you feel very relaxed and happy. You look up at the sky . . . it is a beautiful clear blue . . . little puffy clouds form all kinds of pictures. There is a warm breeze on your face. You feel as if you could stay here forever. Now put yourself back in the restaurant. As the waiter brings the potato chips you feel very good and go ahead and begin to look at them. You are feeling very relaxed and comfortable. You notice the chip's color . . . their texture . . . take a deep breath and notice their odor . . . . Look carefully at the potato chips and study them. As you do, picture yourself once again out in the field of flowers. You are barefoot and you feel the cool soft grass beneath your feet. You have a blanket under your arm and you decide to spread the blanket in this beautiful peaceful field. The breeze is soft. The flowers are delightful and you feel relaxed and very happy . . . .

The importance of practicing these scenes at home was stressed by the therapist, who attempted to convey the same expectations about the treatment sessions as with the covert sensitization group.

No-treatment control condition. Subjects were informed that, because of the unusually large response to the newspaper advertisement, a random selection procedure had to be used to decide who would be selected. They were informed that they were the ones whose treatment had to be temporarily postponed. The same $10 deposit was collected from them as from all other subjects and they were assured that, in 3 weeks, they would be included in the program. They were administered the taste-rating task and the salivary response measure at the same time as subjects in the other two groups.

Following the posttreatment assessment procedures, subjects in all three groups were administered a standardized, group behavior modification treatment program involving the application of a variety of self-control procedures for promoting weight reduction (cf. Romanczyk *et al.*, 1973).

Results

Of the thirty-six subjects initially selected, thirty-five satisfied the attendance criteria and completed the study. One subject (from the CS condition) withdrew for unrelated medical reasons.

Weight. To compensate for individual differences in sex and height, subjects' weights were converted to percentages overweight by subtracting their ideal weights (as determined by the Metropolitan Life Insurance Co. tables) from their pretreatment weights (Table 1).

TABLE 1. Summary Statistics of Treatment Groups: Weight

Treatment group	Percent overweight		Pretreatment weight (lb)		Percent Posttreatment weight (lb)		overweight lost	
	X	SD	X	SD	X	SD	X	SD
Covert sensitization	26.1	16.8	154.3	30.4	153.0	25.5	6.0	9.4
Covert sensitization control	25.3	23.0	155.8	22.9	155.9	35.7	2.9	15.4
No-treatment control	22.9	16.0	148.8	27.6	149.9	28.9	+5.3	30.7

One-way analyses of variance showed that there was no difference among the groups prior to treatment. Similarly, analyses of variance revealed no difference between conditions at posttreatment either in terms of number of pounds lost ($F < 1$; df = 2/32) or percentage overweight lost ($F < 1$; df = 2/32).

Taste-rating task. One-way analyses of variance revealed no difference among the groups at pretreatment on either the specific quantity of chips or total amount of all four foods consumed (Table 2). Similarly, analyses of pre–post difference scores ($F < 1$; df = 2/32) and posttreatment data alone ($F < 1$; df = 2/32) indicated no significant effect of the treatment procedures on either dependent measure.

TABLE 2. Summary Statistics of Treatment Groups: Taste-rating Task

Treatment group	Target food (chips) consumption in grams				Nontarget food consumption in grams			
	Pretreatment		Posttreatment		Pretreatment		Posttreatment	
	X	SD	X	SD	X	SD	X	SD
Covert sensitization	8.7	4.8	11.3	4.7	4.8	2.6	5.1	3.2
Covert sensitization control	6.3	2.4	7.5	4.5	4.6	1.8	6.1	4.1
No-treatment control	7.2	5.7	6.1	4.5	4.5	2.2	4.6	2.5

A one-way analysis of variance of subjects' ratings of both the taste and odor of the target food (chips) revealed highly significant differences (F = 22.37; df =2/32; $p < .001$). Multiple comparisons between means using the Newman–Keuls test (Winer, 1971) showed that both the CS sensitization and CS placebo groups differed significantly from the no treatment control group ($p < .01$). However, the two experimental treatment groups did not differ significantly from each other. Analyses of the non-target foods revealed no significant effect, indicating little influence of either treatment on these foods.

Salivary response measure. One-way analyses of variance showed no significant difference among groups at both pre- or posttreatment assessments.

Questionnaire measures. Subjects' ratings on the Therapy Session Assessment Questionnaire showed no difference between the CS and the CS placebo groups on clarity of imagery. The mean scores for the two groups on a 7-point scale ranging from 1–"very unclear" to 7–"very clear" were 5.3 and 5.6, respectively. Similarly, there was no difference with respect to intensity of affect. The mean scores for the CS and placebo conditions on a 7-point scale ranging from 1–"very weak" to 7–"very intense" were 5.0 and 5.25 respectively. These ratings indicate that most subjects reported clear imagery and experienced relatively high affective arousal in connection with the aversive scenes. Correlations between subjects' imagery and affect ratings during treatment sessions, and posttreatment weights and eating behavior during the taste-rating tasks, were insignificant.

Subjects' responses on the between sessions Progress Assessment Questionnaire revealed no significant difference between the two treatment groups in terms of extratherapeutic rehearsal of scenes. The CS and placebo groups respectively spent a mean of 22.9 and 31.6 minutes practicing aversive scenes during a mean number of 2.2 and 2.3 practices between treatment sessions. Clarity of imagery during these home practice sessions was 5.0 and 4.9 respectively. These questionnaires responses also failed to correlate significantly with posttreatment weight measures or with the quantity of food eaten during the taste-rating task.

Both treatment groups expressed satisfaction with the treatment sessions they participated in on the posttreatment program evaluation. Their mean ratings on a 5-point scale ranging from 1–"very dissatisfied" to 5–"very satisfied" were 4.1 and 4.0 respectively. Subjects' mean scores on a 5-point scale of therapist competence, with 5 = "highly competent", were 4.7 and 4.6 respectively.

Discussion

Covert sensitization procedure, administered under counter-therapeutic demand instructions, failed to produce change on any of the three objective dependent measures of weight loss, amount of food eaten during the taste-rating task, and the salivary response measure. Subjects in the CS group reported a significantly decreased liking for the target food, whereas their ratings of non-target foods remained unaltered. However, the CS control group's data were virtually identical, indicating that the observed changes were a product of suggestion or demand characteristics rather than any differential conditioning effects.

These findings constitute a replication and extension of Foreyt and Hagen's (1973) findings. By virtue of the inclusion of a specific, objective measure of target food consumption, the current study represents perhaps the most relevant and appropriate experimental test of the aversion conditioning rationale of CS to data (Abramson, 1973). And the failure of CS to modify subjects' eating behavior significantly in the laboratory situation strongly suggests that CS is not an effective method of decreasing an individual's intake of specific foods. Whatever effects may be obtained with the standard clinical application of the CS treatment package for obesity may be most plausibly attributed to the role of self-monitoring and/or suggestion influences (Foreyt and Hagen, 1973; Romanczyk et al., 1973).

The absence of any differential effects on the salivary response measure is difficult to interpret. Although Wooley and Wooley (1973) have shown that salivation measured in this manner can reliably reflect differences in state of deprivation, palatability, and subjective feelings of hunger, they also found that the amount of salivation may be significantly attenuated if subjects do not expect subsequently to eat the food they are instructed to imagine. Since subjects undergoing the salivary response test in the present study were not explicitly told that they would have the opportunity to eat, salivation levels were probably attenuated, thereby helping to obscure potential treatment effects.

Cautela (1972) has discussed several factors which might impair the success of CS. Two obvious problems are poor imagery and insufficiently aversive stimuli; Janda and Rimm (1972), for example, found a significant correlation between subjects' self-reported affective arousal during the scenes and weight loss. However, subjects in the present study consistently reported clear imagery and high affective arousal to the aversive scenes which suggests that they were adequate aversive stimuli and that the necessary requirements for the effective application of CS were met. Moreover, in contrast to Janda and Rimm's (1972) results but in line with Lick and Bootzin's (1971) data, there was no correlation between ratings of subjective arousal and weight loss. A third problem listed by Cautela (1972) is incomplete homework. Again, the questionnaire data indicate that this was not a significant factor in the current investigation since subjects did regularly rehearse the treatment procedures at home.

The failure of CS to produce successful results could also be attributed to too few treatment sessions (Wisocki, 1972). While it might be unreasonable to expect significant weight loss in so short a period of time, and with as few sessions as in the present study, the most appropriate index of the effects of CS is target food consumption. The conditioning rationale behind this technique must predict some measurable quantitative suppressant effect on this key dependent measure given the number of treatment trials administered and the completed homework assignments. It is the absence of such an effect which is particularly damaging to the conditioning conceptualization of CS.

These results on the treatment of overeating cannot be generalized to the application of CS to other disorders such as alcoholism and sexual deviance. Indeed, there is reason to believe that CS may be an effective method of modifying inappropriate sexual behavior (Barlow *et al.*, 1972). And logically, it is impossible to prove the null hypothesis that CS is ineffective in treating obesity. What can be concluded is that, in view of the accumulating body of negative experimental evidence with respect to obesity, the onus is squarely on the proponents of this technique to demonstrate its efficacy in appropriately controlled comparative outcome studies.

References

Abramson, E. E. A review of behavioral approaches to weight control. *Behaviour Research and Therapy*, 1973, **11**, 547-556.

Barlow, D. H., Agras, W. S., Leitenberg, H., Callahan, E. J., and Moore, R. C. The contribution of therapeutic instruction to covert sensitization. *Behaviour Research and Therapy*, 1972, **10**, 411-416.

Cautela, J. R. Treatment of compulsive behavior by covert sensitization. *Psychological Record*, 1966, **16**, 33-41.

Cautela, J. R. The treatment of overeating by covert conditioning. *Psychotherapy: Theory, Research, and Practice*, 1972, **9**, 211-216.

Cautela, J. R. Covert processes and behavior modification. *Journal of Nervous and Mental Disease*, 1973, **157**, 27-36.

Foreyt, J. P., and Hagen, R. L. Covert sensitization: Conditioning or suggestion? *Journal of Abnormal Psychology*, 1973, **82**, 17-23.

Harris, M. B. Self-directed program for weight control: A pilot study. *Journal of Abnormal Psychology*, 1969, **74**, 263-270.

Janda, L. H., and Rimm, D. C. Covert sensitization in the treatment of obesity. *Journal of Abnormal Psychology*, 1972, **80**, 37-42.

Lick, J. and Bootzin, R. Covert sensitization for the treatment of obesity. Paper presented at the Midwestern Psychological Association, Detroit, Michigan, 1971.

Manno, B. and Marston, A. R. Weight reduction as a function of negative covert reinforcement (sensitization) versus positive covert reinforcement. *Behaviour Research and Therapy*, 1972, 10, 201-207.

Romanczyk, R. G. Self-monitoring in the treatment of obesity: Parameters of reactivity. *Behavior Therapy*, 1972, 5, 531-540.

Romanczyk, R. G., Tracey, D. A., Wilson, G. T., and Thorpe, G. L. Behavioral techniques in the treatment of obesity: A comparative analysis, *Behaviour Research and Therapy*, 1973, 11, 629-640.

Sachs, L. B., and Ingram, G. L. Covert sensitization as a treatment for weight control. *Psychological Reports*, 1972, 30, 971-974.

Schachter, S., Goldman, R., and Gordon, A. Effects of fear, food deprivation, and obesity on eating. *Journal of Personality and Social Psychology*, 1968, 10, 91-97.

Thoresen, C., and Mahoney, M. J. *Behavioral self-control.* New York: Holt, Rinehart & Winston, 1974.

Wilson, G. T. and Davison, G. C. Aversion techniques in behavior therapy: Some theoretical and metatheoretical considerations. *Journal of Consulting and Clinical Psychology*, 1969, 33, 327-329.

Winer, B. J. *Statistical principles in experimental design.* New York: McGraw-Hill, 1971.

Wisocki, P. A. The empirical evidence of covert sensitization in the treatment of alcoholism: An evaluation. In Rubin, R. D., Fensterheim, H., Henderson, J. D., and Ullmann, L. P. (Eds.) *Advances in behavior therapy*, New York: Academic Press, 1972, pp. 105-113.

Wollersheim, J. P. Effectiveness of group therapy based upon learning principles in the treatment of over-weight women. *Journal of Abnormal Psychology*, 1970, 76, 462-474.

Wolpe, J. and Lazarus, A. A. *Behavior therapy techniques.* New York: Pergamon Press, 1966.

Wooley, S. C. and Wooley, O. W. Salivation to the sight and thought of food: A new measure of appetite. *Psychosomatic Medicine*, 1973, 35, 136-142.

PART IV

COVERANT CONDITIONING

Introduction

The term "coverant", a contraction of *covert operant*, was introduced by Homme in 1965, to refer to mental events such as thinking, imagining, reflecting, and daydreaming. Homme argues that these unobservable private events obey the same laws as nonprivate events and that coverants, like operants, can be manipulated by environmental cues and consequences. The obvious problems involved in trying to measure mental events, according to Homme, have been needlessly exaggerated by researchers since the presence or absence of coverants are easily detected by the individual in whom they are occurring. The key to the control of coverants, like operants, is in the control of reinforcing events (Homme, 1965). To gain control of coverants most effectively and thereby presumably change overt behaviors, Homme suggested using the Premack principle, which states, "For any pair of responses, the more probable one will reinforce the less probable one" (Premack, 1965, p. 132). To lose weight, for example, an obese individual may be required to first think about how ugly she would look when she weighs 300 lb before she permits herself to engage in some highly probable behavior, such as answering her ringing telephone.

In actual practice, the obese individual is first asked to make a list of very unpleasant thoughts that she finds particularly aversive in relation to being obese. These might include thoughts about herself in a tiny bathing suit with fat bulging out all around her, lying on an operating table with the surgeon having to cut through layer after layer of ugly fat to reach her vital organs, dying sooner because her fat contributes to a heart attack, or trying and failing to have sexual intercourse because her rolls of fat interfere. She is then asked to make a list of very pleasant thoughts associated with being slender. These might include thoughts about herself modeling a beautiful dress, becoming a sexual dynamo in bed, feeling healthier, or having fun at a party or on the beach. Third, she is asked to select a reinforcing event, i.e. a high probability behavior (eating behaviors are not allowed) which will occur several times each day, such as answering the telephone, turning on the kitchen faucet, going to the toilet, sitting in a favorite chair, or taking a drink of water. The individual is then told that whenever the urge to perform the high probability behavior occurs (e.g. the telephone rings), she is to first think one of her aversive thoughts (e.g. how ugly she would look in a bathing suit with rolls of fat bulging out around her), then think one of her pleasant thoughts (e.g. how beautiful she would look modeling a dress when she is slender). Only after making these two coverants would she be permitted to engage in the high probability behavior (answering the phone).

It is assumed that experiencing these coverants will lead to changes in eating behaviors, thereby leading to changes in weight. If indeed sufficiently strong aversive consequences of obesity can be created by anti-obesity thoughts and sufficiently strong reinforcing consequences of being slender can be created by pro-slender thoughts, then overeating should be reduced, resulting in weight loss.

The technique, like Cautela's (1966) covert sensitization (Part III), is easily taught to an individual, requires no instrumentation, and can be done at home as often as the individual chooses. However, the problems involved in evaluating the technique are obvious. Since the implicit responses are self-monitored, the contingencies self-prescribed, and the consequences self-produced, the difficulties involved in trying to measure relevant variables, if indeed the technique does work, have to date precluded much experimental research (Mahoney, 1970, 1972).

Since Homme's (1965) original description, use of coverant conditioning in the treatment of obesity, even in case studies, has been sparse. Tyler and Straughan (1970), our first article, used the technique with a group of overweight women and compared it with two other treatments, "breath holding", and relaxation. The results were disappointing, to say the least. The coverant group lost only 0.75 lb over 8 weeks compared to a loss of 0.43 lb for the breath-holding group, and a gain of 0.53 lb for the relaxation group. When almost any treatment technique can produce losses of around 6–9 lb during a 9-week experimental period, these results are particularly discouraging.

Our second study, by Horan and Johnson (1971), fared somewhat better. Starting with ninety-six undergraduate females, the authors assigned each to one of four conditions, the first three being primarily controls for the fourth, the coverant conditioning treatment. Subjects in the coverant treatment lost an average of 5.66 lb, compared with a gain of 0.02 lb for the first control treatment, and losses of 3.13 lb and 2.72 lb for the second and third control treatments, over 8 weeks. Particularly important in this study is the fact that the authors present *individual* data on all subjects. In this case, the data show clearly the striking differences among subjects and how a few subjects who gain or lose large amounts of weight can affect the results. For example, one subject in the coverant conditioning treatment lost 19.25 lb, while one gained 8.50 lb, suggesting that the treatment affected individuals quite differently, that subjects' participation in following the treatment was variable, or that reasons other than the independent variable, coverant conditioning, such as the demand characteristics of the study, including expectancy, therapist and subject enthusiasm, suggestion, etc., contributed significantly to the subjects' weight change.

Our last article (Horan *et al.*, 1975) found that individuals who used only positive coverants before engaging in high probability behaviors lost more weight than those using only negative coverants. Unfortunately, no control groups were used and no follow-up data reported.

Based on these few obesity studies, some conclusions emerge. First, the articles show that subjects who participate in coverant conditioning programs reduce their use of the technique over time (Tyler and Straughan, 1970; Horan and Johnson, 1971; Horan et al., 1975). Indeed, Tyler and Straughan reported that *all* subjects had trouble in consistently performing the technique and that subjects did it only at the instigation of the investigators, not because the technique led to any immediate reinforcement. Horan and Johnson (1971) found that their subjects' average daily use of the technique dropped from 8.1 to 2.0 during the 8-week period of the study.

Second, however one conceptualizes the technique, whether in terms of cognitive dissonance, reciprocal inhibition, immediate vicarious punishment and reward (Horan and Johnson, 1971), or other psychological model, it has yet to demonstrate its effectiveness with weight loss. Reported weight losses are generally minimal and follow-up data have yet to be reported.

Third, some of the subjects in these studies seemed to benefit from the technique and it might be considered by the clinician for use with some of his obese clients although it is not yet known the type of client who might be helped by it. The technique has not yet received enough experimental attention to warrant any definitive statements regarding its efficacy. However, at this stage in its development, Horan et al.'s (1975) conclusion that "At most, coverant control ought to be considered as a highly reactive, albeit short range, treatment component of a comprehensive program which might also include, for example, stimulus control and dietary information", is quite appropriate.

To date, it appears that the technique is too weak to be helpful by itself, ineffective with most individuals (perhaps because subjects do not continue performing the procedure over time) and it is not known whether whatever short-term weight losses are produced are due to nonspecific placebo variables and whether the losses are maintained beyond a few weeks.

References

Cautela, J. R. Treatment of compulsive behavior by covert sensitization. *The Psychological Record*, 1966, **16**, 33–41.

Homme, L. E. Perspectives in psychology: XXIV. Control of coverants, the operants of the mind. *The Psychological Record*, 1965, **15**, 501–511.

Horan, J. J., Baker, S. B., Hoffman, A. M., and Shute, R. E. Weight loss through variations in the coverant control paradigm. *Journal of Consulting and Clinical Psychology*, 1975, **43**, 68–72.

Horan, J. J. and Johnson, R. G. Coverant conditioning through a self-management application of the Premack principle: Its effect on weight reduction. *Journal of Behavior Therapy and Experimental Psychiatry*, 1971, **2**, 243–249.

Mahoney, M. J. Toward an experimental analysis of coverant control. *Behavior Therapy*, 1970, **1**, 510–521.

Mahoney, M. J. Research issues in self-management. *Behavior Therapy*, 1972, **3**, 45–63.

Premack, D. Reinforcement theory. In D. Levine (Ed.), *Nebraska symposium on motivation.* Lincoln, Nebraska: University of Nebraska Press, 1965.

Tyler, V. O. and Straughan, J. H. Coverant control and breath holding as techniques for the treatment of obesity. *The Psychological Record*, 1970, **20**, 473–478.

CHAPTER 20

Coverant Control and Breath holding as Techniques for the Treatment of Obesity[1]

VERNON O. TYLER, Jr.
Western Washington State College

and

JAMES H. STRAUGHAN
Experimental Education Unit University of Washington

Summary— This study tested two techniques for the treatment of obesity. Fifty-seven women volunteers were randomly assigned to three groups matched for age and estimated overweight. The coverant control group was trained in Homme's method. Prior to permitting herself to perform a high probability reinforcing event (e.g., turning on the kitchen faucet or answering the phone), S would emit a negative non-eating coverant (e.g., imagining how ugly her fat was) and a positive non-eating coverant (e.g., visualizing how attractive she would look when she was slim). Ss in the breath-holding group were trained to take a deep breath and hold it when tempted to eat fattening foods. The control group was taught a modified version of Jacobson's relaxation method. The groups were trained in seven sessions over 9 weeks. The coverant control group lost .75 pound, the breath-holding group lost .43 pound, and the relaxation group gained .53 pound. None of these differences were significant. Implications for Homme's theory and further research are discussed.

The present study was designed to test two techniques advocated for the treatment of obesity having in common the training of the obese S in simple, self-initiated behaviors supposed to make it easier for him to avoid eating. The most important of these methods is called *coverant control*, described in several recent papers by Homme (1965, 1966a, 1966b). A second method, breath holding, was suggested by Patterson[2] and studied by Mees (1966) as a possible aid for helping cigarette smokers break the habit. Ss in a control group were taught relaxation methods.

Reprinted with permission from *The Psychological Record*, 1970, 20, 473–478.

[1]This study was in part supported by a grant from the Bureau for Faculty Research, Western Washington State College. The authors wish to express their thanks to Mary Brynes, Northwest Area Supervisor for TOPS, and to the Whatcom County TOPS members who served as subjects in this experiment. Reprint requests should be addressed to V. O. Tyler, Jr., Dept. of Psychology, Western Washington State College, Bellingham, Wash. 98225.

[2]G. R. Patterson, personal communication.

Homme (1965) has described coverant control as being effective with tension, smoking, overeating, undereating, inability to persist at the task of writing research papers, etc. The word *coverant* was coined from a combination of the two words *covert operant*. Homme's thesis is that some operants are seldom socially reinforced because they are unnoticed by other persons. Two examples of these kinds of operants are thoughts and tension states of the body, hence these are called covert operants or coverants.

The problem for the behavior manager becomes one of finding a way to reinforce coverants. Homme argues that he has found the way by the utilization of the *Premack principle* (Premack, 1965). This principle states that any lower probability response will be reinforced if it is immediately followed by a higher probability response. For example, suppose that a child has a high probability of looking at picture books when they are available. The teacher can manage the child's behavior by not permitting picture-book looking to occur until the child has performed some lower probability response, such as doing his arithmetic. The extension of this principle to coverants is more elaborate and demands cooperation from *S*. Suppose that we, as behavior managers, want to reinforce optimistic thoughts in order to help a depressed person. Homme (1965) argues that we should train *S* in a method of self-reinforcement for optimistic thoughts. A response is selected that *S* is likely to make a number of times a day, and that, at certain times discriminable to *S*, has a high probability of occurrence. An example is coffee drinking. Some persons do have the habit of drinking coffee several times a day, and they periodically find the tendency to go for coffee virtually irresistible. This, at the time, is a high probability response. In order to use this high probability response to reinforce the low-probability response of optimistic thinking, *S* is taught to delay his coffee drinking until he has first thought a pre-planned optimistic thought. If this occurs often enough during the day, Homme argues, the depression will change to a more reasonably optimistic mood. He refers to clinical success with the method.

In order to apply coverant control to managing overeating, we make two assumptions: first, that obese persons are rationalizing that being overweight is not so bad after all, and second, that they are not thinking enough about the positive joys of being slender. If these kinds of thoughts are appropriately changed, supposedly the obese person's eating habits will change because tendencies to eat are closely linked to verbal behavior and thoughts.

In the breath-holding method for cigarette smokers (Mees, 1966), *S* is instructed to take a deep breath and hold it either when thinking about smoking on command from *E* or when feeling the normal temptation to smoke at various intervals throughout the day. There is no good explanation of why this method should work, although a couple of plausible hypotheses readily come to mind. One guess is that *S* is essentially punishing himself if he follows the procedure correctly. *S* holds his breath until the feeling is unpleasant while he is thinking about smoking, then he breathes normally while thinking about something else.

A second guess is that a state of tension normally precedes smoking and is the major eliciting stimulus for the act. Taking a deep breath, holding it until uncomfortable and then letting it out may be relaxing and thus reduce the desire to smoke. Whatever the theory, the technique seemed sufficiently promising to warrant a careful test with the problem of overeating.

Method

SUBJECTS

The *S*s were 57 women volunteers from a self-help weight reducing club. They ranged in age from a teenager who came with her mother to a woman in her sixties. Their average was 39.4 years. Their weights ranged from about 140 pounds to well over 200 pounds, with the average being 186.44 pounds. The average of their self-estimated amounts of overweight was 47.02 pounds. The *S*s were randomly assigned to three groups matched for average age and amount of estimated overweight. All *S*s were administered the IPAT 16 PF Test (Cattell, Saunders, & Stice, 1957). Although these data were not used in matching the three groups, the groups were similar on the 16 factors for which the test gives measures.

PROCEDURE

Each of the three groups was seen as a group for an hour once a week. There were seven sessions in all, spread over a period of nine weeks. Two weeks were missed because of Christmas holidays. At each meeting each *S* was weighed without shoes on a medical scale.

Following Homme's suggestions in detail, the following scheme was evolved for the coverant control group. First, each *S* was asked to make a list of *negative non-eating coverants*, highly unpleasant thoughts in relation to overweight. Second, *S*s were asked to make a similar list of very pleasant thoughts about being slender, *positive non-eating coverants*. The items on these lists were very specific memories or fantasies which were reported as being meaningful to *S*. For example, one *S* reported that one of her unpleasant items was the imagined scene of being on the operating table with the surgeon cutting through layer after layer of fat to reach the vital organs. A pleasant thought reported by a *S* was seeing herself in fantasy again modeling an attractive gown that she had once been able to wear. Third, each *S* selected a *reinforcing event*, a high probability behavior which occurred a number of times each day. The stipulation was made that this reinforcing event not be eating. Several *S*s chose as their high probability reinforcing event the act of turning on the kitchen faucet. One used answering the phone when it rang.

The *S*s in the coverant control group were seen together for instruction in the procedures recommended by Homme. First, the intention to perform the reinforcing event would occur; for example, S would decide to turn on the faucet in the kitchen or bathroom. Second, when S became aware of this impulse and before performing the high-probability act of turning on the faucet, she made a negative non-eating coverant, for example, thinking how embarrassing it would be to be injured and, in her "sloppy fat" condition, have to be carried to the ambulance. Third, she made a positive non-eating coverant, for example, thinking how nice it would be to have her husband or boyfriend really admire her. Fourth, she permitted the reinforcing event to occur, i.e., she turned on the faucet and went on about her activities.

The sessions with the coverant control group were spent in several activities. At the first session the method was explained to them and its rationale discussed. Lists of negative non-eating coverants, positive non-eating coverants, and reinforcing events were prepared. At each session there was a general discussion of how the procedure was working, an attempt to refine the procedure, and practice in applying the method. Practice consisted of having Ss imagine that they were about to perform the reinforcing event and then imagine that they were going through the coverant control procedure.

The sessions with the breath-holding group were spent in discussing the rationale of the method, determining how each S was using it, and practicing. Practice consisted of having Ss imagine that they were tempted by some tasty morsel such as a thick, fresh slice of banana cream pie, and then go through the breath-holding procedure.

The control group was taught a modified version of Jacobson's (1939) relaxation instructions over a period of 5 weeks. During the remaining 2 weeks, practice in relaxation was continued, coupled with imagining upsetting scenes around the home or at work. Care was taken not to directly associate the relaxation with any suggestions concerning eating.

Results and Discussion

The outcome of the research was not exciting. The coverant control group showed an average loss of .75 pound for this period of approximately two months. The average member of the breath-holding group lost .43 pound, and the members of the relaxation group gained an average of .53 pound. None of these changes were significant.

What can be said about these results? First, under these conditions neither the coverant-control method nor the breath-holding method is effective by itself. We believe that there are good theoretical reasons to question the effectiveness of each of these methods and that our results confirm a theoretical analysis. Two important considerations are involved. The first and perhaps most important of these is the immediacy of reinforcement. The reward for eating when hungry is immediate and effective. The reinforcements for avoiding food are usually delayed and of doubtful effectiveness. Therefore, self-control methods are handicapped. The second consideration involves the tendency of unnecessary links in a stimulus-response sequence to drop out of the sequence (Bugelski, 1958). With both the breath-holding and the coverant control methods, we are attempting to insert additional s-r links into the sequence between the initial impulse to perform an act and the performance of this reinforcing act. These additional stimulus-response links are not necessary in order to attain the goal of performing the reinforcing act, therefore, they tend to drop out. All *S*s reported that they had trouble in consistently performing the coverant-control or breath-holding acts. In effect, the coverant-control or breath-holding practices were performed only at the instigation of the *E*s and not because the practices led to any immediate reinforcement.

Second, our control group, although intended as a control group, casts doubts on the extent to which overeating may be related to tension. Almost every member of the control group reported gratifying results from the relaxation training. This was the group with the smallest dropout rate. Many brought in stories of better family relations, less concern about upsetting events, and greater self-control. But they continued to eat. This conclusion is consistent with the finding of Schachter (1968) that fear had no relationship to eating by obese *S*s.

Finally, our current speculations are very similar to those with which we began. Initial determinants of obesity may be complex, but overeating is overeating. The act of eating becomes associated with a variety of environmental and internal cues. The reinforcement for overeating is immediate and positive. The positive social reinforcement for not eating may be delayed for months, during which time reinforcement is largely negative. Acts competing with eating must be learned in a variety of situations very much as with smoking. In order, then, to interfere effectively with the act of overeating, these factors should be considered:

1. manipulating the social consequences attendant upon dieting,
2. acquiring reinforced behavior which will conflict with eating, and
3. altering or reducing the cues which typically elicit eating.

References

BUGELSKI, B. R. (1958) *The psychology of learning.* New York: Holt, Rinehart & Winston.

CATTELL, R. B., SAUNDERS, D. R., & STICE, G. (1957) *Handbook for the 16 personality factor questionnaire.* Champaign, Illinois: Institute for Personality and Ability Testing.

HOMME, L. E. (1965) Perspectives in psychology, Vol. XXIV: Control of coverants, the operants of the mind. *Psychological Record* 15, 501–511.

HOMME, L. E. (1966) Coverant control therapy: A special case of contingency management. Paper read at the 1966 Convention of the Rocky Mountain Psychological Association, Albuquerque. (a)

HOMME, L. E. (1966) Contiguity theory and contingency management. *The Psychological Record*, **16**, 233–241. (b)

JACOBSON, E. (1939) *Progressive relaxation*. Chicago: Univ. of Chicago Press.

MEES, H. (1966) Placebo effects in aversive control: A preliminary report. Washington State Psychological Association.

PREMACK, D. (1965) Reinforcement theory. In D. Levine (Ed.), *Nebraska symposium on motivation*. Lincoln: Univ. of Nebraska Press.

SCHACHTER, S. (1968) Obesity and eating. *Science*, **161**, 751–756.

CHAPTER 21

Coverant Conditioning through a Self-management Application of the Premack Principle: its effect on weight reduction

JOHN J. HORAN

Pennsylvania State University

and

R. GILMORE JOHNSON[1]

Michigan State University

Summary— To evaluate Homme's contention that coverants (cognitive behaviors) incompatible with overeating can be reinforced through a self-management application of the Premack principle, 96 women students between 20 per cent and 30 per cent overweight were randomly assigned to one of four individual counseling programs. After 8 weeks the mean weight differences for Treatment 1 (delayed control), Treatment 2 (information and encouragement), Treatment 3 (scheduled coverants), and Treatment 4 (reinforced coverants) were 0.02, −3.13, −2.72 and −5.66 pounds respectively. Analysis of covariance with pretreatment weight as the covariate revealed that Treatment 4 produced more weight loss than Treatment 1, ($p < 0.03$). No other paired comparisons were significant. The efficacy of the Premack principle in a self-management situation was supported but not established.

Etiological views of overeating as a manifestation of biochemical or psychodynamic drives have not proved helpful in the formulation of effective treatment programs for the obese. Recently, however, a number of behavioral approaches to the modification of eating activity have appeared in the literature (Wolpe, 1954; Ferster *et al.*, 1962; Cautela, 1966; Stollak, 1967; Stuart, 1967; Harris, 1969). Operant and respondent techniques have been applied to both overt and covert behaviors, and have met with mixed success. But until our experiment reported here, the effect on weight reduction of coverant conditioning through a self-management application of the Premack principle had not been systematically examined.

Reprinted with permission from *Journal of Behavior Therapy and Experimental Psychiatry*, 1971, 2, 243–249.

[1] Requests for reprints should be addressed to R. Gilmore Johnson, College of Education, 433 Erickson Hall, Michigan State University, East Lansing, Michigan 48823.

Coverant conditioning is a generic term referring to the principles and procedures underlying the modification of cognitive behaviors. Coverants (a contraction of "covert operants" coined by Homme, 1965, p. 502) are cognitive behaviors such as thoughts, images and reflections. An adaptation of the Premack principle — "For any pair of responses, the more probable one will reinforce the less probable one" (Premack, 1965, p. 132) — implies a methodology through which certain coverants might be reinforced. Homme (1965) has suggested that overweight subjects who make the emission of a highly probable behavior contingent upon the experience of coverants which are incompatible with obesity will modify their eating behavior and consequently lose weight.

It might be argued that any successful weight reduction program makes at least informal use of a coverant conditioning mechanism. Consider the woman who finds the thought of her physician's disapproval to be highly aversive. Should she enter treatment for obesity, the dreaded image of "weighing in each week and not losing" occurring on a random basis would undoubtedly influence her daily eating habits. Homme's paradigm forces the repeated occurrence of such anti-obesity coverants.

In addition to the problem of overeating, coverant conditioning technologies can be used to increase the frequency of cognitive behaviors which are incompatible with cigarette smoking, stuttering, depression, possibly even alcoholism, drug addiction and a number of other self-defeating activities as well. Hark (1970), for example, concluded that in conjunction with the presence of a counselor, coverant conditioning was an effective tool for helping motivated groups of clients extinguish their smoking behavior. And Davison (1969) noted that a similar procedure enabled a bright youth with inconsistent parents adaptively to control his rebellious behavior.

The effect of incompatible coverants on specific maladaptive eating habits has been explained in terms of cognitive dissonance, reciprocal inhibition, and immediate vicarious punishment and reward (Horan, 1970). Undoubtedly, a number of other psychological models might also be invoked.

Method

Ninety-six female volunteers, predominantly Michigan State University undergraduates, between 20 per cent and 30 per cent overweight, were recruited through an announcement of a weight-control counseling program in the University newspaper and through referrals from University Health Center physicians. Approximately two-thirds of the subjects were respondents to the newspaper announcement.

The subjects were randomly assigned to one of four treatments. The first was a delayed treatment *control* in which subjects received no treatment between initial and final weighings but were subsequently given counseling after the 8-week experiment. All other subjects had three counseling interviews, each lasting one-half hour. Subjects were seen individually by counselors in offices temporarily established in the University Health Center. The first counseling session followed the initial weighing, the second was scheduled one week later, and the final session was held 8 weeks after the initial session and was used to record posttreatment weights.

Treatment 2 consisted of giving subjects information about weight control including a balanced 1000 calorie diet based on recommendations of the American Dietetic Association. Questions about obesity and weight control were also answered in these individual interviews. Subjects were encouraged to adhere to the diet plan.

Treatments 3 and 4, in addition to giving subjects information on obesity and the 1000 calorie diet, attempted to increase the frequency of coverant pairs which individual subjects identified as being incompatible with their overeating habits. Negative coverants involved the undesirable aspects of being overweight (e.g. "shortened life span"). Positive coverants involved the desirable aspects of being properly proportioned (e.g. "clothes fitting better"). Each subject was helped to identify her own list of coverant pairs.

Subjects in Treatment 3 were exposed to a scheduled coverant treatment designed to determine the necessity of invoking the Premack principle by omitting it as a reinforcement methodology. These subjects were simply told to think of the negative—positive coverant pairs at least seven times a day.

Treatment 4 provided training in coverant conditioning through a self-management application of the Premack principle. These experimental subjects were helped in identifying a specific highly probable behavior (i.e. a non-eating activity occurring at least seven times a day, such as "sitting down on a particular chair"). They were then instructed to make the emission of this behavior contingent upon thinking of a negative—positive coverant pair.

Seven properly proportioned graduate students in counseling conducted the treatment sessions. These counselors were volunteers recruited from a graduate program in counseling at Michigan State University. They were randomly assigned to treatment conditions and given instruction and practice in the administration of treatment sessions. Each subject met with the same counselor throughout the three sessions.

To facilitate coverant identification, an open-ended questionnaire seeking idiosyncratic reasons for losing weight was mailed to all subjects in Treatments 3 and 4 prior to their first counseling interview. Additional questionnaires were used to obtain frequency ratings for experiencing coverant pairs. Pre- and post-treatment weights were taken at the same time of day in street clothes minus shoes on a balance scale to the nearest quarter-pound.

It was hypothesized that:

1. Counseled subjects who received training in a particular type of coverant conditioning (Treatment 4) would exhibit greater weight loss at the end of an

8-week period than would counseled and noncounseled subjects who did not receive such training (Treatments 3, 2 and 1).

2. The frequency of experiencing incompatible coverants in Treatments 3 and 4 would be positively related to weight loss.

3. Subjects who attempted to reinforce their coverants through the use of a self-management application of the Premack principle (Treatment 4) would experience more coverants than would subjects who attempted to follow a predetermined coverant frequency schedule (Treatment 3).

Results

TREATMENT EFFECTS

The effect of the four counseling procedures on weight reduction can be seen in Tables 1 and 2. Average weights before and after treatment and average weight losses of each group are presented in Table 1. Data on individual subjects are presented in Table 2 should a closer inspection be sought. Sixteen of the subjects dropped out of school, moved, or for other reasons were not available for the final weighing and had to be dropped from the experiment.

TABLE 1. Mean pre and post weights and weight losses for groups 1, 2, 3 and 4

	Counseling group	Mean Pre-weight	Mean Post-weight	Mean weight loss
G1:	Delayed treatment	153.80	153.82	+0.02
G2:	Placebo treatment	148.98	145.85	−3.13
G3:	Scheduled treatment	143.26	140.54	−2.72
G4:	Experimental treatment	156.07	150.41	−5.66

No consensus exists in the literature as to the most appropriate method of program evaluation. Success, for example, might be defined in terms of the number of participants losing at least one pound per week. In Treatment 4, 53 per cent of the subjects met such a criterion. This compares quite favorably to the 21 per cent in Treatment 3, the 20 per cent in Treatment 2, and the 5 per cent in Treatment 1 who could be considered successful weight losers.

In this experiment mean weight losses among treatment groups at the end of the 8-week-period were tested using analysis of covariance (ANCOVA) with pretreatment weight as the covariate. The ANCOVA was followed by Scheffe *post hoc* comparisons in order to ascertain which treatment groups differed from each other. It was found that subjects in Treatment 4 lost more weight than those in Treatment 1 ($P < 0.03$). No other comparisons of pairs were significant.

TABLE 2. Pre and post weights, and weight losses of subjects in groups 1, 2, 3 and 4

Subject	Group 1			Group 2			Group 3			Group 4		
	Pre	Post	Loss	Pre	Post	Loss	Pre	Post	Loss	Pre	Post	Loss
A	149.50	149.00	− 0.50	127.00	121.75	− 5.25	149.00	145.50	− 3.50	137.00	129.00	− 8.50
B	131.25	130.00	− 1.25	134.00	132.25	− 1.75	134.25	122.75	−11.75	157.00	146.50	−10.00
C	146.50	147.75	+ 1.25	163.50	166.00	+ 2.50	168.00	164.00	− 4.00	142.25	142.25	−17.50
D	133.25	139.00	+ 5.75	155.00	146.50	− 8.50	116.25	118.50	+ 2.50	123.00	114.50	− 8.50
E	131.00	134.00	+ 3.00	157.25	154.50	− 2.75	122.75	122.00	− 0.75	163.75	148.25	−15.50
F	141.00	145.25	+ 4.25	121.00	114.00	− 7.00	122.50	125.50	+ 3.00	168.25	161.25	− 7.00
G	145.75	142.25	− 3.50	161.25	148.25	−13.00	130.00	129.50	− 0.50	146.25	142.50	− 3.75
H	146.75	147.00	+ 0.25	147.25	148.25	+ 1.50	139.00	137.00	− 1.50	174.75	174.50	− 0.25
I	172.50	158.25	−14.25	134.50	133.50	− 1.00	121.75	119.50	− 2.25	174.50	163.00	−11.50
J	156.50	155.25	− 1.25	121.00	126.50	+ 5.50	126.00	123.50	− 2.50	179.75	160.50	−19.25
K	153.00	151.50	− 1.50	133.50	137.00	+ 3.50	159.00	150.50	− 8.50	162.50	151.25	−11.50
L	136.25	134.50	− 1.75	128.50	126.50	− 2.00	134.75	125.75	− 9.00	145.00	144.00	− 1.00
M	148.25	145.75	− 2.50	151.00	148.50	− 2.50	140.50	135.00	− 5.50	127.00	135.50	+ 8.50
N	152.25	153.50	+ 1.25	141.25	145.50	+ 3.25	174.25	164.25	−10.00	146.75	136.50	−10.25
O	167.50	163.75	− 3.75	164.25	151.50	−12.75	140.25	144.50	+ 4.25	137.50	145.50	+ 8.00
P	169.50	170.00	+ 0.50	138.25	128.50	− 9.75	133.00	135.50	+ 2.50	179.75	185.00	+ 0.25
Q	151.50	153.00	+ 1.50	176.00	176.50	+ 0.50	171.25	169.50	− 1.75	168.25	174.75	+ 6.25
R	165.00	178.00	+13.00	178.00	170.50	− 7.50	198.25	194.50	− 3.75	187.50	179.00	− 8.50
S	144.25	144.75	+ 0.50	183.00	181.50	− 1.50	141.25	142.50	+ 1.25	144.50	141.50	− 3.00
T	167.00	164.25	− 2.75	164.00	160.50	− 3.50						
U	195.50	194.00	− 1.50									
V	179.50	183.25	+ 3.75									

COVERANT FREQUENCY AND WEIGHT REDUCTION

As a result of their counseling, the subjects in Treatments 3 and 4 reported experiencing coverant pairs daily. The frequency of these cognitive behaviors differed between the groups and between subjects. It was expected that the number of coverants elicited each day would be positively related to weight loss. If such coverants were really incompatible with overeating, then subjects who experienced the greatest number would lose the most weight. A Pearson r of 0.27 was found to exist between the two variables. Although the relationship was in the expected direction, it was not significant at the 0.05 level.

EFFECT OF THE PREMACK PRINCIPLE ON COVERANT FREQUENCY

All subjects in Treatment 3 were told to think of the coverant pairs at least seven times per day. The subjects in Treatment 4 were instructed to make the emission of a highly probable behavior (i.e. a non-eating activity identified as occurring at least seven times a day) contingent upon the thinking of a coverant pair. Over the 8-week period, subjects exposed to Treatment 4 reported more coverants than those in Treatment 3 (t test significant at the 0.05 level). Subjects in both treatments exhibited declining frequency of coverants during the course of the 8 weeks. Mean coverant frequencies and standard deviations for subjects in Treatments 3 and 4 for each week are presented in Table 3. Differences

TABLE 3. Mean self-reported daily frequency of coverants

Treatment	Weeks															
	1		2		3		4		5		6		7		8	
	M	SD	M	SD	M	SD	M	SD	M	SD	M	SD	M	SD	M	SD
3	5.4	4.6	4.0	4.5	2.5	3.0	2.2	2.8	1.6	2.5	1.2	2.0	1.2	2.0	1.5	2.2
4	8.1	3.2	6.4	3.7	5.4	3.8	4.8	3.7	3.4	3.8	2.2	2.6	2.2	3.3	2.0	2.8

between treatments for each week were tested separately using t tests and Bonferroni's procedure for partitioning the alpha. No differences at any given week produced a t value large enough to reach the level of significance needed to be within the overall alpha of 0.05.

Discussion

CONCLUSIONS

Apparently, motivation alone (defined as willingness to volunteer for treatment) was not responsible for systematic weight loss. In fact the subjects in Treatment 1 who volunteered but received no counseling showed a slight average gain (0.02 pounds) at the end of the 8 week period. On the other hand, comparable subjects in Treatment 4 who received instruction in coverant conditioning through a self-management application of the Premack principle exhibited a substantial mean weight loss of 5.66 pounds. The difference between these treatments was significant. But perhaps even more noteworthy was the observation that over half of the subjects in Treatment 4 achieved the practical ideal of losing at least a pound per week. (To achieve a maintainable weight loss, some caution should be exercised with respect to encouraging a weight-loss rate greatly in excess of this kind of "ideal".)

Unexpected similarities between the reinforced covarant treatment (Treatment 4) and the informational and scheduled covarant treatments (Treatments 2 and 3) may account for the failure to obtain significant differences between the effects of these procedures. Several successful weight losers in Treatment 2, for example, spontaneously reported using such motivational aids as "I just kept thinking about how nice I would look on my wedding day" or "My roommate and I posted a picture of a fabulously skinny girl on the refrigerator door".

In Treatments 3 and 4 the measured relationship between covarant frequency and weight loss was in the expected direction. Generally speaking, the subjects who experienced the greatest of covarant pairs lost the most weight. However, the correlation of 0.27 between these two variables was much too slight to draw conclusions about the theoretical incompatibility of certain covarants with motor behavior.

Although those in Treatment 4 experienced significantly more covarant pairs than those in Treatment 3, both groups exhibited declining rates. The major changes occurred within the first few weeks of the program. The self-managed covarant-reinforcement system was not maintained by the typical experimental subject.

Essentially, then, covarant conditioning appears to be a viable therapeutic adjunct for the treatment of obesity, probably because the experience of incompatible covarants causes changes in eating behavior. Subjects were helped to give up maladaptive eating habits (i.e. rapid eating, overeating at mealtime, and eating between meals) and to acquire the more adaptive habit of having regularly scheduled, balanced meals of reduced calories. The efficacy of the Premack principle in a self-management situation was not established in this experiment.

LIMITATIONS AND IMPLICATIONS

In view of the recidivism of the obesity problem, a major criticism of this study might be that no long range follow-up was conducted. It was precluded by the transient nature of the student population from which the sample was drawn.

Another limitation was anticipated by Kiesler (1966, p. 111) in his succinct description of the "patient uniformity assumption". This "myth" implies that clients "at the start of treatment are more alike than they are different," and will consequently respond to a given type of therapy in a similar manner. On the contrary, overweight people are probably more different than they are alike. And as might be expected, the experimental treatment was not equally effective with all clients. In fact three Treatment 4 subjects showed conspicuous weight gain. Such "therapeutic failures" naturally lower the average weight loss of the experimental group. But the personal and social variables which might have helped potentially successful subjects were, and remain, unknown.

Many of the subjects in this experiment lived in dormitories and consequently could not plan their own meals. It may be that a substantial fraction of the subjects who did not lose weight (in all treatments) were those who had few, if any, food choice options.

Further study is needed to clarify the nature of the incompatible coverant effect. Perhaps if some reliable scale could be devised which would measure "intensity of experience" it might be shown that the notion of incompatibility is really a function of both coverant frequency and intensity. The oft-repeated fantasy of being "rejected or ridiculed in a sexual situation," for example, might very well effect more changes in eating behavior than would the frequent vicarious experience of being "tired after ascending a flight of stairs".

Researchers in this area might also consider (1) examining the possibly differential effect of negative and positive coverants; (2) using the act of eating as a highly probable behavior; and (3) increasing the number of therapist—client contact hours in order to depend less on the self-management concept.

Coverant conditioning appears to be a promising therapeutic technique. Future research may clarify its impact and increase its effectiveness in the treatment of obesity and other personal problems.

References

CAUTELA, J. R. (1966) Treatment of compulsive behavior by covert sensitization, *Psychol. Rec.* **16**, 33—41.

DAVISON, G. C. (1969) Self-control through "imaginal aversive contingency" and "one-downmanship": Enabling the powerless to accommodate unreasonableness. In *Behavioral Counseling* (Edited by J. D. KRUMBOLTZ and C. E. THORESEN). Holt, Rinehart & Winston, New York.

FERSTER, C. B., NURNBURGER, J. I. and LEVITT, E. E. (1962) The control of eating, *J. Mathetics* **1**, 87—109.

HARK, R. D. (1970) An examination of the effectiveness of coverant conditioning in the reduction of cigarette smoking (Doctoral dissertation, Michigan State University), University Microfilms No. 70—20, 465, Ann Arbor, Michigan.

HARRIS, M. B. (1969) A self-directed program for weight control: A pilot study, *J. abnorm. Psychol.* **74**, (2), 263—270.

HOMME, L. E. (1965) Perspectives in psychology: XXIV Control of coverants, the operants of the mind, *Psychol. Rec.* **15**, 501—511.

HORAN, J. J. (1970) The effect on weight reduction of coverant conditioning through a self-management application of the Premack principle (Doctoral dissertation, Michigan State University), University Microfilms, No. 71—18, 223, Ann Arbor, Michigan.

KIESLER, D. J. (1966) Some myths of psychotherapy research and the search for a paradigm, *Psychol. Bull.* **65** (2), 110–136.

PREMACK, D. (1965) Reinforcement theory. In *Nebraska Symposium on Motivation.* (Edited by D. LEVINE). University of Nebraska Press, Lincoln, Nebraska.

STOLLACK, G. E. (1967) Weight loss obtained under different experimental procedures, *Psychotherapy: Theory, Research and Practice*, **4** (2), 61–64.

STUART, R. B. (1967) Behavioral control of overeating, *Behav. Res. & Therapy* **5**, 357–363.

WOLPE, J. (1954) Reciprocal inhibition as the main basis of psychotherapeutic effects, *Archs. Neurol. Psychiat. Chicago* **72**, 205–226.

CHAPTER 22

Weight Loss through Variations in the Coverant Control Paradigm

JOHN J. HORAN,[1] STANLEY B. BAKER, ALAN M. HOFFMAN,[2] and
ROBERT E. SHUTE

Pennsylvania State University

　　　　Summary— Forty overweight female subjects were randomly assigned to one of
eight treatment combinations in a 2 X 2 X 2 matrix. The use of positive coverants
produced significantly ($p < .005$) more weight loss than negative coverants. No
differences were found between those subjects employing highly probable eating and
noneating behaviors. Group counseling enabled a larger percentage of subjects to lose
at least a pound per week than did individual intervention followed by self-
management. Homme's paradigm should be shortened to three steps when applied to
the problem of weight loss since certain treatment combinations were nearly 100%
effective.

Coverants (a contraction of covert operants) are mental behaviors such as
thoughts, images, reflections, feelings, and the like. The term was coined by
Homme (1965), who suggested that both coverants and operants could be
manipulated by the same kinds of environmental cues and consequences.
Homme further speculated that the subject could serve as his own experimenter.
For instance, to obtain some long-range goal such as losing weight, one might
attempt to increase the frequency of specific coverants that were
"incompatible" with his overeating habits. Incompatible coverants are of two
types. Negative coverants deal with the aversive aspects of being overweight.
Positive coverants focus on the desirable attributes of being properly
proportioned. Examples might include images of an obesity-related coronary
attack versus greatly increased sexual prowess when weight is lost.

Homme recommended a self-management application of the Premack (1965)
principle as a means of coverant acceleration [i.e. "For any pair or responses, the
more probable response will reinforce the less probable one" (Premack, 1965,
p. 132)]. More specifically, overweight subjects might be instructed to
repeatedly engage in the following four-step sequence: (a) detection of an eating

　　Reprinted with permission from *Journal of Consulting and Clinical Psychology*, 1975,
43, 68–72.

[1] Requests for reprints should be sent to John J. Horan, 323 Social Science Building,
Pennsylvania State University, University Park, Pennsylvania 16802.
[2] Alan M. Hoffman is now at Wayne State University.

stimulus; (b) emission of a negative coverant; (c) emission of a positive coverant; and (d) engagement in a "reinforcing" or highly probable behavior. In an important system variation, Homme (1966) acknowledged that highly probable behavior preparatory stimuli could initiate the sequence. Theoretically, with either system variation, the highly probable behavior would reinforce the preceding steps, and the resulting weight loss would ultimately reinforce continued participation in the self-managed coverant control system.

Support for the assumption of coverant incompatibility was recently displayed in a study which found that obese individuals are extremely unwilling to tolerate a reflected image of their bodies (Horan, 1974). Thus, negative coverants are in fact lowly probable. Furthermore, they need not be especially horrifying but simply indicative of the status quo. The "incompatibility" of positive coverants, however, remains to be tested.

Homme's assumptions concerning the technology of coverant acceleration have been subjected to rather penetrating conceptual criticism. Mahoney (1970) offered two revisions based on laboratory and practical considerations, and Danaher (1974) pointed out that in keeping with original Premackian formulations only a special class of highly probable behaviors should ever be employed. The latter criticism is particularly devastating in terms of applying coverant control to problems of weight loss since there are few potential highly probable behaviors that are truly "free", that can occur frequently, and that have hedonic value anywhere near that of eating.

Be that as it may, Homme's coverant control paradigm has proved to be clinically useful (e.g. Horan & Johnson, 1971; Mahoney, 1971; Todd, 1972). The present study was undertaken in a highly inductive frame of reference. Just as systematic desensitization may "work" in spite of the controversy concerning "why" (Evans, 1973), might not certain variations in Homme's paradigm prove to be empirically more effective than others in spite of *a priori* theoretical accoutrements?

The first variable of interest was the possible differential effects of positive and negative coverants. If only one type is particularly reactive, the four-step sequence could be streamlined to three, thus minimizing the "frustrative nonreward" issue raised by Mahoney (1970).

A second experimental concern evolved from Homme's emphatic protestation that the highly probable behavior should not be the problem behavior. Admittedly, one might question the logic of using an unwanted behavior to reward thinking about not engaging in that behavior. On the other hand, with the obese, eating *per se* is not the problem. Overeating — that is, excessive consumption in response to external rather than internal stimuli — is the undesirable activity. Furthermore, might not the quantity of calories ultimately consumed be considerably diminished after thinking about the potential consequences of continued imbibing? Finally, if in fact the highly probable behavior really serves to cue rather than reinforce the sequence (a legitimate alternative explanation), perhaps the repeated pairing of food stimuli with incompatible coverants would reduce the attractiveness of probability of eating.

The last experimental issues concern the reality of Homme's self-management assumption, the potential differential effects of individual versus group counseling modes, and the question of cost effectiveness. Specifically, if therapist time and caseload are held constant, are weekly group meetings more effective than intensive individual intervention followed by self-management?

Method

Forty female respondents to newspaper announcements of a weight control program were randomly assigned to one of eight treatment combinations in a 2 X 2 X 2 matrix. The independent variables were (a) coverant type (positive or negative); (b) highly probable behavior type (eating or noneating); and (c) counseling mode (individual or group). Five subjects, for example, were counseled on an individual basis and used the act of eating to reinforce the emission of positive coverants. Since the experimental questions specifically and exclusively concerned comparisons between variations of an already established therapeutic procedure, placebo controls were considered superfluous.

All of the subjects placed a $20 deposit which was refunded (contingent upon mere attendance) in gradually increasing amounts over the course of the 8-week program. Two subjects withdrew for valid reasons shortly after enrolling (one became pregnant, the other was hospitalized for thrombosis). They were replaced by subjects randomly selected from a waiting list. Three other subjects, who participated in the study for at least 4 weeks, dropped out of the program for reasons unknown. Their weights at the time of withdrawal were used in the final analysis.

The subjects were seen by one of two properly proportioned male counseling psychologists with earned doctorates. A booklet (Horan, 1971) containing a behavioral explanation of obesity, suggestions for stimulus control, and an optional 1000-calorie per day food exchange diet was given to all subjects. Losses of between 1 and 2 pounds (.45 and .90 kg) per week were to be considered ideal. Weights were taken at the outset of every counseling session at approximately the same time of day, on the same balance-type scale, in street clothes minus shoes, to the nearest ¼ pound.

To facilitate coverant identification, open-ended questionnaires seeking idiosyncratic reasons for losing weight were mailed to all subjects prior to their first counseling interview. After potential coverants were identified, the subjects were given approximately 10 minutes of imagery training (Phillips, 1971). A credit-card-type display packet in which cue words for specific coverants could be stored and viewed was also provided. The subjects were urged to develop a clear image instead of simply reading the words prior to participation in a highly probable behavior.

TABLE 1. Individual percentage weight loss and summary statistics for each treatment combination

Counseling	Sub-ject	Positive covarant					Sub-ject	Negative coverant				
		Pre-weight (lbs.)	Post-weight (lbs.)	% loss	Mean cell loss (%)	Cell SD (%)		Pre-weight (lbs.)	Post-weight (lbs.)	% loss	Mean cell loss (%)	Cell SD (%)
Individual												
Highly probable eating behaviors	1	225.00	216.25[1]	-3.9	-4.50	1.77	21	160.50	164.00	+ 2.2	-1.60	3.04
	2	154.50	146.00[1]	-5.5			22	192.00	188.00	- 2.1		
	3	173.50	170.50	-1.7			23	182.75	178.00	- 2.6		
	4	172.75	162.00[1]	-6.2			24	168.50	169.00	+ .3		
	5	173.25	164.25[1]	-5.2			25	146.00	137.50[1]	- 5.8		
Highly probable noneating behaviors	6	165.25	158.00	-4.4	-4.50	1.43	26	155.75	140.00[1]	-10.1	-4.80	3.94
	7	131.00	126.50	-3.4			27	159.50	158.00	- .9		
	8	205.00	192.00[1]	-6.3			28	191.50	186.25	- 2.7		
	9	190.25	179.50[1]	-5.6			29	161.00	148.50[1]	- 7.8		
	10	146.50	142.25	-2.9			30	171.25	167.00	- 2.5		
Group												
Highly probable eating behaviors	11	224.50	214.25[1]	-4.6	-7.40	1.61	31	163.50	146.50[1]	-10.4	-3.00	4.20
	12	130.00	119.50[1]	-8.1			32	143.00	141.25	- 1.2		
	13	119.50	110.25[1]	-7.7			33	151.00	151.00	0.0		
	14	135.75	124.50[1]	-8.3			34	165.50	162.00	- 2.1		
	15	158.75	145.25[1]	-8.5			35	252.25	249.00	- 1.3		
Highly probable noneating behaviors	16	154.00	144.75[1]	-6.0	-6.80	1.45	36	224.25	216.25[1]	- 3.6	-3.30	2.78
	17	141.25	129.25[1]	-8.5			37	152.50	143.25[1]	- 6.1		
	18	175.00	162.00[1]	-7.4			38	162.75	153.00[1]	- 6.0		
	19	159.75	152.00	-4.8			39	136.25	135.50	- .6		
	20	172.50	159.50[1]	-7.5			40	142.75	142.25	- .4		

[1] Indicates a loss of at least 1 pound per week.

Half of the subjects received a questionnaire in the mail designed to identify potential highly probable noneating behaviors. (Use of eating as a highly probable behavior for the remaining half was predetermined.) All subjects were instructed to self-monitor the frequency and clarity (McCullough & Powell, 1972) of coverant emission on a daily basis. However, since the data derived from such self-report forms is highly influenced by experimental demand characteristics, no analyses were planned. Self-monitoring was simply expected to increase the reactivity of each treatment combination.

Subjects in the individual counseling mode met with their counselor for three ½-hour sessions. The first session took place several days after the subject applied for the program, placed her deposit, and received an initial weighing. The second and third sessions followed the first by 1 and 8 weeks, respectively. Subjects receiving good counseling ($n = 5$ per group) met for approximately 55 minutes each week throughout the 8-week program. Therapist time and caseload were thus held constant for each counseling mode.

Results

A $2 \times 2 \times 2$ (Coverant Type $\times$ Highly Probable Behavior $\times$ Counseling Mode) analysis of variance was performed on the subjects' "percentage lost" scores [(pre-post)/pre $\times$ 100%]. Table 1 depicts individual losses as well as group means and standard deviations for each treatment combination.

A highly significant main effect was found for coverant type, $F(1, 32) = 9.29$, $p < .005$. The use of positive coverants, regardless of counseling mode or highly probable behavior type, produced considerably more weight loss than did negative coverants. In practical terms, 75% of the subjects experiencing positive coverants lost at least a pound a week, compared to 35% of the subjects experiencing negative coverants who met such a criterion.

No significant differences were found between those subjects using the act of eating to reinforce coverant elicitation and those subjects using highly probable noneating behaviors, $F(1, 32) = 2.36$, $p < .14$. Each reinforcement methodology enabled 55% of its participants to lose a pound a week.

Many of the subjects in the individual counseling mode expressed a preference for more frequent meetings. Only one subject in the group counseling mode appeared dissatisfied with the format. Although 65% of the group counseled subjects compared to 45% of the individually counseled subjects met the pound per week criterion, the analysis of variance on individual scores was not significant, $F(1, 32) = 2.25$, $p < .14$.

No significant interactions occurred, possibly because of the small cell ns; however, it should be noted that the least effective treatment combinations involved pairing the act of eating with negative coverant elicitation. Only three subjects in the study did not lose weight. Two "gainers" were found in the negative-eating–highly probable behavior-individual cell; one "no loss" occurred in the negative-eating–highly probable behavior-group cell.

Group counseling involving positive covarant elicitation produced the most weight reduction. Here, the highly probable behavior type was of no consequence. All but one subject in these two cells lost in excess of 1 pound (.45 kg) per week. The lone "failure" missed this mark by a mere 4 ounces (113 g).

Discussion

The twofold problem of weight loss and maintenance is far more complicated than the literature on covarant control would imply. Demand characteristics notwithstanding, the seriously obese individual who faithfully follows Homme's original paradigm for a sustained period of time is a rarity. In an earlier test of this paradigm, Horan and Johnson (1971) reported that the average daily frequency of covarant–highly probable behavior pairing declined over the 8-week experimental period from 8.1 to 2.8. For this reason, no long-term follow-up was conducted in the present study. At most, covarant control ought to be considered as a highly reactive, albeit short-range, treatment component of a comprehensive program that must also include, for example, stimulus control and dietary information (Horan, 1973).

Since most individuals assigned to delayed or no-treatment control groups rarely lose and indeed often gain weight, the fact that 55% of the subjects in this study achieved the success criterion of a pound per week would suggest that covarant control regardless of format is better than nothing at all. More important, however, is the finding that the use of positive covarants produces significantly (and practically!) greater weight loss than the use of negative covarants. Clinicians employing Homme's (1965) original paradigm now ought to give serious consideration to dropping the second step in the sequence. Positive covarants are not only substantially more reactive than negative covarants, but their exclusive use also seems to produce much less variability in subject responsiveness (a difficulty that characteristically plagues covarant control and obesity research). In this study, group counseling involving the use of positive covarants was nearly 100% effective.

Homme (1965) anticipated the finding that pairing negative covarants with the target behavior is a "most treacherous . . . error" (p. 507). This may be true, but possibly not for the reasons Homme provided. Instead of the expected "adaptation to the aversiveness of the covarant" (p. 506), many subjects apparently resisted or at least did not sustain this rather uncomfortable form of self-management. For example, one subject reported "Thinking about all those awful images made me depressed; I found myself eating more, so I just cut it out entirely." Other subjects expressed similar views. Although posttreatment interviews such as the foregoing lack credibility as data sources, it is significant to note that similar "treatment avoidance behavior" was manifested in two analogue studies on the effects of negative coverants that were conducted concurrently with the present experiment (Horan, Smyers, Dorfman, & Jenkins, in press).

The use of eating to reinforce positive coverants, however, was not similarly problematic. After thinking about the desirable aspects of being properly proportioned, the subjects were seemingly content to limit themselves to a relatively small amount of food. Oftentimes the subjects would follow eating stimuli with the positive coverant and not eat at all. Perhaps positive coverants — coupled with the knowledge that weight loss is in fact occurring — are reinforcing in their own right.

Essentially this study has found that Homme's (1965) original paradigm might prove to be more beneficial if it is shortened to three steps when applied to the problem of weight loss. After detection of an eating or highly probable behavior stimulus, overweight individuals ought to reinforce only positive coverants.

References

Danaher, B. G. The theoretical foundations and clinical applications of the Premack principle: A review and critique. *Behavior Therapy*, 1974, 5, 307–324.

Evans, I. M. The logical requirements for explanations of systematic desensitization. *Behavior Therapy*, 1973, 4, 506–514.

Homme, L. E. Perspectives in psychology: XXIV control of coverants, the operants of the mind. *Psychological Record*, 1965, 15, 501–511.

Homme, L. E. Contiguity theory and contingency management. *Psychological Record*, 1966. 16, 233–241.

Horan, J. J. *Sense and nonsense about obesity*. State College, Pa.: Counselor Education Press, 1971.

Horan, J. J. Obesity: Toward a behavioral perspective. *Rehabilitation Counseling Bulletin*, 1973, 17, 6–14.

Horan, J. J. Negative coverant probability: An analogue study. *Behaviour Research and Therapy*, 1974, 12, 265–266.

Horan, J. & Johnson, R. G. Coverant conditioning through a self-management application of the Premack principle: Its effect on weight reduction. *Journal of Behavior Therapy and Experimental Psychiatry*, 1971, 2, 243–249.

Horan, J. J., Smyers, R. D., Dorfman, D. L. & Jenkins, W. W. Two analogue attempts to harness the negative coverant effect. *Behaviour Research and Therapy*, 1975, in press.

Mahoney, M. J. Toward an experimental analysis of coverant control. *Behavior Therapy*, 1970, 1, 510–521.

Mahoney, M. J. The self-management of covert behaviors: A case study. *Behavior Therapy*, 1971, 2, 575–578.

McCullough, J. P., & Powell, P. O. A technique for measuring clarity of imagery in therapy clients. *Behavior Therapy*, 1972, 3, 447–448.

Phillips, L. W. Training of sensory and imaginal responses in behavior therapy. In R. D. Rubin, H. Fensterheim, A. A. Lazarus, & C. M. Franks (Eds.), *Advances in behavior therapy*. New York: Academic Press, 1971.

Premack, D. Reinforcement theory. In D. Levine (Ed.), *Nebraska Symposium on Motivation*. (Vol. 13) Lincoln: University of Nebraska Press, 1965.

Todd, F. J. Coverant control of self-evaluative responses in the treatment of depression: A new use for an old principle. *Behavior Therapy*, 1972, 3, 91–94.

PART V

THERAPIST REINFORCEMENT TECHNIQUES

Introduction

The studies in this section involve the use of operant reinforcement or punishment procedures to effect weight loss. The majority of them were carried out in institutions with patient populations, allowing the therapist fairly extensive control over the relevant reinforcers in the lives of his subjects. To date, the use of these operant techniques in institutions primarily has been confined to clinical case studies.

Our first four articles are case studies dealing with psychiatric populations. Dramatic in terms of weight loss is the first case study in which Bernard (1968) describes the use of a hospital token economy with a severely obese schizophrenic. Placing her on a diet, restricting food from her family and hospital canteen, and paying her 10 tokens for each pound lost, the patient's weight dropped from 407 lb to 305 lb in just 26 weeks. Upper and Newton (1971), using tokens, off-ward privileges and social approval as reinforcers, report weight losses of 63 lb and 31 lb in two chronic paranoid schizophrenics over 28 and 26 weeks, respectively. Also using tokens, Klein et al. (1972) describe a mean weight loss of 10.8 lb for five schizophrenics after 26 weeks. Unfortunately, no initial weights, individual weight data, or follow-up weights are reported. Using social approval as a reinforcer, Moore and Crum (1969) achieved a 35-lb weight loss in a schizophrenic female during a 26-week treatment period. The patient weighed each day; if she lost weight the therapist immediately reinforced her verbally; if she had not lost weight, he simply shook his head in a negative manner and pointed out the weight difference to the patient.

Taken as a whole, these four reports show clearly that schizophrenic patients will lose weight inside a hospital when their environment is programmed in such a way so that it is to their advantage to reduce themselves. No one argues anymore about the effectiveness of such a program with psychiatric patients. Questions now revolve around the permanence of the changes.

The next two studies describe weight-loss programs with retardates. Foreyt and Parks (1975) developed a treatment program in a day-care training center involving the use of a manual of weight loss techniques for parents of retardates, use of colored tokens to represent food groups, monetary payments for pounds lost, and daily weighings. Even though their three clients were severely retarded, with IQ scores of 26, 30, and 35, they were able to learn to control some of their eating behaviors and managed to achieve an average weight loss of 15.2 lb after 40 weeks. Foxx (1972), using social attention as reinforcement, reported a 79 lb weight loss in a mildy retarded institutionalized female over 42 weeks. Foxx tried to demonstrate the effect of the social reinforcement on weight loss by removing and reinstating it during the treatment period.

Our seventh study is a case report describing the use of a behavioral contract with an immature, emotionally disturbed 10-year-old boy (Dinoff, Rickard, and Colwick, 1972). The boy lost 30 lb over a 7-week camping period by following three written contracts which permitted him to look through a one-way mirror, operate a video-tape machine, and use the camp dictaphone.

Articles eight and nine represent studies utilizing experimental designs in attempts to isolate the variables leading to weight loss. Harmatz and Lapuc (1968) compared three treatments for weight loss with twenty-one institution-alized schizophrenic patients: (a) diet only, (b) diet plus group therapy, and (c) diet plus behavior modification. The effective treatment, diet plus behavior modification, consisted of placing patients on 1800 calories a day and requiring them to forfeit part of a regular weekly $5.00 allotment for not losing weight. The patients in this group not only lost weight during the 6-week treatment period, but continued losing during a 4-week follow-up, averaging 15 lb of weight loss over the 10 weeks of the study. The diet only condition resulted in no weight loss, while the diet plus group therapy treatment showed an initial drop in weight but patients began regaining the lost pounds as soon as the treatment ended. Mann (1972) required his obese subjects to turn over to him valuable possessions including money, jewelry and clothing. The subjects signed contracts stipulating that they would earn these valuables back by losing weight or forfeit the items if they gained weight. Using a reversal design, he found most subjects lost weight while the contingencies were in effect and gained weight during the reversal period, when the contingencies were not in effect. He also found that the punishing contingency, the permanent loss of valuables for not losing weight, was a necessary component of the treatment.

Our final article in this section (Jeffrey, Christensen and Pappas, 1973) presents a detailed step-by-step account on how to set up a behavioral program using contingency contracting and other techniques with obese subjects. The authors cite two studies, one a pilot and one an experimental investigation, supporting the effectiveness of their program. Their experimental study compared a behavior therapy group to a "willpower" treatment and a no-treatment control. The behavior therapy group lost an average of 16.38 lb during 18 weeks compared to 5.09 lb for the willpower group, and 1.7 lb for the controls. A 12-week follow-up on the behavior therapy group only showed no significant weight gain.

Overall, many of the studies in this section reported impressive weight losses. However, there are several problems using therapist controls. The first one involves the extent of control a therapist can realistically achieve. Six of the studies in this chapter were carried out in institutions (Bernard, 1968; Upper and

Newton, 1971; Klein *et al.*, 1972; Moore and Crum, 1969; Foxx, 1972; Harmatz and Lapuc, 1968) and two in somewhat restrictive environments, a daycare center (Foreyt and Parks, 1975) and a summer camp (Dinoff, Rickard and Colwick, 1972). Environmental controls are much easier to develop inside institutions where therapists can set up artificial programs in which they are able to manipulate reinforcers and arrange contingencies in their subjects' daily lives. It is extremely difficult (and costly if the therapist is going to supply the reinforcers) to gain experimental control over variables outside of this institutional setting. Behaviors reinforced with tokens on a hospital ward will not be reinforced with tokens when the patient leaves the institution. No one is going to pay the ex-patient ten tokens for each pound he continues to lose. Therapists have to make use of techniques such as contracts (Mann, 1972; Jeffrey, Christensen and Pappas, 1973) which, unless individuals are highly motivated, oftentimes lead to the development of patterns of behavior aimed at circumventing, rather than following, the contingencies of the contract.

The second serious problem involves the techniques themselves. That is, the techniques generally reinforce *weight loss* (and/or punish weight gain) but fail to teach subjects *how* to most effectively achieve that loss. In Mann's (1972) study using contingency contracting, for example, he said, "Unsolicited anecdotal reports from some of the subjects indicated that they had used extreme measures at various times to lose weight rapidly and temporarily in order to avoid aversive consequences. These measures, reportedly, included taking laxatives, diuretics, and doing vigorous exercises just before being weighed" (p. 108). This idea, "lose weight fast, any way possible", cannot be expected to lead to any permanent, stable weight pattern, or change in eating habits, the goal of weight-loss programs.

The third problem involves the reporting of follow-up data, i.e. what happens to the patient when he leaves the institution or the program and the contingencies are no longer in effect. Many of the studies in this chapter report no follow-up data at all. Of the few that do, the data are generally short term, e.g. 4 weeks (Harmatz and Lapuc, 1968), 6 weeks (Bernard, 1968), or with equivocal results, e.g. Jeffrey *et al.* (1973) reported that of the four patients who stayed in their 6-month pilot program, a 6-month follow-up showed that one subject had regained all of his lost weight, another had regained a portion of his lost weight, and two had still maintained their losses.

Studies employing a reversal design (e.g. Foxx, 1972), in which reinforcers are withdrawn and then reapplied face a problem regarding the appropriateness of such a design with obese human subjects. This issue is a broad one, involving not only weight-loss studies, but all outcome research with humans, and includes the question of whether or not no-treatment groups, "delayed treatment" groups, and placebo groups should be used. Nevertheless, it is probable that a reversal design is not the most appropriate experimental design for use with obese subjects, because of the nature of the problem and because the usual dependent variable, weight, is not a particularly sensitive measure in such a design.

In summary, therapist reinforcement techniques have demonstrated rapid, impressive, sometimes dramatic (Ayllon, 1963; Bernard, 1968) weight losses with institutionalized patients during a treatment period. Whether these losses are maintained when patients leave the institution (or the treatment program) is still an open question since follow-up data have generally not been reported. The contingency contracting technique has been used with a few subjects and shows some promise for short-term weight loss. Long-term data are needed to assess the permanence of the losses. The most difficult problem to overcome with these therapist reinforcement techniques may be their inability to generalize from the institution to the natural environment.

References

Ayllon, T. Intensive treatment of psychotic behavior by stimulus satiation and food reinforcement. *Behaviour Research and Therapy*, 1963, 1, 53–61.

Bernard, J. L. Rapid treatment of gross obesity by operant techniques. *Psychological Reports*, 1968, 23, 663–666.

Dinoff, M., Rickard, H. C., and Colwick, J. Weight reduction through successive contracts. *American Journal of Orthopsychiatry*, 1972, 42, 110–113.

Foreyt, J. P. and Parks, J. T. Behavioral controls for achieving weight loss in the severely retarded. *Journal of Behavior Therapy and Experimental Psychiatry*, 1975, 6, 27–29.

Foxx, R. M. Social reinforcement of weight reduction: A case report on an obese retarded adolescent. *Mental Retardation*, 1972, 10, 21–23.

Harmatz, M. G. and Lapuc, P. Behavior modification of overeating in a psychiatric population. *Journal of Consulting and Clinical Psychology*, 1968, 32, 583–587.

Jeffrey, D. B., Christensen, E. R., and Pappas, J. P. Developing a behavioral program and therapist manual for the treatment of obesity. *Journal of the American College Health Association*, 1973, 21, 455–459.

Klein, B., Steele, R. L., Simon, W. E., and Primavera, L. H. Reinforcement and weight loss in schizophrenics. *Psychological Reports*, 1972, 30, 581–582.

Mann, R. A. The behavior-therapeutic use of contingency contracting to control an adult behavior problem: Weight control. *Journal of Applied Behavior Analysis*, 1972, 5, 99–109.

Moore, C. H. and Crum, B. C. Weight reduction in a chronic schizophrenic by means of operant conditioning procedures: A case study. *Behaviour Research and Therapy*, 1969, 7, 129–131.

Upper, D. and Newton, J. G. A weight-reduction program for schizophrenic patients on a token economy unit: Two case studies. *Journal of Behavior Therapy and Experimental Psychiatry*, 1971, 2, 113–115.

CHAPTER 23

Rapid Treatment of Gross Obesity by Operant Techniques

J. L. BERNARD

Memphis State University

Summary– This paper reports the application of operant techniques in the treatment of a case of gross obesity. The patient weighed 407 lbs. at the initiation of the program, was schizophrenic, and probably had metabolic and/or endocrine dysfunction as contributing factors. Over a period of 6 mo., of which the last 6 wk. were an extinction period, she lost 102 lbs. at a relatively stable rate. At the end of the extinction period, the loss rate had slowed somewhat but showed no indications of reversal. The rapid weight loss, compared to that in earlier studies, is attributed to positive reinforcement for weight lost, in addition to control of caloric intake.

American society seems almost morbidly preoccupied with problems of real, or imagined, obesity (cf., consumer demand for such products as Metrecal, dietetic soft drinks, and "No-Cal Pizza"). Successful application of behavioristic techniques to the problem of anorexia nervosa has been reported by several writers, e.g. Ayllon *et al.* (1964), Bachrach *et al.*, and Lang (both in Ullmann & Krasner, 1965), yet Ferster *et al.* (1964) have noted that the problem of obesity has received considerably less attention. Ayllon (1963) does report one behavior modification program in which a hospitalized schizophrenic lost 17% of her original body weight over a 14-mo. period when her chronic food stealing was established as a discriminative stimulus for her being removed from the dining room. Ferster *et al.* (1964) have reported what they describe as a "pilot program" for weight reduction, in which they note, however: "We cannot state whether the program we carried out is suitable for severely obese individuals (particularly those who have medical or psychiatric complications)." This paper describes the treatment of obesity in an individual who appears to meet all of Ferster's specifications: (a) "severely obese" [the patient weighed 407 pounds at the beginning of the program], (b) "medical complications" [she had been previously diagnosed as having a metabolic disturbance and was believed by the staff to have indications of endocrine disturbance as well], and (c) "psychiatric complications" [she was hospitalized, and diagnosed as Schizophrenic Reaction, simple type]. Ferster *et al.* (1964) also note: "The central issue is the development of self-control in eating which will endure and become an available part of

Reprinted with permission from *Psychological Reports*, 1968, **23**, 663–666. ©Southern Universities Press 1968.

the individual's future repertoire." This paper also reports the results of a 6-wk. extinction period subsequent to the treatment procedure.

The patient, a white female in her mid-twenties, was first admitted to a psychiatric hospital in 1963. She was then diagnosed as Chronic Brain Syndrome, associated with disturbance of metabolism, and discharged (against advice) 6 wk. later. While no record of her weight at that time is available, the writer recalls her as being grotesquely obese. Her second admission was in 1965, at which time her diagnosis was changed to Schizophrenic Reaction, simple type, and she was placed on a chronic ward. Her weight at that time was 350 lbs.

In 1966, the writer established an experimental behavior modification ward in the hospital and arranged to have the patient transferred there. The treatment program to be described was not initiated until after she had been on the ward for several months, by which time her weight had risen to 407 lbs., in spite of the fact that the ward physician had tried her on 1800- and 1000-calories diets. This was probably attributable (as noted by the ward personnel) to the fact that the patient's family brought her large amounts of "goodies" every time they visited, took her on outings that seemed to amount to nothing more than going from candy store to soda fountain to bakery to candy store (at the patient's request) and gave her a liberal allowance, most of which she spent on candy, cookies, cokes, etc.

Procedure

In essence, the program involved controlling caloric intake. This was accomplished by placing her on an 1800-calorie diet, notifying the family that she would no longer be allowed to receive "goodies" (a restriction with which they complied after a token testing of limits), and restricting her "store privileges" in order to control her consumption of high-calorie sweets. It should be noted at this point that, while such tight controls are relatively easy to maintain on a behavior modification ward, one loophole remained to be plugged.

Experience on the ward had shown that, when a patient was restricted from a privilege (e.g., cigarettes, candy, etc.), she could often induce sympathetic friends to smuggle the restricted item to her or, if this failed, purchase it from other patients on a "black market" basis, using the ward's token currency. Thus, as an additional incentive for weight loss, the patient was told that she would be weighed regularly and paid 10 tokens for each pound lost. While she was restricted from using these tokens at the ward store, they could be exchanged for such things as "walkout privileges", telephone calls, admission to dances, recreational events and movies, and for rent on a semi-private, or private room on the ward. During the months the ward had been in operation before the procedure was initiated, these tokens had gained clear status as a powerful secondary reinforcer, and the patient's earning power had thus far been relatively undistinguished.

The patient was weighed (a procedure that necessitated her standing on a board stretched across two 300-lb. capacity medical scales) just prior to breakfast three days a week (Monday, Wednesday, and Friday) and paid on the spot for weight lost; payments often amounted to as much as 50 tokens at a time, on a ward where the average patient's "income" was about 25 tokens per day.

The extinction procedure involved returning her store privileges, while terminating payment for weight lost. The 1000-calorie diet initiated at Week 18 was continued, and the family was not informed that they might once more bring "goodies". (To have reinstated this aspect of the pre-treatment situation would have only served to confuse the family, and parenthetically, they had already informed the ward personnel that the patient no longer asked to be taken to candy stores, etc., when on outings.) Further, the patient was given a brief pep talk on the morning extinction began, informing her that she would continue to be weighed but would no longer be paid for weight lost. She was advised that her store privileges were being returned and encouraged to assume responsibility for controlling her own weight. This eliminated the most significant restrictions on caloric intake, and all reinforcement for weight loss, aside from the social reinforcement of compliments from ward personnel and other patients. The return of store privileges, while removing the patient's major source of income, may seem a hollow gesture, but it should be noted that she had accumulated several hundred tokens during the treatment period, and thus was one of the "wealthiest" patients on the ward.

Results

As Fig. 1 indicates, during the first 17 wk. of the procedure the patient's weight dropped from 407 to 337 lbs., a loss of approximately 20% of her initial body weight, at a rate of almost 4½ pounds per week. It is notable that this matches the weight lost by Ayllon's patient over a 14-mo. interval. As no adverse physical reactions (e.g., dehydration) had been noted, her diet was reduced to 1000 calories per day, and the procedure continued. During the next 3 wk., she dropped to 318 lbs.; a loss of 19 lbs. at a rate of over 6 lbs. per week. This brought the total weight lost during the 20-wk. treatment period to 89 lbs.; a loss of 22% of initial body weight at a rate of 4½ lbs. per week.

Extinction began on the first Monday following the Friday on which the treatment procedure was terminated, by which time the patient's weight had risen from 318 to 323 lbs. Over the subsequent 6 wk. she dropped to 305 lbs., representing 18 lbs. lost over 6 wk. at a rate of 3 lbs. per week. Fig. 1 indicates that while the rate during this period was more erratic than during the treatment period, there is no apparent tendency toward reversal of the trend.

The results obtained appear to indicate that the possibility of endocrine or metabolic dysfunction need not contraindicate a weight control program of this kind. Further, they reinforce Ayllon's (1963) finding that severe obesity and

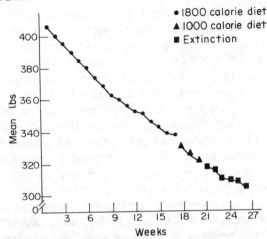

FIG. 1. Mean weight loss by weeks

"psychiatric complications" are not barriers to this approach. The fact that this patient lost weight at a rate almost 4 times that of Ayllon's patient may be attributable in part to the fact that her initial weight was considerably higher, but it also suggests that a program including positive reinforcement for weight loss is more effective than one which only controls caloric intake. Once this program was established, it required very little attention from staff or ward personnel. Since the diets in many state hospitals contain a preponderance of starchy foods, and weight control is a common problem, it seems that this sort of program might easily be adapted for larger populations (i.e., all patients on the ward who are overweight).

References

AYLLON, T. Intensive treatment of psychotic behavior by stimulus satiation and food reinforcement. *Behav. Res. & Ther.*, 1963, 1, 53–61.

AYLLON, T., HAUGHTON, E., & OSMOND, H. Chronic anorexia: a behavior problem. *Canad. J. Psychiat.*, 1964, 9, 147–154.

BACHRACH, A. J., ERWIN, W. J., & MOHR, J. P. The control of eating behavior in an anorexic by operant techniques. In L. P. Ullmann & L. Krasner (Eds.), *Case studies in behavior modification.* New York: Holt, Reinhart, & Wilson, 1966. Pp. 153–164.

FERSTER, C. B., NURNBERGER, J. I., & LEVITT, E. E. The control of eating. *J. Mathetics*, 1962, 1, 87–109.

LANG, P. J. Behavior therapy with a case of nervous anorexia. In L. P. Ullmann & L. Krasner (Eds.), *Case studies in behavior modification.* New York: Holt, Reinhart, & Wilson, 1966. Pp. 217–222.

CHAPTER 24

A Weight-Reduction Program for Schizophrenic Patients on a Token Economy Unit: two case studies

DENNIS UPPER[1] and JUDITH G. NEWTON
V. A. Hospital, Brockton, Massachusetts

Summary— Overweight patients on a token economy psychiatric ward were reinforced with tokens, off-ward privileges and social approval for meeting a weight-loss criterion of 3 lb. per week. The progress of two subjects, both chronic paranoid schizophrenics, is described. One subject began at 263 lb. and consistently lost weight until he had reached a target weight of 200 lb. in 28 weeks. The other began at 201 lb. and reached his target weight of 170 lb. in 26 weeks. The procedure appears to be an effective means of modifying the behavior of overweight psychiatric patients.

Overeating and obesity are problems which occur with a high incidence in the general population. Kennedy and Foreyt (1968) cite actuarial evidence, compiled by the Metropolitan Life Insurance Company, which indicates that one person in twenty weighs at least 20% above his "best" weight. Among chronic hospitalized schizophrenics, who are relatively inactive physically and whose eating habits are relatively unrestricted, obesity may be a problem of even greater magnitude than in the population in general. Traditional treatment procedures have been largely unsuccessful in alleviating obesity and habitual overeating. In a comprehensive review of the treatment of obesity, covering the medical literature for the previous 30 years, Stunkard and McLaren-Hume (1959) found that only 25% of treated patients lost a significant amount of weight. A number of recent behavior therapy studies, however, suggest that learning-theory-based treatment techniques have been at least moderately effective when applied to the problems of obesity and habitual overeating.

Among the techniques which have been employed are aversive or avoidance conditioning (Kennedy and Foreyt, 1968; Wolpe, 1954; Meyer and Crisp, 1964); covert sensitization (Cautela, 1966); stimulus control (Ferster, Nurnberger and Levitt, 1962; Stuart, 1967); and operant reinforcement (Moore and Crum, 1969; Harmatz and Lapuc, 1968). The present study was carried out within the

Reprinted with permission from *Journal of Behavior Therapy and Experimental Psychiatry*, 1971, 2, 113—115.
[1] Requests for reprints should be addressed to Dennis Upper, Veterans Administration Hospital, Brockton, Massachusetts.

context of a ward-wide token economy program and involved the administration of tokens, off-ward privileges, and social approval as reinforcing agents following the weekly loss of weight.

Subjects

S1 was a 36-year-old single male with a diagnosis of chronic paranoid schizophrenia who had been hospitalized in mental institutions almost continuously for 18 years. At the time of his transfer to the present hospital 8 years before the start of the weight-control program, he weighed 233 lb. During the 8 years following his transfer, he gained weight steadily and had reached 280 lb 10 months before beginning the weight program. His beginning program weight was 263 lb, and, following consultation with the patient and his ward physician, a weight of 200 lb was chosen as a reasonable goal.

S2 was a 45-year-old divorced male who also was diagnosed as a chronic paranoid schizophrenic. He had been hospitalized almost continuously for 12 years before the start of the weight program, and he had increased in weight from an admission weight of 166 lb to a maximum weight of 240 lb 2 years before starting on the weight program. When the weight-reduction program began, he weighed 201 lb and following consultation with the patient and ward physician, a target weight of 170 lb was chosen.

Method

Patients on the token economy program of the Brockton V.A. Hospital may use tokens to purchase (among other things) four types of off-ward privileges: meal privileges (an hour at each mealtime to go to the main dining hall), work privileges (meal privileges plus two hours each morning and afternoon to attend a work assignment), partial privileges (from 7 a.m. to 6.30 p.m.), and full privileges (from 7 a.m. to 9.30 p.m.). Each patient pays tokens for his privileges once a week at ward rounds, during which patients are seen individually by the assembled ward treatment term. Because the ward rounds provide the only occasion during the week when the entire treatment team meets with each patient and because the patient's off-ward privilege status is reviewed at this time, it was decided to monitor the subjects' weight and to reinforce them for weight loss during rounds. Subjects on the weight-reduction program were placed on a 1500-calorie reduction diet and were weighed each week immediately before rounds.

When a weight-reduction subject came into rounds, he was told what his current weight was and whether or not he had met the previously-established criterion of a 3 lb loss per week. If he had lost 3 lb or more, he was advanced to the next-highest privilege step (e.g. from meal to work privileges); he was also given one token refund on the price of privileges for each pound he had lost that week and was praised by the team members for having met the criterion. If the patient had not lost weight during the week, he received no token refund and was told he must remain at the same privilege step. If he had gained weight during the week, the subject dropped one step in the privilege hierarchy and received neither token nor social reinforcement from the treatment team.

Results

$S1$ started at 263 lb and began to lose weight quickly. In the first 3 weeks, he lost 19 lb and moved from non-privileged status to that of having work privileges. Throughout the program, he lost weight relatively consistently (although not without some temporary weight gains), and he reached the target weight of 200 lb on the 28th week of being on the program. During this 28-week period, he lost some weight during 19 of the weeks, stayed at the same weight one week, and gained weight during only eight of the weekly periods. He met the 3 lb criterion for reinforcement on 11 of the 19 weeks during which he lost weight, and his largest weekly loss was 10 lb. His average loss per week was 2.29 lb.

$S2$ started at 201 lb and also began to lose weight relatively consistently, although at a lower rate than did $S1$. $S2$ met the criterion of a 3 lb loss per week only twice during the first 4 weeks, although he lost 11 lb during this period. He reached his target weight of 170 lb in 26 weeks, losing an average of 1.19 lb per week. He lost some weight on 16 of the 26 weeks, although he met the 3 lb criterion on only eight of these weeks; he remained at the same weight during 5 weeks and gained weight during 5 other weeks. The largest weekly weight loss for $S2$ was 5 lb.

Discussion

Apparently the reinforcement procedure as outlined above was an effective means of reducing the subjects' body weight within the context of a ward token economy program. While it is true that they were on reduction diets during the reinforcement period, it is significant to note that both Ss had been on similar diets in the past without noticeable reductions in weight occurring. In fact, $S1$ is quoted in his clinical record as stating that he had had so much trouble following his pre-program diet that he wanted ward personnel to confine him to the ward and to force him to follow it. This was never done, however.

It is felt that reinforcing subjects for weekly weight *loss*, rather than for emitting specific responses (e.g. picking up the special diet card prior to meals, avoiding snacks between meals), served to focus their attention on the primary goal of the procedure — reduction in body weight. The weekly monitoring of weight and the feedback they received weekly in rounds provided them with much more information about the success of their own weight-reduction efforts

1

than they typically would have received in the course of more traditional hospital weight-reduction procedures. In fact, rather than externally imposing the type of control that S1 had requested, the procedure presented here was designed to bring the subjects' eating behavior under their own control. Since reinforcement was made contingent upon weight loss itself, rather than upon behaviors that (hopefully) would lead to weight loss as a by-product, the operant most successful for achieving weight reduction in the particular individual would be reinforced. Traditional weight-loss programs "force" on the individual an operant which may not be effective for him. On the present program, adherence to the diet was presented as one means of achieving the desired goal, but if the subject chose to meet the weight-loss criterion by eating a lot on some days and only a little on others he was still reinforced for losing weight.

The cue value of the reinforcement should not be overlooked either. Subjects were reinforced by social approval, tokens, and privileges for relatively small losses of weight, and reinforcement occurred early and often in the weight-reduction program. A problem with traditional hospital procedures for promoting weight loss is that the potential benefits resulting from losing weight are often vaguely-defined (e.g. "better health"), long-delayed (e.g. "longer life"), and unrelated to the problems of surviving in the hospital or preparing for discharge.

Frequent, consistent and contingent reinforcement for weight loss, combined with a restriction of off-ward privileges for not losing weight, makes the issue of weight reduction a much more relevant and potent one for the patient. The indications are that this is an effective procedure for producing weight loss among institutionalized patients.

References

CAUTELA, J. R. (1966) Treatment of compulsive behavior by covert sensitization, *Psychol. Record* 16, 33–41.
FERSTER, C. B., NURNBERGER, J. I. and LEVITT, E. E. (1962) The control of eating, *J. Mathetics* 1, 87–109.
HARMATZ, M. G. and LAPUC, P. (1968) Behavior modification of over-eating in a psychiatric population, *J. Consulting & Clin. Psychol.* 32, 583–587.
KENNEDY, W. A. and FOREYT, J. P. (1968) Control of eating behavior in an obese patient by avoidance conditioning, *Psychol. Reports* 22, 571–576.
MEYER, V. and CRISP, A. H. (1964) Aversion therapy in two cases of obesity, *Behav. Res. & Therapy* 2, 143–147.
MOORE, C. W. and CRUM, B. C. (1969) Weight reduction in a chronic schizophrenic by means of operant conditioning procedures: a case study, *Behav. Res. & Therapy* 7, 129–131.
STUART, R. B. (1967) Behavioral control of overeating, *Behav. Res. & Therapy* 5, 357–365.
STUNKARD, A. J. and McLAREN-HUME M. (1959) The results of treatment of obesity: A review of the literature and report of a series, *Arch. Internal Med.* 103, 79–85.
WOLPE, J. (1954) Reciprocal inhibition as the main basis of psychotherapeutic effects, *A.M.A. Arch. Neurol. & Psychiat.* 72, 205–226.

CHAPTER 25

Reinforcement and Weight Loss in Schizophrenics

BERNARD KLEIN[1]
Eastern State Hospital, Williamsburg, Va.

RICHARD L. STEELE
College of William and Mary.

WILLIAM E. SIMON
Southampton College

and

LOUIS H. PRIMAVERA
St. Francis College.

   Summary— Weight loss for 5 schizophrenics was effected during 90 days of a 180-day period in a token-economy paradigm using tokens as reinforcers for weight loss.

A recent development in the modification of socially unacceptable behavior involves use of secondary reinforcement to effect positive behavioral change. A number of studies have reported the elimination of undesirable behavior in chronic institutionalized patients by operant conditioning procedures, [2,3,4]. Atthowe and Krasner [1] provided positive reinforcement in the form of cardboard tokens for adaptive behavior by patients on a token-economy ward. The tokens could be exchanged for candy, drinks, clothing, leaves, and other social privileges. The method was successful in modifying behavior previously resistant to conventional psychotherapeutic techniques. Applying the same procedure, the present study explored the effects of secondary reinforcement on weight loss with 5 obese female schizophrenics from a functioning token-economy program at Eastern State Hospital. Cardboard tokens, redeemable for commodities at a location within the unit, were used as reinforcers. Ss were told that they would receive one token for each pound of weight lost each week and would have to pay E one token for each pound gained

Reprinted with permission from *Psychological Reports*, 1972, 30, 581–582.
[1] Reprints available from the first author at 3206 Clubhouse Road, Merrick, New York 11566.

during that period. They neither acquired nor lost tokens if their weight remained constant. Weights for all Ss were recorded every 7 days over 180 days.

The average weight loss was 10.8 lb. (SD = 6.5). Sandler's A-statistic, a derivation of Student's t for use with correlated samples (Runyon & Haber, 1967, pp. 171–172) showed a significant difference among Ss in total amount of weight lost over the 180 days (A = 0.272, df = 4, $p <$ .05). Figure 1 shows

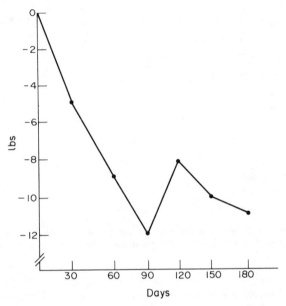

FIG. 1. Mean weight fluctuation over days for 5 schizophrenics.

that the greatest weight loss for the group occurred during the first 90 days. Thus, the token-economy paradigm, through use of secondary reinforcers, was effective in facilitating weight loss. Although 5 Ss are few, data are consistent with the literature, showing operant procedures to be effective in shaping desired patterns of behavior.

References

1.   ATTHOWE, J. M. & KRASNER, L. Preliminary report on the application of contingent reinforcement procedures (token economy) on a "chronic" psychiatric ward. *Journal of Abnormal and Social Psychology*, 1968, 73, 37–43.

2.   AYLLON, T. Intensive treatment of psychotic behavior by stimulus satiation and food reinforcement. *Behavior Research and Therapy*, 1963, 1, 53–61.

3.   KING, G. F., ARMITAGE, S. G., & TILTON, J. R. A therapeutic approach to schizophrenics of extreme pathology: an operant-interpersonal method. *Journal of Abnormal and Social Psychology*, 1960, 61, 273–286.

4.　MARTIN, P. L. & FARISH, D. L: Behavioral control of early morning rising of hospital wards for the mentally ill. *California Mental Health Research Digest*, 1967, 5, 109–110.

5.　RUNYON, R. P. & HABER, A. *Fundamentals of behavioral statistics*. New York: Addison-Wesley, 1967.

CHAPTER 26

Weight Reduction in a Chronic Schizophrenic by means of Operant Conditioning Procedures: a case study

C. H. MOORE and B. C. CRUM

School of Medicine, University of North Carolina, University of Georgia

Summary— Obesity and excessive eating are complex problems that traditional treatment procedures have been largely unsuccessful in alleviating, but recent behavior therapy studies suggest that the treatment of these problems by learning theory techniques has been moderately successful. Ferster, Nurnberger and Levitt (1963) reported on the possible application of operant conditioning principles to the modification of eating behavior and described a chaining procedure which was developed to inhibit eating while Stuart (1967) demonstrated that a graduated behavioral curriculum which governed the frequency, rate and amount of food ingested was successful in causing a weight loss. In addition, Ayllon (1963) has shown that a weight loss in the form of removing excess clothing is possible by having the S meet a decreasing weight criterion with access to food used as a reinforcing agent. The present paper is an extension of the latter study in that actual body weight rather than excessive clothing was the dependent variable and social reinforcement and approval were used as reinforcing agents contingent upon a daily demonstration of weight loss.

Case History

The S was a 24-year-old white female resident of a large mental institution who had been hospitalized for three years with a diagnosis of schizophrenic reaction, chronic undifferentiated type. The S mother was described as a dominating, complaining woman who had been a semi-invalid since the S was 12 yr old, while her father was described as a passive, submissive individual who, in addition to his work as a book-keeper, was responsible for running the house and preparing the meals. The S siblings were an older brother and a younger sister, both of whom were extremely successful in academic and social affairs. In contrast, the S was seen as a rather physically unattractive individual who had a long history of academic and social difficulties.

Her lack of achievements was continually compared with the successes of her brother and sister and because of her ineptness the S was continually castigated by her family. Her attempts to gain acceptance from her family through performing menial tasks typically ended in failure. The one area in which the S

Reprinted with permission from *Behaviour Research and Therapy*, 1969, 7, 129–131.

could gain acceptance was in eating, behavior desirable tó her family because it demonstrated to them that the S was well cared for. As a result of this, the S had a long history of excessive eating and had been overweight since the age of 15.

At the age of 19, the S married a man whom she had known for 4 weeks and during the first year of marriage became pregnant. At the same time her ability to function at home began to deteriorate. Her behavior became progressively bizarre, and she was hospitalized just prior to giving birth to a daughter. Immediately after the birth, the S began to consume more food and within the next year her weight increased to 168 lb, a level which was maintained for the next 1½ yr. During this time, she was on a low calorie diet under the care of a physician, but this was largely unsuccessful in controlling her weight problem.

At the time of the project, the S spent her day in varied activities which consisted of wandering aimlessly around the ward, sitting in a rocking chair and rocking vigorously for several hours, and laughing in a silly manner. Her affect was typically blunted and she rarely spoke spontaneously, never changed facial expression and would not respond to amusing or fear-provoking situations. In addition, at times she would become agitated, speak incoherently, seem to respond to voices, and develop ideas of being God and the Queen of England.

Procedure

From the history, it was inferred that rejection led to a lack of development of social skills in the S behavioral repertoire. This was associated with her becoming a rather compliant and passive person who had a great need for social approval and acceptance. From this analysis, it was concluded that social approval and acceptance perhaps could be used as reinforcing agents to help inhibit eating. Thus, the E began to see the S frequently and attention and verbal reinforcement were provided so that the E was discriminated by the S as a socially reinforcing agent.

The S ward chart was consulted and her periodic weight checks indicated that she maintained a weight of from 165–170 lb over a period of at least 1 year. As an additional check, the S was weighed at 3-day intervals for a period of 2 weeks by an attendant to establish a reliable base line. Once the base line weight had been ascertained, the S was seen and the following procedure was initiated: the S was escorted to the ward chart room where she was met by the E. The E then weighed the S and recorded the daily weight on a wall chart. If the S had lost weight from the previous day, the E immediately responded by reinforcement which consisted of indicating approval and acceptance for the weight loss. If there was no weight loss or weight increase, the E would simply shake his head in a negative fashion, record the weight, point out the difference to the S and ask her to return to her ward. The actual time spent with the S amounted to about 5 min per session. At the end of 2 weeks, the S began to report to the chart room on her own initiative, without encouragement from staff members.

This procedure continued for the next four and one-half months with weighing-sessions occurring every week day. Following the initial 5-month period, the S was weighed on an indeterminate but less frequent basis for a 1-month period with no significant increases or decreases in weight. The S was then returned to the usual ward weighing schedules without reinforcement.

Results

The day-to-day weight recordings were plotted and appear in Fig. 1. Analysis of these data indicates that a total weight loss during the entire period amounted to 35 lb with a mean daily weight loss over the period of 0.20 lb. During the eighth week, the reinforcement contingencies were discontinued and the S was allowed to visit home for 1 week. This period permitted the Es to observe the effects of discontinuing the ward reinforcement schedule since the subject was

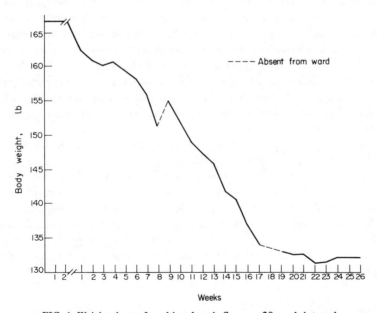

FIG. 1. Weight chart of a schizophrenic S over a 28-week interval.

placed in a different social environment. As seen in Fig. 1, there was a reversal effect in the 56-day trend of weight loss and the S demonstrated an approximate ½ lb per day weight increase for the seven-day period. Eight weeks later, the S was again removed from the ward environment for a period of 2 weeks. It should be noted that the reversal effect did not take place at this point and the S maintained her approximate current weight level throughout the visit. This was taken as an indication that the S had gained some measure of self-control and was no longer totally reliant on external reinforcement.

Discussion

The final goal of all learning theory approaches to weight reduction is the attainment of control on the part of the S so that his eating behavior can be self-monitored and ultimately self-controlled. Ferster, *et al.*, (1962) and Stuart (1967) suggested a wide variety of mechanisms which were designed to limit the range of external stimuli which control the eating response. These procedures were designed to make each response in the eating chain more discrete and consequently more amenable to control. In contrast, the present work used a rather global social reinforcement which was limited to the actual daily weight recording sessions. This procedure was established so that the S might learn the ultimate consequences of both over-and-appropriate eating and eventually gain control of her eating behavior through self-reinforcement. Support for the hypothesis that the S actually gained self-control is demonstrated in the seventeenth week on the weight chart when the S maintained the weight loss trend in the absence of reinforcement while she was unable to do so at the eighth week. Additional support is presented in the form of the overall weight loss and the maintenance of the loss over a 5-month unreinforced period. These findings become even more impressive when one remembers that the S had a severely debilitating behavioral disorder of long standing which predisposed her to poor self control.

Finally, previous review articles concerning obesity which utilized the more traditional diet control programs, programs involving medication, or a combination of these two, suggest that weight reduction is a difficult task and, furthermore, not usually considered permanent. Stunkard (1959) in a review article, suggested that the loss of more than 20 lb of body weight was very rare and the maintenance of such a weight loss had a very low success ratio. A comparison of Stunkard's findings with those of the present study suggests the operant conditioning procedure utilized here was at least as successful as, and possibly superior to, the existing programs for the control of obesity.

References

AYLLON, T. (1963) Intensive treatment of psychotic behavior by stimulus satiation and food reinforcement. *Behav. Res. & Therapy* 1, 53–61.

FERSTER, C. B., NURNBERGER, J. I. and LEVITT, E. E. (1962) The control of eating. *J. Mathetics* 1, 87–109.

STUART, R. B. (1967) Behavioral control overeating. *Behav. Res. & Therapy* 5, 357–365.

STUNKARD, A. J. (1959) Eating patterns and obesity. *Psychiat. Quart.* 33, 284–295.

CHAPTER 27

Behavioral Controls for Achieving Weight Loss in the Severely Retarded[1]

JOHN PAUL FOREYT and JIM T. PARKS

Florida State University

Summary— A weight loss program for several retarded adults based on behavioral controls consisted of: (1) a manual for parents of retardates, (2) colored tokens to represent food groups, (3) monetary payments for weight lost, and (4) daily weighings. Despite very limited intellectual capacities, subjects were able to develop new eating behaviors resulting in weight losses that were maintained at follow-up.

Ferster, Nurnberger and Levitt (1962), Stuart (1967, 1971), Stuart and Davis (1972), Harris (1969), Harris and Bruner (1971), Stunkard, Levine and Fox (1970), Penick *et al.* (1971), Stunkard (1972), Wollersheim (1970) and others have developed weight loss programs based on behavioral controls. Although these techniques are successful with many subjects, they require considerable re-education of eating habits and development of self-control behaviors, and have not been systematically applied to obese retarded subjects.

This report describes an adaptation of these behavioral techniques, especially Stuart and Davis (1972), for use with three severely retarded adults. The program was designed to help these obese subjects achieve an initial weight loss and to teach them new eating habits to maintain their losses.

Method

SUBJECTS

The subjects, three severely retarded women attending a daycare training facility for retardates, were identified as obese by an examining physician and were more than 10 per cent above their best weight as defined by the New Weight Standards for men and women (Metropolitan Life Insurance Company,

Reprinted with permission from *Journal of Behavior Therapy and Experimental Psychiatry*, 1975, 6, 27–29.

[1] Requests for reprints should be addressed to John Paul Foreyt, Baylor College of Medicine, Fondren and Brown Building #B 202, 6516 Bertner, Houston, Texas 77025.

November–December, 1959). Each subject agreed to participate in the program and permission was also obtained from the subjects' parents.

Subject 1, 36-yr-old, weighed 243 lb, and had an I.Q. of 26; subject 2 was 19, weighed 161, with an I.Q. of 35; subject 3 was 21, weighed 126, and had an I.Q. of 30.

APPARATUS

A manual by J.T.P. entitled "A guide for parents of an overweight son or daughter" was given to the parents of each subject. Subjects used colored tokens in a plastic box to account for all food eaten daily. A physician's balance beam scale was used to weigh subjects.

PROCEDURE

Baseline weights were taken for 13 weeks, subjects being weighed each morning at the Training Center and the weight posted on a large chart. No instruction in weight loss was given during this period, but the subjects were told that they would be helped to lose weight later.

The treatment program consisted of: (1) a weight loss manual for the parents, (2) colored tokens for the subjects to help make them aware of their daily food intake, (3) a payment of 50¢ per week for a weekly weight loss of at least 1 lb, and (4) daily weighings.

The parents met with the investigator and staff members from the center to discuss the program. The manual the parents received was written in simple, easy to understand language and included short chapters on the cause of weight changes, eating habits, importance of a balanced diet, how their daughters were to use the colored tokens, helpful hints about weight loss, sample low calorie recipes, etc. Its main purpose was to help the parents establish behavioral controls over eating in the home and understand a basic weight loss program. Each parent was contacted at least once a month and encouraged to telephone at any time help was needed.

The colored tokens in plastic boxes had a threefold purpose. First, they served as a means of communication between the center and the home about the amount and kinds of food eaten each day. Second, they served as a guide for a balanced diet and third, they eliminated the need for counting calories.

Servings in the various food groups (meats, vegetables, fruits, etc.) based on the food exchanges from Stuart and Davis (1972), were used rather than require subjects to count calories, a task far beyond the capacities of these women and some of their parents. The colored tokens represented the different food groups: red tokens for meats, green for cooked vegetables, yellow for breads, cereals, and some vegetables such as beans or potatoes, orange for fruits, white for milk or milk products, and brown for miscellaneous foods such as oils and sweets.

The plastic boxes had two compartments, in one of which the appropriate number of different colored tokens was placed in the morning, and moved to the other compartment as the various foods were eaten during the day. The tokens served as an estimate of what had already been eaten and the amount and types of food that could still be eaten that day. This communication was necessary since the subjects ate a snack and lunch at the center and the rest of their meals at home.

Each subject was also paid 50¢ per week during the 11-week treatment period for weekly weight losses of at least 1 lb.

Results

Average weight loss for subjects at the end of the 11 week treatment period was 8.5 lb with subject 1 losing 10 lb; subject 2, 11 lb; and subject 3, 4.5 lb.

Average weight loss for subjects at the end of the 29-week follow-up period was 15.2 lb, with subject 1 losing 21.5 lb; subject 2, 18.75 lb; and subject 3, 5.75 lb.

Figure 1 presents the weekly mean weight change in pounds for the three subjects during 13-week baseline, 11-week treatment, and 29-week follow-up.

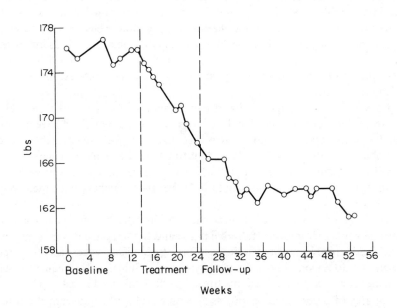

FIG. 1. Mean weight change in pounds per week for the three subjects during
13 week baseline, 11-week
treatment, and 29-week follow-up.

Discussion

All three subjects lost weight during the 11-week program, as expected. Each continued to lose during the 29-week follow-up period when they were no longer paid 50¢ per week for weight losses.

Observations by the investigator, the center's staff, and reports from parents suggested that each of the program's four components was important to the subjects, but the order of importance differed.

The manual was a useful means of giving the parents the information needed to implement the program and provided a reference source to help them as questions arose. It also lessened the need for lengthy meetings with the parents. The family of subject 2 particularly used the manual extensively and the whole family began changing their eating habits. Subject 2's mother and sister lost several pounds during this period. Subject 3's family also made considerable use of the manual.

The boxes of tokens were important and helpful to all subjects. They were carried to the center and home again each day and served as an easy way to communicate with the parents concerning the amount and types of foods which had been eaten at the center each day. The subjects seemed proud to carry their boxes with them.

The importance of the money varied according to the economic situation of the home, with those from poorer homes more concerned with money. The slower rate of weight loss during the follow-up period, when payments were no longer made, suggests that some kind of monetary reinforcer is useful at least initially when starting a weight loss program. Subject 1 maintained her rate of loss during follow-up, even though she showed the most interest in being paid during treatment.

Daily weighing appeared to be of equal importance to subjects since they all wanted to be weighed immediately after arrival at the center and have it posted on the chart. Staff attention and verbal praise for lost weight enhanced the desirability of the weighings. It is doubtful that the subjects understood the numerical amounts involved, but they knew that losing weight was an accomplishment to be proud of and would tell other staff members when their weight was down.

The relationship of the subjects with the investigator and their classroom instructor was very important. Verbal praise and encouragement were generously given and apparently were quite reinforcing. Subjects were eager to report weight loss to the one who had not weighed them. Subjects also frequently made statements such as "I didn't eat my bread" or "I didn't eat any cake today".

An area of particular concern was how much subjects could learn about food choices and to what extent they could become self-monitoring, since all were classified as functioning within the range of severe mental retardation. The subjects did not attain complete control of the mechanics of the program but did control some eating behaviors. They all gradually began voluntarily to refuse snacks of sweetrolls and doughnuts. During afternoon breaks, they bought only "diet colas" even though other drinks were available. They also quit buying candy and potato chips from the center's store.

In addition to applying their learning to their eating behavior, the subjects also learned to verbalize somewhat the requirements of weight loss. For example, when a new trainee said he wanted to lose weight, the instructor would ask subject 1 to tell him how to do it. Subject 1 answered, "Eat less. Can't have no cokes, no candy, no cake, no ice cream, no potato chips". When asked how to eat fried chicken, subject 1 said, "Take the skin off first".

During the follow-up period, subjects continued to carry the token boxes, weigh each morning, and eat together at the center. Parents reported that they were continuing to rely on the manual even though the investigator gradually withdrew from active participation in the program.

Although it is difficult to ascertain just how much the subjects have learned, observation of their changed eating habits at the center and reports from parents indicate that there has been some knowledge gained and some self-control instituted.

This adaptation of a program to gain behavioral control of obesity in retarded subjects by working with them and with those individuals who control portions of the subjects' lives appears to have a good chance of success. Further research is needed to identify the most effective components of a weight loss program for retardates.

References

FERSTER, C. B., NURNBERGER, J. I. and LEVITT, E. E. (1962) The control of eating. *J. Math.* **1**, 87–109.

HARRIS, M. B. (1969) Self directed program for weight control: a pilot study. *J. abnorm. Psychol.* **74**, 263–270.

HARRIS, M. B. and BRUNER, C. G. (1971) A comparison of a self-control and a contract procedure for weight control. *Behav. Res. & Therapy* **9**, 347–354.

Metropolitan Life Insurance Company (1959) New weight standards for men and women. *Stat. Bull.* **40**, 1–4.

PENICK, S. B., FILION, R., FOX, S. and STUNKARD, A. J. (1971) Behavior modification in the treatment of obesity. *Psychosom. Med.* **33**, 49–55.

STUART, R. B. (1967) Behavioral control of overeating. *Behav. Res. & Therapy* **5**, 357–365.

STUART, R. B. (1971) A three-dimensional program for the treatment of obesity. *Behav. Res. & Therapy* **9**, 177–186.

STUART, R. B. and DAVIS, B. (1972) *Slim Chance in a Fat World*, Research Press, Champaign, Illinois.

STUNKARD, A. J. (1972) New therapies for the eating disorders. *Archs gen. Psychiat.* **26**, 391–398.

STUNKARD, A. J., LEVINE, H. and FOX, S. (1970) The management of obesity: patient self-help and medical treatment. *Archs Int. Med.* **125**, 1067–1072.

WOLLERSHEIM, J. P. (1970) Effectiveness of group therapy based upon learning principles in the treatment of overweight women. *J. abnorm. Psychol.* **76**, 462–474.

CHAPTER 28

Social Reinforcement of Weight Reduction:
a case report on an obese retarded adolescent

RICHARD M. FOXX

Behavior Research Laboratory, Anna State Hospital, Illinois

Summary— Social reinforcement in the form of attention and praise by the experimenter was delivered to an obese, mildly retarded, adolescent female for weight loss per week at or below a specified level. Her initial weight was 239 pounds. Over a period of 42 weeks, of which the first 15 weeks involved reinforcement, the next 15 weeks an extinction period and the last 10 weeks the reinstatement of reinforcement, she lost 79 pounds. Weight loss per week was greatest during the two reinforcement phases; weight loss per week decreased below the baseline period during extinction. Rapid weight loss was attributed to social reinforcement delivered by the experimenter as other environmental aspects were unaltered during the experiment.

Successful treatment of obesity through behavior modification has fallen into several categories: self-control (Ferster, Nurnberger, & Levitt, 1962; Stuart, 1967; Harris, 1969); payment of tokens for weight loss coupled with a low calorie diet (Bernard, 1968); payment of tokens paired with social reinforcement for leaving portions of food at mealtimes (Schaeffer & Martin, 1969); social reinforcement for daily weight loss (Moore & Crum, 1969); removal from the dining room for chronic food stealing (Ayllon, 1963); aversive counter-conditioning with shock (Wolpe, 1958); symbolic aversive counter-conditioning with nausea (Cautela, 1966); and operant conditioning with shock (Meyer & Crisp, 1964). Many studies with more traditional treatments have reported little success: dietary instruction (Young *et al.*, 1955; Franklin & Rynearson, 1960); group discussion of physical and emotional factors (Harmon, Purkonen & Rasmussen, 1958); psychotherapy (Shipman & Plesset, 1963); appetite depressants and other drug therapy (Silverstone & Solomon, 1965).

Social reinforcement appears to be a most desirable form of treatment for obese mildly retarded individuals whose potential for developing self-controlling behaviors may require support from the environment. Social reinforcement does not require the strict programming contingencies of other forms of behavior modification and is easily dispensed by individuals in the patient's "natural" environment, provided they represent reinforcing situations to the obese person. Aversive conditioning as a treatment tactic may be limited, as the fear produced by aversive conditioning may extinguish should the behavior occur a sufficient

Reprinted with permission from *Mental Retardation*, 1972, **10**, 21–23.

number of times without a subsequent programmed aversive consequence; a situation which can occur once treatment is discontinued (Eysenck, 1960). This is especially true in cases of obesity because food is readily available, as are the stimuli which prime eating behaviors.

Social reinforcement has been used successfully in the treatment of anorexic and obese individuals. Bachrach, Erwin, and Mohr (1965) treated an anorexic female by programming all social interaction contingent upon eating behaviors, while Ayllon and Haughton (1962) treated an anorexic by withdrawing social interaction for food rejection. Social reinforcement was paired with the payment of tokens to overweight hospitalized chronic schizophrenics for leaving portions of a meal on the plate (Schaeffer & Martin, 1969). Moore and Crum (1969) relied exclusively on social reinforcement delivered by the experimenter for daily weight loss in treating an obese female schizophrenic, but did not systematically remove and reinstate social reinforcement so as to clearly identify its effect upon their subject's weight loss. The present research made social reinforcement contingent on a specified weekly minimum weight loss under conditions of both social reinforcement and extinction.

Method

SUBJECT

The subject was an institutionalized 14-year-old mildly retarded girl. Standing 5 feet 3 inches tall, she weighed 239 pounds, a combination making her physical appearance unattractive to others. She was institutionalized when she had become sullen, argumentative, fought with her siblings, and refused to help around the house. She had Jacksonian seizures and an "orthopedic disorder of her right lower extremity," a great bowing of her right leg resulting in a decidedly noticeable right-sided limp. An orthopedist had suggested corrective surgery provided that a sufficient amount of weight could be lost. The girl had been assigned to a token economy ward in which efforts were made to bring under control her behavior and weight problems. In 6 months of residency, her behavior problems had improved, but she had lost only 23 pounds despite having been placed on a diet and required to purchase low calorie food stuffs from the hospital canteen. Several factors appeared to be retarding weight loss: (1) She had frequently earned (in exchange for tokens) trips home and off hospital grounds where her eating was completely unchecked resulting in weight gains of several pounds. (2) She was working (as part of her ward behavioral program) at the sheltered workshop and would frequently stop at the canteen on her way back to steal or beg food. (3) She stole food on the ward whenever possible.

PROCEDURE

The tactic selected was to try and control excessive eating by providing an effective reinforcer contingent upon losing weight. Confinement to the ward seemed impossible and inappropriate. In preparation for placement back in her home or in the community, it was important to expose her to environments outside the ward where she might acquire skills commensurate with successful community adjustment. Controlling her weight by confinement might effect weight loss but would not alter the external stimuli which set the occasion for overeating. Additionally, the girl expressed little desire to have corrective surgery to straighten her leg or to lose weight. Praise, the stressing of the therapeutic benefit of having her leg straightened, and a promise of new clothes, although commonly regarded as reinforcers, did not serve as such for her and had not been effective in promoting weight loss.

One element in her environment which seemed highly reinforcing was the attention paid her by the experimenter. Based upon this observation, the following procedure was instituted: the girl would receive attention from the experimenter provided she had lost weight during the previous week. Prior to beginning this program, she was taken to the hospital canteen on several occasions by the experimenter; a low calorie soft drink was purchased for her, and the two sat down and talked. After 10 minutes, she was accompanied back to the ward. This procedure approximated "magazine training" or reinforcer sampling (Ayllon & Azrin, 1968a; Ayllon & Azrin, 1968b).

The sampling procedure was successful inasmuch as the girl would frequently ask for additional canteen trips. These frequent requests suggested that the trips were reinforcing; therefore, a weekly trip to the canteen with the experimenter became contingent upon loss of at least 1½ pounds in the preceding week. The girl was informed of this contingency. The canteen trip was the afternoon following the weekly weighing of all ward residents. In addition to neutral conversation during the trip, the experimenter stressed the advantages of the girl's losing weight.

The experimental design was A B A with an extinction phase in which weight loss was ignored by the experimenter and canteen trips with him stopped, counter-balanced between two social reinforcement phases. All other conditions existing prior to the experiment were to remain in effect; i.e. her diet, opportunity to steal or beg food, a weekly trip by herself to the canteen to purchase a soft drink, and the girl's ward behavioral program.

Results

Table 1 presents the mean weight loss per week during her residency before the experiment, and during three experimental phases. Before the experiment, weight loss had been .9 pound per week; during social reinforcement weight loss accelerated to 2.9 (Phase A_1) and 2.8 (Phase A_2) pounds per week, while the

TABLE 1. Comparison of weight change during particular phases of treatment

Phase	Number of weeks	Beginning wt.	Ending wt.	Wt. change (lbs.)	X̄-Loss per wk. (lbs.)
Before experiment	25	264	239	−23	.9
Social reinforcement (A₁)	15	239	196	−43	2.9
Withdraw reinforcement (B)	15	196	188½	− 7½	.5
Social reinforcement (A₂)	10	188½	160	−28½	2.8

withdrawal of social reinforcement (Phase B) retarded weight loss to only .5 pound per week.

The girl's recorded weight at the beginning of the experiment was 239 pounds. In the 15 weeks of social reinforcement contingent upon weight loss (Phase A₁) her weight dropped to 196 pounds, a loss of 43 pounds. During Phase A there was an increase in weight of 1½ pounds following a home visit; however, this was the only instance of weight gain during either social reinforcement phase. In the 15 weeks of Phase B, canteen trips with the experimenter were stopped. During Phase B there was a net weight loss of 7.5 pounds. There were 4 weeks in Phase B in which weight gains over the previous week were recorded. The reinstatement of social reinforcement in Phase A₂ produced a weight loss of 28 pounds in 10 weeks

Discussion

In 42 weeks the girl lost 33% of her pre-experimental body weight. This compares favorably with the reported results of other investigators. Ayllon's (1963) subject lost 17% body weight in 14 months; Bernard (1968) reports a 407 pound female schizophrenic lost 22% of her initial body weight in 20 weeks; Moore and Crum's (1969) patient lost 22% initial body weight in 26 weeks.

Greatest weight losses were a consequence of contingent social reinforcement as illustrated by the girl's behavior throughout the experiment. During the social reinforcement phases she bragged to the other girls about her escort, asked many times during Phase B why she was no longer being accompanied to the canteen, and frequently searched for the experimenter as soon as weighings were over to tell him exactly how much weight she had lost. The mere passage of time was not responsible for the weight loss, since the girl's weight loss accelerated or remained relatively static depending upon whether or not social reinforcement by the experimenter was available. The general applicability of this search may depend upon the degree to which one individual is reinforcing for another and suggests that preferences indicated by a retarded resident for a particular member or members of a ward treatment staff may be a helpful cue when designing behavioral programs.

The orthopedic surgeon reports that surgery for this girl is now a possibility in the immediate future. There was no sudden increase in weight following completion of the experiment, the girl's weight continuing to drop to 155 pounds. Eating behavior has now come under the control of a wide variety of social reinforcers, since generous amounts of praise and attention from others (including a new boyfriend) allowed the experimenter to fade out as the controlling stimulus.

References

Ayllon, T. Intensive treatment of psychotic behavior in stimulus satiation and food reinforcement. *Behavior Research and Therapy*, 1963, **1**, 53—61.

Ayllon, T. & Haughton, E. Control of the behavior of schizophrenic patients by food. *Journal of the Experimental Analysis of Behavior*, 1962, **5**, 343—352.

Ayllon, T. & Azrin, N. H. Reinforcer sampling: A technique for increasing the behavior of mental patients. *Journal of Applied Behavior Analysis*, 1968a, **1**, 13—20.

Ayllon, T. & Azrin, N. H. *The token economy: A motivational system for therapy and rehabilitation.* New York: Appleton-Century-Crofts, 1968b.

Bachrach, A. J., Erwin, W. J. & Mohr, J. P. The control of eating behavior in an anorexic by operant conditioning techniques. In L. Ullmann and L. P. Krasner (Eds.), *Case studies in behavior modification*. New York: Holt, Rinehart and Winston, 1965.

Bernard, J. L. Rapid treatment of gross obesity by operant techniques, *Psychological Reports*, 1968, **23**, 663—666.

Cautela, J. R. Treatment of compulsive behavior by covert sensitization, *Psychological Record*, 1966, **16**, 33—41.

Eysenck, H. J. *Handbook of Abnormal Psychology*. New York: Basic Books, 1960.

Ferster, C. B., Nurnberger, J. I. & Levitt, E. E. The control of eating. *Journal of Mathetics*, 1962, **1**, 87—109.

Franklin, R. E. & Rynearson, E. H. An evaluation of the effectiveness of dietary instruction for the obese. *Staff Meetings of the Mayo Clinic*, 1960, **35**, 123—131.

Harmon, A. R., Purkonen, R. A. & Rasmussen, L. P. Obesity: A physical and emotional problem. *Nursing Outlook*, 1958, **6**, 452—456.

Harris, M. B. A self-directed program for weight control: A pilot study. *Journal of Abnormal Psychology*, 1969, **74**, 263—270.

Meyer, V. & Crisp, A. H. Aversion therapy in two cases of obesity. *Behaviour Research and Therapy*, 1964, **2**, 143—147.

Moore, C. H. & Crum, B. C. Weight reduction in a chronic schizophrenic by means of operant conditioning procedures: A case study. *Behaviour Research and Therapy*, 1969, **7**, 129—131.

Schaeffer, H. & Martin, P. L. *Behavior Therapy*. New York: McGraw-Hill, 1969.

Shipman, W. G. & Plesset, M. R. Anxiety and depression in obese dieters. *Archives of General Psychiatry*, 1963, **8**, 530—535.

Silverstone, J. T. & Solomon, T. The long-term management of obesity in general practice. *British Journal of Clinical Practice*, 1965, **19**, 395—398.

Stuart, R. B. Behavioral control of overeating. *Behaviour Research and Therapy*, 1967, **5**, 357—365.

Wolpe, J. *Psychotherapy by Reciprocal Inhibition*. Stanford: Stanford University Press, 1958.

Young, C. M., Moore, N. S., Berresford, K., Einset, B. McK. & Waldner, B. G. The problem of the obese patient. *Journal of the American Dietary Association*, 1955, **31**, 1111—1115.

CHAPTER 29

Weight Reduction through Successive Contracts

MICHAEL DINOFF, HENRY C. RICKARD, and JOHN COLWICK
University of Alabama

Summary— Through ongoing improvement of contractual agreements, a 30-pound weight loss was obtained with a bright, emotionally disturbed 10-year-old boy. Contracts, specifying goals and rewards, were rewritten after each loss of 10 pounds. The weight loss, accomplished over 7 weeks, suggests that the contracts were able to reverse his increasing obesity.

Factors related to obesity have been described by other investigators. [5,9,11,12] Recently, interest has shifted from description and explanation to the treatment of obesity through procedures based upon behavioral principles [4,8] The use of contracts, as a behavioral approach to the modification of unwanted responses, has been employed in the control of a wide variety of behaviors. [3,6,13] The following case study describes the successful application of behaviorial contracts in a weight reduction program [10] for an obese boy attending a therapeutic summer camp.

Subject

Tom was a 10-year, 4-month old white male, described by the referral source as an extremely bright but immature youngster who attempted to manipulate his parents through hypochrondriasis and whining behavior. He was 5ft 2in. in height and weighed 194 pounds. Large rolls of fat hung from his waist and neck, and though he was strong, he found it extremely difficult to keep up with his group in the many camp activities that demanded physical exertion. His gross obesity immediately was made a target for derision by some of his more aggressive cabin mates.

Observation of the youngster's manipulative behavior in the presence of his parents, and perusal of the available case history information, suggested a number of hypotheses concerning the etiology of his excessive eating behavior and concurrent weight gains. However, the decision to implement a program of weight loss was based primarily upon the assumption that weight reduction

Reprinted with permission from *American Journal of Orthopsychiatry*, 1972, **42**, 110–113.

would result in immediate and favorable environmental feedback (e.g. greater ease and participation in activities, more acceptance from the cabin group, and the opportunity for self reinforcement).

Contract Criteria

Dinoff[2] has indicated that behavorial contracts must meet several criteria in order to be successful:

1. The contract must actively involve both parties. A contract between an adult and a child, which specifies only what the child agrees to contribute, is no contract at all.
2. Behavorial contracts should be written, at least in the early stages of negotiation. When criteria are vague, unstated, or poorly attended to, there is a distinct risk that an inappropriate behavior might be reinforced.
3   The terms of the contract must be exactly specified and understood by the two participants. If either of the participants does not understand what is expected he cannot successfully complete the contract.
4. The contract must be perceived as fair and honorable to both parties. As a result of changing situations the contract needs to be re-assessed from time to time to make sure that the parties still believe it to be fair and that their goals are still mutually agreed upon.
5. The contract must be reasonable, i.e. it must be within the capabilities of both parties.

As Sulzer[13] has pointed out, in making a contract, it is extremely important first to determine what objectives or activities are meaningful enough to the individual to act as reinforcing events. It is also important that these events be re-evaluated or re-chosen by the patient as the treatment continues because of changes in what constitutes an effective reinforcer. [1]

Procedure

Weight reduction was approached by first introducing a written contractual agreement in which the subject and his counselor (who was also overweight) agreed to reduce their food intake to one normal serving per meal as opposed to the two or three servings that each normally ate at each meal. In return for this reduction in food intake it was contracted that the boy would be allowed to look through a one-way mirror in the research area (about which he was very curious) when he had reduced his weight by 10 pounds.

The subject's weight was checked each morning before breakfast in a serious manner. This weighing ritual served to reinforce the honoring of contracts, and served as well as a daily check on weight loss or gain. After about 1 week it became apparent that problems were arising concerning not only what constituted a normal serving, but also concerning the types of food eaten. It was observed, for example, that the boy would take larger servings of starchy foods, which he liked best, and pass over proteins and fresh fruits. However, he reduced his weight by 10 pounds and received permission to examine the equipment and look through the one-way mirror, as per the contract.

As a result of the problems encountered in this first contract, a new contract was constructed in which he was required to show his serving to one of the two camp directors at each meal. A director would approve or disapprove the serving, in terms of the conditions of the new contract, and in a matter-of-fact way. In addition to the type and size of servings, desserts were restricted to one of his choosing per week.

Additionally, one of the camp directors offered to allow the boy to operate a video-tape machine that was being used in experimental work at the camp, after he had reduced his weight by another 10 pounds. At the negotiation of this second contract a video-tape of the subject was made showing him in various poses. He was then allowed to see himself in a more life-like fashion than when simply posing before a mirror. This life-like confrontation seemed to surprise him and he exclaimed that he did not know he looked that fat.

Weight loss after negotiation of the second contract was steady until about the fifth week, when he began to hover around the weight of 178 pounds for several days. When this static phase appeared, it was observed that he began to take added pains to reduce his caloric intake. Several times he purposely denied himself meals and requested to remain in the cabin while the other campers were eating. To minimize the possibility of his being perceived as a special or privileged member of the cabin group, he was told that he did not have to eat the meal if he so chose, but that he must sit at the table with the group. Interpersonal interaction seemed to deteriorate somewhat during this static phase. After about 3 days he began again to lose weight at a steady rate, his temperament improved, and he began to exercise (on his own volition) to increase his weight loss.

After the subject had fulfilled the terms of the second weight reduction contract, a third contract was negotiated. For the third loss of 10 pounds he was to be allowed to operate the camp dictaphone. This contract was fulfilled on the last day of the 7-week camping session. Total weight loss at the termination of all contracts amounted to 30 pounds.

Tom was treated in a manner that allowed an immediate reinforcing event to follow each weight loss (the weighing-in sessions each morning) as well as a major reinforcing event that occurred after a ten-pound loss. The major reinforcing events were chosen by the subject when each contract was negotiated between himself and a camp director. The use of a separate contract for each 10-pound loss allowed an opportunity for the subject to make any revisions he felt fair or necessary as time progressed. He was free at all times to revise his contract and allow himself more food; however, he did not do so. Although he was somewhat unhappy at times during the diet weeks, he was never forced or verbally coerced into staying on his contracted diet. No attempt made to discover or point out any dynamic factors underlying the subject's obesity. His problem was attacked as a single maladaptive piece of behavior which could be approached by modifying the behavior itself. It is difficult to give full credit to the contracts for controlling this youngster's obesity, since he was in a total treatment program, but it is felt that these procedures need to be explored systematically in future research.

References

1.   CLEMENTS, C. AND McKEE, J. (1968). Programmed instruction for institutionalized offenders. *Psychol. Reports* 7, 957–964.
2.   DINOFF, M. (1966). Therapeutic contracts. Paper presented at Southeastern Psychological Association meeting, April 1966.
3.   DINOFF, M. AND RICKARD, H. (1969). Learning that privileges entail responsibilities. In *Behavorial Counseling: Cases and Techniques*, J. Krumboltz and C. Thoresen (Eds). Holt, Rinehart and Winston, New York.
4.   FERSTER, C., NURNBERGER, J. AND LEVITT, E. (1962). The control of eating. *J. Mathetics* 1, 87–109.
5.   HAMBURGER, W. 1951. Emotional aspects of obesity. *Med. Clinics of North America* 35, 483–499.
6.   KRUMBOLTZ, J. (1966). Behavioral goals for counseling. *J. Couns. Psychol.* 13, 153–159.
7.   MENNINGER, K. (1958). *Theory of Psychoanalytic Technique*. The Academy Library.
8.   MEYER, V. AND CRISP, A. (1964). Aversion therapy in two cases of obesity. *Behav. Res. Therapy* 2, 143–147.
9.   NICHOLSON, W. (1946). Emotional factors in obesity. *Amer. J. Med. Sci.* 2221 443–447.
10. RICKARD, H. AND DINOFF, M. (1971). Behavior modification in a therapeutic summer camp. In *Behavioral Intervention in Human Problems*, H. Rickard, (Ed.). Pergamon Press, New York.
11. SIMON, R. (1963). Obesity as a depressive equivalent, *JAMA* 3, 208–210.
12. STUNKARD, A. (1959). Eating patterns and obesity. *Psychiat. Quart.* 33, 284–295.
13. SULZER, E. (1962). Reinforcement and the therapeutic contract. *J. Couns. Psychol.* 9, 271–276.

CHAPTER 30

Behavior Modification of Overeating in a Psychiatric Population

MORTON G. HARMATZ and PAUL LAPUC

University of Massachusetts

Summary— The present study presents and evaluates a procedure for controlling overeating through reinforcement. Overweight psychiatric patients were placed on an 1800-calorie-a-day diet for regular meals but were not restricted in their use of the canteen or vending machines. Three groups were employed: (a) a behavior modification condition in which S lost money (the source of cigarettes, beverages, supplies, food, etc.) for failure to lose weight; (b) a group therapy condition in which S was under social pressure and social reinforcement for weight loss; and (c) a control group which was only on the diet. Weight loss was evaluated for 6 wk. of treatment and 4 follow-up nontreatment wk. The findings indicated that both behavior modification procedures and group therapy produced weight loss during the treatment phase. The behavior modification group, however, continued to lose weight during the follow-up period while the group therapy Ss regained the weight they had lost.

Overeating is a form of maladaptive behavior with serious medical and psychological consequences. It is also a problem with an extremely high incidence in the American culture. Despite these facts there have been few studies concerned with the control of overeating. Ferster, Nurnberger, and Levitt (1962) noted "that specific techniques for changing an individual's eating behavior are given little attention in published reports" [p. 87]. This may be due to the fact that the predominant views on the etiology of overeating are psychoanalytic, in which the overeating is only a symptom of a deeper disturbance (Bruch, 1961; Kaplan & Kaplan, 1957), and a complete restructuring of the personality is the recommended treatment (Blum, 1953).

A learning theory approach would focus on the overeating not as a symptom, but as a learned behavior controlled by its immediate consequences. In such a system overeating is an example of behavioral excess—a normal behavior with too high a frequency of occurrence. Viewed in this manner, overeating is similar to other examples of behavioral excess such as alcoholism, smoking, drug

Reprinted with permission from *Journal of Consulting and Clinical Psychology* 1968, *32*, 583–587.

[1] This study was supported in part by a Faculty Research Grant (FR-J21) from the Graduate School, University of Massachusetts. The authors are indebted to the staff of the Northampton Veterans Administration Hospital where the research was conducted, and especially to Saul Rotman, Chief of the Psychology Service.

addiction, fetishism, etc. The predominant behavior modification approach to the control of such behaviors has been aversive conditioning procedures, in which the stimuli for the pleasurable behavior are paired with noxious stimuli until they elicit avoidance behavior by themselves. Such a procedure has been attempted with overeating in which only two cases were treated, one without results and one with some control over weight (Meyer & Crisp, 1965). On theoretical grounds, however, this would appear to be an inappropriate treatment for overeating. In treating alcoholism or drug addiction, the goal is to extinguish the behavior entirely and aversive conditioning procedures would be appropriate to the complete suppression of the behavior. In dealing with the behavior of overeating, the goal is not to extinguish eating, but only the excessive aspects of the eating response. The only way this could successfully be accomplished is to train S to monitor and control his own eating behavior by making reinforcement contingent upon such control. The present study presents and evaluates a possible procedure for reinforcing S's self-controlling response.

Obese hospitalized psychiatric patients were used as the population for assessment of the procedure. There were two reasons for this choice: (a) Control over reinforcement events is more feasible in the hospital setting, and (b) the concern of the hospital dietetic service with the overeating and resulting obesity of a number of patients at the Veterans Administration Hospital.

The procedure employed was to completely control the patient's intake during mealtime while leaving the patient free to overeat at other times. Weight gain or loss over the period of a week was the behavior positively or negatively reinforced. The reinforcer was money, which is a potent reinforcer in the hospital since it is used to purchase most other reinforcers, for example, cigarettes, magazines, food, drinks, etc. It is, in fact, a generalized reinforcer for all pleasurable stimulation other than that supplied by the hospital. The conditioning involved the use of a shaping procedure where, if the patient did not lose weight since the last weigh-in he lost part of his weekly allotment. If he continued to not lose weight by the next week, he lost an additional amount from that week's allotment, and so on. In this way he was initially helped to lose by having less money to spend, but had to continue his weight loss when he was reinforced in order to continue to receive his full allotment of money. The patient had to control his own behavior between weigh-in periods.

Weight was obtained at the end of each of the 6 treatment weeks. However, of greater importance to the project was the assessment of the patient's ability to generalize his self-control beyond the treatment phase. For this reason the patients were weighed weekly for 4 weeks after the last week of treatment.

A type of behavioral control of overeating which has become popular, with some anecdotal evidence of success, is a group therapy type of situation, for example, the Weight Watchers Society. It would seem fruitful to compare the behavior modification approach to such a group treatment to evaluate relative efficiency of treatment methods and to provide a control for the attention and effect of talking with someone about the weight problem. A third group used for control purposes was a group of patients who were on the same diet as the other two groups but received no additional treatment.

It is hypothesized from work on other habit disturbances that the behavior modification procedure would be more effective in amount of weight lost and would show the greatest generalization of the nonovereating behavior during the follow-up phase. The group therapy group may show some initial weight loss but should be less effective than the behavior modification group. The diet-only group, it is predicted, will show no weight loss.

Method

SUBJECTS

Twenty-one male psychiatric patients, who were adjudged to be overweight by the Hospital Dietetic Service, constituted the S pool for this study. These men ranged in age from 29 to 48. All carried a diagnosis of Schizophrenic Reaction, Chronic Undifferentiated type. The length of hospitalization varied from 5 to 7 years. The level and type of medication that each received was relatively equal.

TREATMENT CONDITIONS

The Ss were randomly assigned to the three treatment groups: the diet-only group, the therapy group, and the behavior modification group.

The design provided that each S would participate in 6 weeks of treatment and a 4-week follow-up period. The therapist informed each individual that since he was overweight he was being placed on a treatment regimen designed to help him lose weight.

Each S in the study was given a $5.00 or $10.00 per week allowance money. This allotment, which was in cash, could be used for any purpose. Individuals in the diet-only group and group therapy group did not have their money allotments affected by their gaining weight or losing weight while the behavior modification group did.

DIET-ONLY CONDITION

The Ss in the diet-only condition were given reduced portion meals which limited their calorie intake to 1800 calories per day. In addition to the smaller mealtime portions, Ss were required to use salt and sugar substitutes. There was no supervision of these men other than at mealtimes. Therefore, it was possible that the men could purchase food between meals. The Ss were weighed once a week on a counterbalance scale. At the weigh-in, the therapist would note Ss weight in a neutral tone of voice, for example, "You weigh 200 pounds this week." The S was then free to go without further comment.

GROUP THERAPY CONDITION

These Ss were also put on an 1800-calorie-a-day diet in the same manner as described above. In addition, they were required to attend a group session which met once a week for an hour. The therapist suggested that talking about overeating and some of its underlying causes might be beneficial in helping the patient understand his problem and to do something about it. The general format of these sessions consisted of a weigh-in at the onset of the therapy hour. A wall chart depicting lost weight was maintained. If an S lost weight, the therapist made positive comments, for example, "Very good, you lost _____ pounds since last week." If S exhibited no improvement, the therapist was nonpunitive, supportive, and reaffirmed his belief that S could lose weight. Discussion of why and how some individuals lost weight and others gained was the general focal point of the meetings.

BEHAVIOR MODIFICATION CONDITION

This group was similarly placed on the 1800-calorie-per-day diet and were weighed weekly. In addition to the basic diet, they were subject to the following restriction. If they gained weight or stayed the same weight, they would forfeit some of their allotment money. Each S started out with the basic $5.00 allotment. His weight was recorded at the beginning of treatment. When he was weighed the next week and if he had not lost weight, he would forfeit $1.00 of his allotment. Thus instead of receiving $5.00, he would receive $4.00. For each successive week that he gained weight he would lose another dollar, so that 3 successive weeks of no weight loss would result in a $2.00 allotment.

If the patient were to gain weight 1 week and thus forfeit a dollar, putting him at the $4.00 level, he would have to lose enough weight to put him below his original weigh-in weight to receive his $5.00 allotment. Once below his initial weight, he was judged on a week-to-week basis. This allowed S to be reinforced immediately for weight loss even after a temporary loss in control. Weight loss carried no other reward than insuring the patient of his $5.00 allotment.

SEMANTIC DIFFERENTIAL

To assess any change in patient attitudes as a result of treatment, the patients were administered the semantic differential scale each week through treatment and rated the concepts *myself* and *the therapist*. Also, each week the therapist rated the concept, Mr. (*patient's name*). These concepts were rated on nine 7-point polar scales. These scales were: large-small, fair-unfair, active-passive, clean-dirty, strong-weak, slow-fast, light-heavy, and good-bad. These scales were chosen because of their high loading on one of the three semantic differential factors: activity, potency, or evaluative, and their negligible loading on the other two factors (Osgood, Suci, & Tannenbaum, 1957).

Results

The average weight for each group prior to treatment was: diet-only, 195.8 lbs.; group therapy, 196.3 lbs.; and behavior modification, 195.1 lbs. There were no differences between these groups.

The dependent measure consisted of weekly percentages based on the weeks of experimental interest and the initial base-line week prior to treatment. The base-line week was taken to be 100% and improvement consisted of any percentage less than 100%.

Figure 1 presents the weekly percentages of weight for each of the treatment groups. The first 6 weeks are treatment weeks, while the last 4 weeks constitute the follow-up period.

The most direct way to examine these data is to evaluate the groups at the end of treatment. An analysis of variance was performed on the data for Week 6

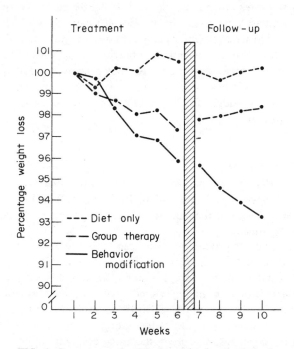

FIG. 1. Percentage of original weight for the behavior modification group, group therapy group, and the control group for each week of the 6-week treatment and 4-week follow-up periods.

(last week of treatment). This analysis showed a main effect for treatment $(F = 3.65, df = 2/18, p < .05)$. A Duncan's multiple-range test indicated that both the group therapy and behavior modification groups were significantly below the diet-only group $(p < .05$ and $p < .01$, respectively), but were not significantly different from one another.

The analysis of the data after the follow-up period similarly showed a significant treatment effect $(F = 7.3, df = 2/18, p < .01)$. The multiple-range test demonstrated that the behavior modification group was significantly different from both the group therapy and diet-only group $(p < .01)$. Of major importance was the fact that the group therapy condition did not differ from the diet-only condition at the end of the follow-up period. As Fig. 1 demonstrates, Ss in group therapy regained weight they had previously lost and were approaching their original weight levels.

A repeated measurements analysis of variance was performed on the weekly treatment percentages for the 10 weeks of the experiment. A significant main effect for treatment $(p < .05)$ indicated that the behavior modification group was significantly different from both the diet-only and group therapy groups. The significant Treatment X Weeks interaction $(p < .001)$ resulted from the divergence of the three groups (see Fig. 1). Initially the group therapy condition exhibited the greatest weight loss. In the second treatment week all but two of these patients had lost weight, and by the third week all but one had lost weight. This is in contrast to the behavior modification group where four Ss gained weight in the second week; this dropped to three persons by Week 3; and one by Week 4. Figure 1 also indicates the trend for the group therapy Ss, who initially matched the behavior modification Ss in weight loss, to gain back the lost weight during the follow-up period.

SEMANTIC DIFFERENTIAL

Analyses of variance were performed for each of the three factors for each of the concepts, "myself" and "the therapist," which S had rated, and the therapist's rating of each of the patients. These ratings were made each week for the 6 weeks of treatment.

None of the analyses produced a significant effect with the exception of S's rating of the therapist's potency. A significant Treatment X weeks interaction $(p < .001)$ indicated that the behavior modification and group therapy groups differed in their ratings of therapist's potency. The group therapy Ss, after showing an initially high potency level for the therapist, had a negative slope for the 6 weeks. The behavior modification group, on the other hand, after an initially negative slope, rose sharply in the rating of therapist potency in Week 4 and stayed at a high level until the end of the treatment phase. It is interesting to note that Week 4 in Figure 1 is the first point which clearly shows the behavior modification group exceeding the group therapy group in weight loss.

Discussion

The results support the hypothesized superiority of the behavior modification procedure over the control procedures in producing and maintaining weight loss. The behavior modification group showed a consistent weight loss for each week of measurement. At the end of treatment this group was significantly lower in weight than the diet-only control and, at the end of the follow-up period, was significantly below both the diet-only and the group therapy condition. The continuation of weight loss after the treatment phase of the experiment supports the conclusion of greater generalization by the behavior modification procedures.

The Ss in the behavior modification condition appear to have gained control of the overeating response. It would appear that reinforcing the end product of an extended behavioral sequence (controlling eating behavior for a week) can be effective in modifying behavior. It should be kept in mind that money is a very potent reinforcer in this situation. The S had to maintain his new behavior through self-reinforcement—in a sense he had to learn and maintain "self-control" procedures. The result was the striking generalization of the non-overeating behavior during the 4 weeks of follow-up. A study is planned which seeks to examine the self-control procedure actually employed by different Ss.

One of the most intriguing findings of this study relates to the results from the group therapy condition. This treatment was as effective in producing weight loss as behavior modification procedures until the first week of the no-treatment follow-up period, where they demonstrated a positive trend back to the original weight levels. The positive effects of group therapy during the treatment phase is supported by the notion that dieting is aided by group therapy participation. However, the results from the follow-up phase of the experiment support anecdotal accounts that when the group contact is no longer available, the person returns to former modes of responding and gains back the lost weight.

The question arises as to why group therapy does not generalize once the group stops meeting. From interviews with the Ss, the view emerged that Ss in the group therapy condition were embarrassed to come to meetings and not exhibit any weight loss when the others had lost weight. The weight-losing behaviors thus appear to be maintained by the verbal behavior of the other group members both at the meeting and perhaps between meetings. The control is thus entirely externally based and once removed, the former modes of behavior return. The result is the lack of generalization during the follow-up phase.

Dramatic weight loss was neither a goal nor a result of this study. The behavior manipulation group averaged about 180 pounds at the end of the 10 weeks from a base level of 195 pounds, an average loss of 15 pounds per S. As was demonstrated in Fig. 1, this was a relatively steady weight loss averaging approximately 1.5 pounds per week decrease. Since drug doses were not reduced

K

nor physical exercise increased, the loss occurred in spite of the adverse effects of these ongoing conditions. The manipulation of these two variables should easily increase the weight loss without further reduction of calorie intake.

The semantic differential did not show major differences in the patient's attitudes toward themselves. The behavior modification group did, however, dramatically raise the rating of the therapist's potency during the treatment phase while the group therapy Ss lowered these ratings. It is possible that the fact that they were losing weight indicated to the behavior modification Ss that the therapist was knowledgeable and helping them lose weight. Conversely, they may have felt the controlling aspects of the situation and were rating the potency scales in a negative sense.

References

BLUM, G. S. *Psychoanalytic theories of personality.* New York: McGraw-Hill, 1953.

BRUCH, H. Transformation of oral impulses in eating disorders: A conceptual approach. *Psychiatric Quarterly*, 1961, 35, 458–481.

FERSTER, C. H., NURNBERGER, J. I., & LEVITT, E. E. The control of eating. *Journal of Mathetics*, 1962, 1, 87–109.

KAPLAN, H. I., & KAPLAN, H. S. The psychosomatic concept of obesity. *Journal of Nervous and Mental Disease*, 1957, 125 181–201.

MEYER, V., & CRISP, A. H. Aversion therapy in two cases of obesity. *Behavior Research and Therapy*, 1964, 2, 71–82.

OSGOOD, C. E., SUCI, G. J., & TANNENBAUM, P. H. *The measurement of meaning.* Urbana: University of Illinois Press, 1957.

CHAPTER 31

The Behavior-therapeutic use of Contingency Contracting to Control an Adult Behavior Problem: weight control[1]

RONALD A. MANN

The University of California at Los Angeles

Summary— Items considered valuable by the subject and originally his property were surrendered to the researcher and incorporated into a contractual system of prearranged contingencies. Each subject signed a legal contract that prescribed the manner in which he could earn back or permanently lose his valuables. Specifically, a portion of each subject's valuables were returned to him contingent upon both specified weight losses and losing weight at an agreed-upon rate. Furthermore, each subject permanently lost a portion of his valuables contingent upon both specified weight gains and losing weight at a rate below the agreed-upon rate. Single-subject reversal designs were employed to determine the effectiveness of the treatment contingencies. This study demonstrated that items considered valuable by the subject and originally his property, could be used successfully to modify the subject's weight when these items were used procedurally both as reinforcing and as punishing consequences. In addition, a systematic analysis of the contingencies indicated that punishing or aversive consequences presumably were a necessary component of the treatment procedure.

Comparatively few therapeutic techniques displaying generality in natural settings have been developed to deal with the behavior problems of normal non-institutionalized adults. Two major reasons for this are suggested. First, it is difficult for a therapist to discover and/or gain systematic control over relevant consequences of an adult's behavior in its natural settings. Second, even if a therapist did have such control, it would still be difficult to maintain reliable measurement of the behavior. Without reliable measurement, it would be

Reprinted with permission from the *Journal of Applied Behavior Analysis*, 1972, 5, 99–109.

[1] This investigation was partially supported by PHS Training Grant 00183 from the National Institute of Child Health and Human Development to the Kansas Center for Research in Mental Retardation and Human Development. This study is based upon a dissertation submitted to the Department of Human Development, University of Kansas, in partial fulfillment of the requirements for the degree of Doctor of Philosophy. The author expresses deep appreciation and indebtedness to Dr. Donald M. Baer for his encouraging support, insightful advice, and helpful suggestions. Special thanks to Drs. L. Keith Miller and James A. Sherman for their critical evaluations and suggestions in preparing the manuscript. Reprints may be obtained from the author, Department of Psychology, University of California, Los Angeles, California 90024.

difficult to deliver relevant consequences at appropriate times. Similarly, it would be difficult to assess any changes that might occur in the behavior. Thus, an applied demonstration of a therapeutic change in behavior could be made, but with difficulty.

A recently discussed procedure that may have potential as a technique to remediate adult behavior problems in their natural settings is that of contingency contracting (Homme, 1966; Homme, Csanyi, Gonzales, and Rechs, 1969; Tharp and Wetzel, 1969; Michael, 1970). Its applications as a therapeutic technique, however, have been suggested mainly for use in school settings with children (Homme et al., 1969; Cantrell, Cantrell, Huddleston, and Woolridge, 1969) and in home settings to remediate the behavior problems of pre-delinquent adolescents (Tharp and Wetzel, 1969; Stuart, 1970).

The term "contingency contracting", as it has most commonly been used has meant an explicit statement of contingencies (i.e., a rule), usually agreed upon by two or more people. In other words, it has been a specification of a number of behaviors whose occurrence would produce specified consequences, presumably to be delivered by parents or teachers. It has been amply demonstrated that contingencies can, in fact, change behavior. Nevertheless, little evidence has been gathered to support the notion that the use of contingency contracts will facilitate the remediation of child or adult behavior problems.

The present study attempted to develop a therapeutic technique that would effectively remediate the behavior problems of normal non-institutionalized adults. The basic technique used was that of contingency contracting. The contingency contract used in this study was similar to others that have been discussed, in that it too was an explicit statement of contingencies. However, this contract incorporated a number of additional techniques that were considered necessary to accomplish effectively an applied behaviour analysis, and which were relevant to the problems both of gaining systematic control of effective consequences and of maintaining reliable measurement.

In brief, this study attempted to test the applicability of contingency contracting with adult subjects, and to assess the effects of various treatment contingencies on weight reduction. Weight was used as the dependent variable for two reasons: (1) It is a convenient and reliably measurable "behavior", and (2) weight control is a socially important behavior problem.

Method

SUBJECTS

Seven women and one man, 18 to 33 yr old, had responded to an advertisement for a "behavior therapy research program of weight reduction". Each subject was required to give to the researcher a signed physician's statement indicating that it would be medically safe for him or her to lose the specified weight agreed upon for this research over the agreed-upon time and at the agreed-upon rate. Furthermore, the physician's statement included an entry indicating whether the subject's physician had prescribed a diet for him. It was made clear to every subject, both verbally and as a written clause included in each contact, that any diet or foods that the subject selected or his physician prescribed would be ultimately the subject's responsibility. With one exception, only those individuals agreeing to lose 25 pounds or more and who had their physician's approval were accepted as subjects. (The one exception was a subject who agreed to lose 16 pounds.)

THE CONTINGENCY CONTRACT

The Contingency Contract was a legal document that incorporated as separate clauses all of the procedures in the weight control program. First, the contract required each subject to surrender a large number of items considered to be valuable to himself. These items were retained by the researcher (a similar technique has been discussed by Tighe and Elliott, 1968). Secondly, the contract prescribed the manner in which the subject could earn back or permanently lose his valuables (i.e., the statement of contingencies). Third, the contract required the subject to be weighed by the researcher at regular intervals. Fourth, the contract stipulated that the researcher, at his discretion, would change the procedures from baseline, to treatment, to reversal, and back to treatment conditions. Thus, the contingencies of the contract could be either continued or temporarily discontinued in order to assess experimentally the causal variables and the efficacy of the contract itself. The details of the experimental conditions were also specified in the contingency contract.

In brief, the contract was a guarantee to the subject that valuables supplied by him would be returned contingent upon meeting the specified requirements, or would be permanently lost if those requirements were not met. It was also a guarantee to the researcher that the subject would be available for measurements and the delivery of consequences at specified intervals.

All individuals interested in losing weight were shown a copy of a contingency contract and given a detailed prescription of the procedures to be used. The procedures were explicitly characterized as being extremely rigid and severe. The researcher then answered any questions raised by the prospective subjects. Each subject was encouraged to take as much time as he needed to consider whether he should sign the contract. When an individual decided to be a subject in the program, he was asked to nominate a number of objects he considered valuable to himself, either in the form of money and/or personal items (e.g. medals and trophies, clothes, jewelry, etc.). It was emphasized to all subjects that the items should be as valuable as possible. The contract was then tailored to each subject's personal specifications, with reference to intermediate and terminal requirements of the program: (1) the minimum number of pounds to be lost cumulatively by the end of each succeeding 2-week period (i.e. the minimum rate for losing weight), and (2) the terminal weight requirement. The number of valuables obtained from each subject to be used as consequences depended in part upon the amount of weight that the subject agreed to lose, and the minimum rate at which he agreed to lose it. Finally, the researcher, subject, and one witness signed two copies of the contract. The researcher and the subject retained one copy each.

Three sets of contingencies were specified in the contract: (1) Immediate Contingencies; (2) Two-week Contingencies; and (3) Terminal Contingencies.

The Immediate Contingencies were applied to each cumulative 2-pound gain or loss of weight that occurred during the treatment conditions. Any time the subject cumulatively lost two pounds with reference to the final weight measurement of baseline, he received one valuable from the researcher. Each additional two-pound weight loss below the previous weight loss was rewarded with one more valuable, and so on. On the other hand, each cumulative two-pound weight gain (above the subject's lowest recorded weight) was punished by the loss of one valuable. The weight of each subject was always recorded to the nearest half-pound.

The Two-week Contingencies required the subject to lose a minimum number of pounds by the end of each successive 2-week period during the treatment conditions. The 2-week periods and their associated minimum weight losses were calculated from the last baseline weight measurement and date. Every two weeks, if this requirement was met, the researcher delivered a bonus valuable. If this requirement was not met, the subject lost that valuable as a punishing consequence. The Immediate and the Two-week Contingencies were each a single valuable selected unsystematically by the researcher. Subjects never knew in advance which valuable would be used as a consequence.

The Terminal Contingency was a portion of the valuables (or money) delivered to the subject *only* if and when his terminal weight requirement was met. These particular valuables were itemized in the contract as specifically for this purpose, and consequently were never in jeopardy of being lost as penalties (i.e. for weight gains or for not meeting a Two-week Contingency) nor available to be regained before reaching terminal weight. In addition, the researcher agreed to deliver to the subject all of the other remaining valuables that had not been regained or lost as penalties, whenever the subject reached his terminal weight. However, if at any time the subject decided to terminate the program, then all remaining valuables in the possession of the researcher, including the Terminal Contingency, became the property of the researcher. Thus, the Terminal Contingency helped to ensure that the subject would remain in the program until his terminal weight requirement was met.[2] A clause in the

---

[2] Although the contingency contract did not specify the possibility, the researcher, in fact, would dissolve the contract with the mutual agreement of the subject for special circumstances, and return to the subject the remainder of his valuables.

contract stipulated that all items that became the property of the researcher would be disposed of in a manner not personally profitable or beneficial to the researcher. These items were subsequently donated to various charities.

It should be stressed that the terminal contingencies were always in effect during every phase of the program (i.e. during baseline, treatment, and reversal conditions). In other words, they were long-term consequences that presumably would operate against the usual outcome of a reversal.

MEASUREMENT AND RELIABILITY

The contract stipulated that the subject be weighed at a specific time and place every Monday, Wednesday, and Friday of each successive week until his terminal weight was reached. The subjects were weighed on the same medical-type scale throughout the experiment. Both the subject and the researcher independently recorded the subject's weight to the nearest half pound. However, the consequences were delivered in accordance with the researcher's weight determinations.

Reliability determinations were made on each of the days that the subject was weighed by subtracting the subject's notation of his own weight from the researcher's notation. The range of differences of weight occurring throughout the program was the measure of reliability.

The differences between the subject's and the researcher's weight determinations ranged from plus or minus half a pound. Both the subject and the researcher were in agreement on 95% of the weight determinations.

PROCEDURES

The procedures followed a single-subject reversal design (cf. Baer, Wolf, and Risley, 1968). The design included sequential baseline, treatment, reversal, and treatment conditions (i.e. an ABAB design).

During the baseline condition, the subject's weight was regularly measured; there were no scheduled consequences for weight, except the Terminal Contingency. Baseline data were recorded for approximately 2 to 5 weeks, depending upon the stability of the subject's weight. The criterion for stability was a 2-week period in which either a subject gained weight, remained stable, or lost no more than 1 pound per week. The final 2-week criterion period was considered baseline.[3] At a time unknown in advance to the subject, the researcher notified the subject that the treatment procedure was beginning. The weight of the subject and the date at the time of this notification were considered the final weight measurement and date of the baseline condition.

During the treatment condition, all three contingencies were in effect: The

---

[3] Use of the last 14 days of baseline gives each subject a uniform baseline to facilitate comparisons to other subjects. Fourteen days was the shortest baseline of any subject.

Immediate, Two-week and Terminal Contingencies. Both the Immediate and the Two-week Contingencies were calculated from the final weight measurement and the date of the baseline condition. The treatment condition was maintained at least for four weeks, and often longer, depending upon the stability of the subject's rate of losing weight. At a time unknown in advance to the subject, the researcher notified the subject that the reversal procedure was beginning and that until told otherwise, he could continue losing weight but he would neither receive back valuables for losing weight nor lose valuables for gaining. He was also told that whenever he reached terminal weight, the remaining valuables would be returned. The weight of the subject at the time of this notification was considered the final weight measurement of the treatment condition.

During the reversal condition, the subject continued to be weighed regularly, but there were no scheduled consequences, except the Terminal Contingency, regardless of whether the subject lost weight, gained weight, or remained stable. The reversal condition was maintained for approximately 2 to 4 weeks. At a time unknown in advance to the subject, the researcher notified the subject that the second treatment procedure was beginning. The weight of the subject and the date at the time of this notification were considered the final weight measurement and date of the reversal condition.

The second and first treatment procedures were identical. During the second treatment condition, however, both the Immediate and the Two-week Contingencies were calculated from the final weight measurement and date of the reversal condition.

In summary, items considered valuable by the subject and originally his property were surrendered to the researcher and incorporated into a contractual system of prearranged contingencies. The contract prescribed the manner in which the subject could earn back or permanently lose these items. This complex of contingencies, presumably both of reinforcing and of punishing consequences, was in effect during the treatment conditions. Experiment I assessed the effects of the whole complex of treatment contingencies on weight reduction.

Results and Discussion

EXPERIMENT I

Six of the eight subjects who were in the weight-reduction program participated in Experiment I. The data of one of these subjects have been selected to exemplify the procedures and are presented in Fig. 1a and 1b. In these figures, each open circle (connected by the thin solid line) represents a two-week minimum weight loss requirement. Each of the solid dots (connected by the thick solid line) represents the subject's weight on each of the days that he was measured. Each triangle indicates the point at which the subject was penalized by a loss of valuables, either for gaining weight, or for not meeting a 2-week minimum weight loss requirement. Only the data of the first four conditions (i.e. baseline, treatment, reversal, and treatment) are considered as Experiment I (Fig. 1a). A subsequent experimental manipulation was made with this subject (Fig. 1b) and those data were considered as part of Experiment II. This is discussed later. As the data of Fig. 1a indicate, this subject gained weight (slightly) during baseline, lost weight during treatment conditions, and gained weight during reversal.

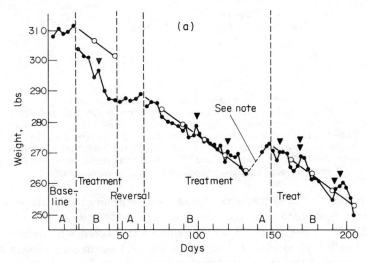

FIG. 1a. A record of the weight of Subject 1 during all conditions. The first four conditions (i.e., Baseline, Treatment, Reversal, and Treatment) were considered as Experiment I. During the Baseline and Reversal conditions, the subject's weight was regularly measured; there were no scheduled consequences. During both Treatment conditions the contingencies of the contract, presumably both of reinforcing and of punishing consequences, were in effect. Each open circle (connected by the thin solid line) represents a 2-week minimum weight loss requirement. Each of the solid dots (connected by the thick solid lines) represents the subject's weight on each of the days that he was measured. Each triangle indicates the point at which the subject was penalized by a loss of valuables, either for gaining weight or for not meeting a 2-week minimum weight loss requirement. Experiment II begins with the third Treatment condition (continued in Fig. 1b). *Note:* the subject was ordered by his physician to consume at least 2500 calories per day for 10 days, in preparation for medical tests.

Although the data of this subject were selected as the most orderly to exemplify the procedures, it was representative to the extent that the data of the other subjects, similarly, suggested that the researcher's control of the treatment contingencies were responsible for all losses in weight. That is, most of the subjects gained weight or remained stable during baseline, lost weight during treatment conditions, and gained weight or remained stable during reversal.

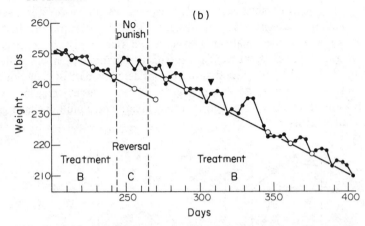

FIG. 1b. A record of the weight of subject 1 (continued from Fig. 1a). The last three conditions (i.e. Treatment, No Punishment Reversal, and Treatment) were considered as Experiment II. The Treatment conditions of Experiment II were procedurally identical to those of Experiment I. The No Punishment Reversal condition was identical to the Treatment conditions with the following exception: the punishing consequences were removed; only the reinforcing consequences continued to remain in effect.

A comparison of each subject's rate of losing or gaining weight during each of the first four conditions (i.e. baseline, treatment, reversal, and treatment conditions) is presented in Table 1. These data were calculated for each specified condition (except baseline) by subtracting the final weight measurement of the preceding condition from the final weight measurement of the specified condition. The difference was then divided by the number of weeks that the specified condition was in effect. The baseline data were calculated by subtracting the first weight measurement from the final weight measurement of baseline. This difference was then divided by the two weeks considered as baseline. These calculations yielded an average estimate of the number of pounds lost or gained per week by each subject during each of the four conditions. Only the data from baseline and the first treatment condition are presented for Subjects 5 and 6. Subjects 5 and 6 each initially lost approximately 20 pounds during treatment. However, a continuation of scheduled consequences seemed to have no effect on decreasing their weight further. Therefore, both of these subjects were terminated from the program, by mutual agreement.

In all cases except one, the subjects either gained weight or remained stable during the baseline condition. The exception, Subject 3, lost weight during baseline. All of the subjects gained weight during the reversal condition and lost weight during the treatment conditions. Subject 3 lost weight at a greater rate during each of the treatment conditions than during the baseline condition.

A summary assessment of the functions of each of the first four conditions of the program are presented in Fig. 2. These data represent the mean weight

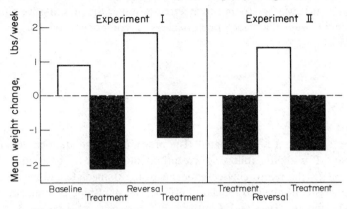

FIG. 2. Summary assessment of the functions of each condition of Experiment I and Experiment II for all subjects. These data represent the mean weight change in pounds per week gained (+) or lost (−) by all subjects during each of the conditions. They were calculated by taking the means of the average number of pounds lost or gained per week by each subject during each of the conditions of Experiments I and II.

change in pounds per week that were gained or lost during each of the four conditions. They were calculated by averaging the rates of each subject as listed in Table 1. The baseline and first treatment condition data of Subjects 7 and 8 (Experiment II subjects) were included in these calculations because the baseline and first treatment condition procedures of these subjects were identical to those of Experiment I subjects. The reversal and second treatment condition data of Subjects 7 and 8 were not included, because the reversal condition of Experiment II differed from that of Experiment I. As Fig. 2 shows graphically, the mean weight change during baseline and reversal conditions was +0.9 and +1.9 pounds per week, respectively. Figure 2 also shows the mean weight change during the two treatment conditions was −2.1 and −1.2 pounds per week, respectively.

In summary, Experiment I investigated the applicability of contingency contracting with adult subjects, and assessed experimentally the effects of a complex of contingencies on weight reduction. A single-subject reversal design was used. Almost all of the subjects gained weight or remained stable during the baseline condition, lost weight during treatment conditions, and gained weight or remained stable during the reversal condition. The results suggest that items considered valuable by the subject and originally his property, can be used successfully to modify the subject's weight when these items are surrendered to the researcher and incorporated into a contractual system of prearranged contingencies. Both intra- and inter-subject replications support the generality of these findings. However, Experiment I did not analyse whether the reinforcing consequences, the punishing consequences, or both, were necessary components of the treatment procedure.

Experiment II was an attempt to ascertain whether the presumptive punishing consequences were, in fact, functional as a component of the treatment procedure.

Method

EXPERIMENT II

Subjects 1, 7, and 8 participated. The procedures were identical to those of Experiment I, with the following exception: during the reversal condition of Experiment II, the reinforcing components of the Immediate and the Two-week Contingencies continued to remain in effect. The punishing components of the Immediate and the Two-week Contingencies, however, were removed. In other words, during the reversal condition of Experiment II, the researcher continued to deliver to the subject one valuable contingent upon each cumulative two-pound weight loss. However, if the subject gained weight, he did not lose any of his valuables as a punishing consequence. In addition, the subject continued to receive a bonus valuable contingent upon meeting each 2-week minimum weight loss requirement. Nevertheless, no valuables were lost by the subject if he did not meet this requirement. At a time unknown in advance to the subject, the researcher notified the subject that the second treatment procedure was beginning. The weight of the subject and the date at the time of this notification were considered the final weight measurement and date of the reversal condition. During the second treatment condition, both the Immediate and the Two-week Contingencies were calculated from the final weight measurement and date of the reversal condition.

It should be noted that Subject I was used in both Experiments I and II, and consequently was exposed to both types of reversals.

Results and Discussion

Only the treatment-reversal-treatment portions of the data were considered as Experiment II. The last reversal condition in which Subject I participated was procedurally identical to those of Subjects 7 and 8 (see Fig. 1a and 1b). Therefore, the last treatment-reversal-treatment condition data of this subject were similarly included in the analysis of this experiment.

During the first and second treatment conditions, all of the subjects lost weight with reference to the final weight measurement of the preceding conditions (i.e. baseline and reversal). During the reversal condition, all of the subjects gained weight with reference to the final weight measurement of the preceding condition.

A comparison of each subject's rate of losing or gaining weight during each of the three conditions (i.e. treatment, reversal, treatment) is presented in Table 1.

These data were calculated (in the same manner as for Experiment I) for each specified condition by subtracting the final weight measurement of the preceding condition from the final weight measurement of the specified condition. The difference was then divided by the number of weeks that the specified condition was in effect. These calculations yielded an average estimate of the number of pounds lost or gained per week by each subject during each of the three conditions. In all cases the subjects lost weight during both treatment conditions and gained weight during the reversal condition.

TABLE 1. The average number of pounds lost or gained per week by each subject during each condition of Experiment I (i.e. Baseline, Treatment, Reversal and Treatment) and Experiment II (i.e. Treatment, No Punishment Reversal, and Treatment). *Subjects 5 and 6 were terminated from the program before a Reversal and second Treatment condition.

Experimental condition	Experiment I							Experiment II			
	S–1	S–2	S–3	S–4	S–5	S–6	X̄	S–&	S–8	S–1	X̄
Baseline A	1.4	0.0	−1.0	0.0	1.0	3.2	0.9	1.5	1.2	–	–
Treatment B	−6.1	−1.7	−2.0	−1.6	−1.3	−1.1	−2.1	−1.5	−1.4	−2.2	−1.7
Reversal A-C	0.8	2.1	4.1	0.4	*	*	1.9	0.4	2.6	1.2	1.4
Treatment B	−2.6	−0.2	−0.5	−1.4	*	*	−1.2	−1.4	−1.5	−1.8	−1.6

A summary assessment of the functions of each condition are presented in Fig. 2. These data represent the mean weight change in pounds per week gained or lost during each of the three conditions. They were calculated (in the same manner as for Experiment I) by averaging the rates of each subject (i.e. Subjects 1, 7, and 8) as listed in Table 1. As Fig. 2 shows graphically, the mean weight change during the reversal condition was +1.4 pounds per week. The mean weight change during each treatment condition was −1.7 and −1.6 pounds per week, respectively. As can be seen in Fig. 2, the functions of the reversals in Experiment I and in Experiment II were almost identical.

In summary, Experiment II attempted to ascertain whether the permanent loss of a subject's valuables contingent upon either specified weight gains or losing weight at a rate lower than an agreed-upon rate, was a punishing or aversive consequence. Subjects 1, 7, and 8 lost weight during the two treatment conditions and gained weight during the reversal condition. When the presumably punishing consequences were removed from the procedure (i.e. during reversal), the subjects gained weight even though positive contingencies for losing weight remained in effect (Table 1). The data suggest that the permanent loss of the subject's valuables, when used as consequences are a necessary component of the treatment procedure.

General Discussion and Summary

The present research investigated the applicability of contingency contracting with adult subjects, and the effects of a complex of treatment contingencies on weight reduction.

The results suggest that properly designed contingency contracts may be an effective means to control some behavior problems of normal non-institutionalized adults. In this case, being overweight was treated as the behavior problem.

This study demonstrated that items considered valuable by the subject and originally his property, could be used successfully to modify the subject's weight when used as reinforcing and as punishing consequences. Furthermore, a systematic analysis of the contingencies indicated that punishing consequences were a necessary component of the treatment procedure for the three subjects of Experiment II.

The contingency contract used differed from those previously discussed by other investigators (Homme *et al.*, 1969; Cantrell *et al.*, 1969; Tharp and Wetzel, 1970). Those contracts were essentially an explicit statement of contingencies, usually agreed upon by two or more people. The contingency contract used in this study was also an explicit statement of contingencies, but it incorporated a number of additional features salient to its effectiveness.

First, the contract required each subject to surrender a large number of his valuables to the researcher. The subject then could earn back portions of those valuables contingent upon meeting the specified behavioral requirements (i.e. weight losses), or lose valuables if those requirements were not met.

Second, the subject signed the contract in front of witnesses, thus further legalizing the researcher's authority to control the delivery of those valuables as consequences. The researcher also signed the contract, thus obligating him to abide by the terms of the contract.

Third, the contract required the subject to be available for behavioral measurement and the delivery of consequences at specified intervals.

Fourth, the contract included a clause stipulating that the researcher could, at his discretion, experimentally manipulate the treatment variables. Thus, the contingencies of the contract could be continued or temporarily discontinued in order to assess experimentally the causal variables.

Last, the contract was designed as a "behavior trap". A behavior trap, as discussed by Baer and Wolf (1970, p. 321) and Baer, Rowbury, and Goetz (1971), is basically a situation in which, "only a relatively simple response is necessary to enter the trap, yet once entered, the trap cannot be resisted in creating general behavioral change".

In this study, the subject's surrendering of his valuables to the researcher and signing the contract can be conceptualized as the "relatively simple response" required of the subject to enter the behavior trap. Once these responses were made, the subject was in the program (i.e. in the behavior trap), and was required to lose weight steadily (at the agreed-upon rate) or be penalized by the permanent loss of portions of his valuables. Furthermore, the subject could terminate the program, before reaching his terminal weight, only if he forfeited all of his remaining valuables. Thus, the contingencies of this contract presumably acted as a behavior trap by facilitating the subject both to lose weight steadily and to remain in the program until his terminal weight was reached. Still, it should be emphasized that the behavior trap principle was functional only to the extent that the subject did, in fact, surrender items of value.

Although each subject verbally reported which items he considered valuable before surrendering them to the researcher, the definition of valuable in this procedure was still in terms of the effects those items had on the subject's weight. In other words, the items surrendered to the researcher by some of the subjects, could have been valuable (i.e. reinforcing) with respect to affecting some behaviors, but not necessarily as effective with respect to losing weight. This may account, in part, for the variability in the effectiveness of this procedure.

Variability in the effectiveness of this type of procedure may have other sources as well. For example, as a subject steadily loses weight, presumably because of dieting, the probability of consuming larger quantities of food may increase. This increase in probability can then compete with the aversive effects of losing valuables. This type of effect may be facilitated further because the reinforcing effects of eating are immediate while the aversive effects of losing valuables are minimized by the delay in time imposed by this type of procedure.

Before concluding, it should be pointed out that this procedure had some problems, especially as it related to weight control. Unsolicited anecdotal reports from some of the subjects indicated that they had used extreme measures at various times to lose weight rapidly and temporarily in order to avoid aversive consequences. These measures, reportedly, included taking laxatives, diuretics, and doing vigorous exercises just before being weighed. This problem may have occurred because the contract specified that the treatment contingencies be delivered contingent upon specified weight changes rather than the behaviors that can produce those changes. Weight, as a measure, is the result of various other behaviors. The contract neither specified, controlled, nor prescribed the manner in which the subject could arrive at changes in his weight. Therefore, any one of a number of behaviors could have resulted in a reduction of weight. These included appropriate dieting, an increase in exercise, or both, as well as extreme measures such as laxatives or diuretics which could avoid aversive consequences, at least on a temporary basis.

Consequently, contingency contracting and other techniques should be used with caution to the extent that these techniques place effective contingencies on the outcomes of various behaviors. It is difficult for a researcher or therapist to anticipate all of the behaviors that can produce a specified outcome or result. And some of the behaviors that can produce such an outcome may be socially undesirable or even dangerous in some cases.

In summary, properly designed contingency contracts may be an effective technique to facilitate remediation of some behavior problems of non-institutionalized adults. The probability of this is increased to the extent that such techniques can facilitate a therapist both in gaining systematic control of effective consequences and in maintaining reliable measurement of the behavior to be changed. The present study met these two criteria and thereby demonstrated the application of contingency contracting with adult subjects. The dependent variable of this study was both a convenient and reliably measureable "behavior". Other behavior problems do not lend themselves as readily to reliable measurement. Smoking, drinking, and stealing are examples of behaviors that are much more difficult to measure reliably. Nevertheless, as better methods of surveillance and monitoring of these types of behaviors develop, so may an increase in the use of contingency contracting with adult subjects.

References

Baer, D. M., Wolf, M. M., and Risley, T. R. Some current dimensions of applied behavior analysis. *Journal of Applied Behavior Analysis*, 1968, 1, 91-97.

Baer, D. M. and Wolf, M. M. The entry into natural communities of reinforcement. In R. Ulrich, T. Stachnick, and J. Mabry (Eds.), *Control of human behavior*. Glenview, Illinois: Scott, Foresman and Company, 1970, Pp. 319–324.

Baer, D. M., Rowbury, T., and Goetz, E. The pre-school as a behavioral trap: a proposal for research. In C. Lavatelli (Ed.), *The natural curriculum of the child*. Washington, D. C.: National Association for the Education of Young Children 1971.

Cantrell, R. P., Cantrell, M. L., Huddleston, C. M., and Woolridge, R. L. Contingency contracting with school problems. *Journal of Applied Behavior Analysis*, 1969, 2, 215–220.

Homme, L. Human motivation and the environment. In N. Haring and R. Whelan (Eds.), *The learning environment: relationship to behavior modification and implications for special education*. Lawrence: University of Kansas Press, 1966.

Homme, L., Csanyi, A. P., Gonzales, M. A., and Rechs, J. R. *How to use contingency contracting in the classroom*. U.S.A. Research Press, 1969.

Michael, Jack L. Principles of behavior usage. In R. Ulrich, T. Stachnik, and J. Mabry (Eds.), *Control of human behavior*. Glenview, Illinois: Scott, Foresman and Company, 1970. Pp. 28–35.

Stuart, R. B. *Behavioral contracting within the families of delinquents*. Paper delivered at the American Psychological Association Convention Miami Beach, 1970.

Tharp, R. G. and Wetzel, R. J. *Behavior modification in the natural environment*. New York: Academic Press, 1969.

Tighe, T. J. and Elliott, R. A technique for controlling behavior in natural life setting. *Journal of Applied Behavior Analysis*, 1968, 1, 263–266.

CHAPTER 32

Developing a Behavioral Program and Therapist Manual for the Treatment of Obesity[1]

D. BALFOUR JEFFREY,[2] EDWIN R. CHRISTENSEN,[3] and JAMES P. PAPPAS[3]
University of Utah

Obesity is a common clinical problem that psychodynamically oriented psychotherapy has been largely unsuccessful in treating, according to Stunkard and McLaren-Hume.[1] Recently there have been a number of studies suggesting that a variety of learning theory approaches have been successful in helping patients to obtain a reduction in weight. Stuart, using a three-dimensional model which included environmental manipulations, nutrition management, and energy expenditure, effected significant weight loss in women.[2] Mann has used a behavioral contract procedure for losing weight. In this technique, a patient signs a written contract whereby he agrees to deposit money or valuable objects with the therapist. He earns back part of the deposit each week if he loses weight, or loses part of the deposit each week if he does not lose weight.[3] Harris has developed self-control procedures for losing weight.[4] Wollersheim has used group therapy based upon learning theory principles in the treatment of overweight.[5]

The assumptions common to these studies are that: (a) most obesity occurs because of inappropriately learned eating and energy expenditure habits, (b) for these cases, the problem is basically a learning problem and not an inherent physical problem, and (c) the work of experimental learning psychology has direct implications for the development of a treatment program.

The purpose of this paper is to provide an overview of a behavioral program and a therapist manual that have been developed from a series of research projects conducted at the University of Utah Counseling Services over the last 3 years.[6]

Reprinted with permission with the *Journal of the American College Health Association*, 1973, 21, 455—459.

[1]Presented before the General Sessions as part of the Research Symposium, American College Health Association, Fiftieth Annual Meeting, Atlanta, Georgia, April 5, 1972.

[2]Counseling and Psychological Services, University of Utah. Reprints may be obtained from D. Balfour Jeffrey, Department of Psychology, University of Utah, Salt Lake City, Utah 84112.

[3]Counseling and Psychological Services, University of Utah.

Clinical and Research Projects

A pilot study with four patients was developed to test procedures hypothesized to be effective in a weight loss program.[7] The treatment involved a written contract (see Mann above), loss of deposited funds for failure to lose weight, graphing and keeping charts relative to weight loss, displaying reminder symbols (for example, a "piggy" key chain) during meals, some energy expenditure or exercise, and group support via verbal reinforcement. The pilot group (three males and one female) met for 22 weekly 45-minute sessions and for 10 weekly 5-minute sessions over a 6-month time span. During the baseline or pretreatment phase, the Maudsley Personality Inventory and a treatment questionnaire were administered to patients. This latter consisted of demographic data items (age, sex, occupation) and questions about a patient's commitment to, and belief about, amount of control or responsibility he perceived himself to have in losing weight. Patients responded to these on a continuum from 1 to 9.

All four patients stayed in treatment for the 6 months and had a mean weight loss of 27 pounds. Follow-up, 24 weeks later, indicated that two patients had maintained their weight loss, one had regained a portion of his weight loss, and one had returned to his original weight. The data also indicated that patients falling within one standard deviation of the norm group mean on the Maudsley Personality Inventory and those reporting a high commitment to change had a better weight loss and maintenance.

The next step was to conduct a research study using an experimental design which compared the relative efficacy of behavior therapy, "willpower" treatment, and no-treatment control procedures.[8] In this study, forty-three adult university students and staff were randomly assigned to these three categories. The behavioral treatment was similar to that described in the pilot study but with more emphasis on specific "shoulds" and "should nots" in terms of changing eating habits. The behavior therapy patients met twice a week for an 18-week period, once in a 45-minute group therapy session, and later in a second 5-minute session. The willpower patients were given the same instructions as the behavior therapy patients. However, instead of meeting regularly in a group they were told to apply self-control or willpower to their problem as this was "the most important aspect of losing weight." The therapist indicated he would check with them on their progress in a few months. The third group was a standard control group who were offered no treatment at that time, but were placed on a waiting list.

The results indicated that the behavior therapy group lost significantly ($p < .005$) more weight than the willpower and control groups. The mean losses were: behavior therapy, 16.39 pounds; willpower, 5.09 pounds and no treatment, 1.70 pounds. A 12-week follow-up on the behavior therapy group indicated that there was no significant weight gain from the end of treatment to follow-up. Because of practical and ethical considerations (for example, lack of willingness of the "willpower" groups to be weighed, and starting the waiting list control group with therapy) no follow-up data were available for the other groups.

Behavioral Program and Therapist Manual for the Treatment of Obesity

From these studies a behavioral program and therapist manual for the treatment of obesity have been developed. These procedures provide a program that can be implemented in a variety of settings, such as in health services, counseling centers and clinics.

The therapist manual is divided into six sections: intake, baseline, standardized treatment, individualized treatment, maintenance follow-up, and a special section on therapist behaviors.

INTAKE PHASE

The system used for intake of clients need not be altered from the normal system used in an agency. However, clinical and research experience with these types of patients suggested that it is profitable to be sensitive to some unique "cues" during this phase. These cues are: (1) patient characteristics which hinder weight reduction treatment such as fears in connection with becoming attractive to the opposite sex, or having a restricted diet because of stomach ulcers, (2) patient characteristics which aid in weight reduction treatment such as a genuine desire to be attractive to the opposite sex or the desire to lose weight in order to decrease the risk of heart failure, (3) past or present performance in other programs for weight reduction, (4) the length of time a patient has been overweight, (5) the patient's desired weight, and (6) the patient's commitment to losing weight.

BASELINE PHASE

In the first session an overview of the program is given. The patient is told that this program is designed to help him reduce to his weight goal and then maintain that weight by conditioning a change in his eating habits. This is done by his earning rewards of money or other items of value previously deposited with the therapist as he reaches weekly weight loss goals, attends therapy sessions, does the necessary tasks, such as cutting caloric intake, graphing daily weight, and attaining the final desired weight.

If the program is being conducted using a group format, attempts at building cohesion should be implemented by standard group procedures such as the group members dividing into pairs for a few minutes to learn about each other and subsequently introducing their partners to the group.

The patients and therapist should also establish meeting times so that there are two separate sessions each week, one 45-minute group discussion and reward session, and a second short "weigh-in" session of about 5 minutes.

Food Intake Monitoring Sheets (FIMS) are given each patient on which items and amounts eaten are recorded during the week. They also receive a daily weight graph to record their weight each day. At this time the contracts are not yet filled out, but patients are encouraged to think about weight goals. Instructions are given that they must obtain a physician's approval (certified on a prepared form) for participating in the program and his suggestion for a possible diet.

Each patient is then asked to bring either money or objects of value to him for deposit with the therapists to be used as rewards (reinforcers) as he loses weight.

At the second session, instructions are given about calculating average daily caloric intake for each of six eating time periods, representing the three meals and the times between meals, which are on the FIMS. Alterations to patterns of timing and amount of caloric intake can be suggested from the data on the FIMS. For example, obese individuals often eat very little in the morning, and then overeat in the evenings. Also, if more calories are used through increased physical activity there will be an additional weight loss.

In this session the patients are asked to make an overtly stated commitment to the group concerning their desire to lose weight.

During the baseline sessions enough learning should occur so that the following self-monitoring behaviors are conditioned: (1) the patient weighs himself daily, (2) he records his weight daily on a graph and, (3) he attends both weekly meetings regularly.

Because of this monitoring, patients often become so aware of how much they eat that they begin to lose weight. This should be verbally encouraged (reinforced) but monetary rewards or other formal devices are not appropriate until the next phase of the program begins.

STANDARDIZED TREATMENT PHASE

In the third weekly session physician approval forms are returned, final weight goals are set, patient weight loss contracts are signed, and deposits are collected. Often the tendency at this point is for the patient to set his goals too high. Some patients will try to establish their final weight goal at an unrealistic level, for example, the same weight they were when in high school. To avoid this, interim goals should be encouraged for any desired weight loss exceeding 20 pounds. After this goal has been reached, a new goal can be set. Experience has shown that setting goals that are too far away from the patient's pre-treatment weight can be discouraging, seem unattainable, and may result in early termination of treatment. At this time, rewards may or may not be established for the attainment of the final weight goal, depending on individual preferences.

Rewards are given or lost in each 45-minute weekly session in accordance with whether or not the patient has attained his weight loss goal for that week. It is important that these weekly goals encourage a gradual weight loss. Sudden losses are not usually accompanied by permanent changes in eating habits; thus, the loss is not maintained. A weekly loss of 1 or 2 pounds is usually appropriate. Obese individuals will lose more weight per week initially than those who are not so heavy.

During this phase the following week's goal should be clearly established and recorded on both the patient's and therapist's copies of the daily weight graph. Rewards or punishments for attaining the weight loss should be clearly stated and understood between both parties. Reminders of both the goal and rewards should be given at the short weigh-in session.

A suggested routine for the two separate weekly sessions is listed below:

45-MINUTE SESSION

(1) Weigh-in (in groups, or in private if desired).
(2) Therapist transcribes daily weights from patient's graph to his copy.
(3) Next week's goal is indicated on the graph.
(4) Appropriate verbal reinforcements are given in the group.
(5) Monetary or other reinforcements are given for attendance at both meetings during the week for weight loss.
(6) Progress and problems in lowering caloric intake and altering eating patterns are discussed.

As final goals come nearer to being reached, a gradual reduction of the number of group meetings and reinforcements becomes appropriate; this can be accomplished by changing this meeting to biweekly meetings until termination.

5-MINUTE WEIGH-IN

(1) Weigh-in (privately).
(2) Therapist transcribes weight from patient's graph to his copy.
(3) Therapist gives a reminder of next week's goal and how much weight has to be lost to make it by the next 45-minute session.
(4) Verbal reinforcements given, but no monetary rewards unless individually contracted.

As final goals come nearer to being reached a phone call and finally termination of these meetings becomes appropriate.

A "dropout" punishment should also be negotiated. The authors use a method whereby all money or objects deposited are lost if a patient drops out before attaining his goal without first having a private interview with the therapist.

Initially, neither patient nor therapist knows how much weekly reinforcement or loss of reinforcement in monetary terms will be enough to condition weight loss behavior. For students with small incomes, we have used amounts which varied between $2 and $8 per week earned back out of their deposits. For someone working full time larger amounts may be more appropriate; for some, earning back physical objects has more reinforcement value. The objects should be amenable to being earned back piecemeal. Such things as record collections, golf clubs, favorite books, or favorite items of clothing are examples of objects which may be deposited with the therapist. In addition to being used for weekly reinforcements these and other objects can also be used as reinforcements when the final weight goal is attained. Experience indicates that changes in the nature or amount of reinforcement become appropriate as individual preferences become obvious.

INDIVIDUALIZED TREATMENT PHASE

Assessment and a shift to more individualized treatment occurs as the therapist and patient observe and respond to the following:

(1)   Total weight loss since the beginning of the program.
(2)   The *weekly* weight loss as recorded on the therapist's *weekly* weight graph.
(3)   Attendance, daily graphing and the implementation of therapist's instructions for the changing of eating habits.
(4)   What is and is not reinforcing for the individual. (Careful observation, questioning, and responses to a form with choices of reinforcements are helpful in this assessment.)
(5)   The effect of timing and different amounts of reinforcement.

Experimentation, assessment and altering of various aspects of the program are expected to occur in order to facilitate weight loss. Increased or decreased weekly goals may be desirable, or alternative structuring of weekly goals may become appropriate. One alternative method is to negotiate the amount of weight to be lost for the following week at each 45-minute weekly session. This may be helpful if it is noticed that someone has lost weight in widely varying amounts because of intervening factors. For example, a woman may be able to lose more during some weeks and less during others because of water retention at certain times in her menstrual cycle.

With some individuals the use of materials, such as statements of consequences for losing or not losing weight are useful, for example, "I will be more attractive to the opposite sex if I lose weight" or "If I don't lose weight I will have heart failure". Also, "ugly" photographs of oneself or small toys (pigs) have been used as stimuli to remind clients of their commitments. Where, when, and how these objects will be displayed can be written into the patient–therapist weight loss contracts.

MAINTENANCE–FOLLOW-UP PHASE

This phase is perhaps the most important because it is here that the permanence of the changed eating behavior and the patient's control is tested. It is, therefore, important that follow-up maintenance sessions be conducted. The procedures used here are essentially extensions of the individualized treatment phase with a significantly reduced frequency of meetings. The monetary rewards are dropped unless requests are made for "booster" sessions and it seems that they are necessary. Usually resetting goals, recommitment and verbal reinforcement are all that are necessary. The spacing and timing of sessions during this phase are individually determined. Some individuals in groups desire to meet together; others do not. Some individuals may wish to meet less often than others. It is probably best to set dates and times when the sessions will be held before this phase is begun so that there is precommitment to meet after long lapses of time.

One way to set maintenance goals during this phase is to draw a horizontal line across the weight graphs at the point which the client desires to maintain and then base reinforcement on whether or not the weight is kept above or below this line. A patient's commitment should be obtained in the same manner for this phase as for the earlier phases.

THERAPIST BEHAVIORS

There are certain therapist behaviors that are essential to the treatment process:

The therapist should give verbal reinforcement which is viewed as positive. This need not always means direct approval or encouragement. He should be direct and candid in presenting what a client's performance has been, or is at present. Visual presentation of daily and weekly weight graphs with an accompanying discussion is a prime example of such behavior. Indicating successes or failures in performance, if well-timed and presented, is reinforcing in most cases.

Sensitivity to competing variables is important. Patients will sometimes receive reinforcement antithetical to weight loss from outside sources. These competing reinforcements can be more powerful than those the therapist might impose, for example, a boyfriend who says he likes "plump" girls, or eating to "feel good" when a person is lonesome.

Obviously the setting of goals is an important part of this program and the therapist is the negotiator in this process. It is helpful to allow renegotiations of goals. Often initial goals tend to be set too high, and there will be a need to make interim goals or to renegotiate the goals later.

To lose weight the patient needs certain basic information about dieting and high caloric foods. The therapist should serve as a resource for such information.

The therapist also needs to be constantly up to date with his graphs and other assessments of a patient's progress so that he can be sensitive to any changes in behavior or environment which might alter performance.

In summary, it is important for the environment to be such that patients can learn to control their weight and it is equally important that therapists behave in ways that create such an environment.

The research data indicate that a behavioral therapy approach, such as outlined here, offers the most promising approach so far in the treatment of obesity.[9] Therapies based on learning theory, however, are no panacea. Obesity is a complex problem about which much is unknown. Consequently, there is a continuing need for more research into understanding and treating obesity.

References

1. Stunkard, A. and McLaren-Hume, M. The results of treatment for obesity, *Arch. Intern. Med.* **103**, 79–85, 1959.
2. Stuart, R. B. A three dimensional program for the treatment of obesity. *Behav. Res. Ther.* **9**, 177–186, 1971.
3. Mann, R. A. The use of contingency contracting to control obesity in adult subjects. Paper presented at the Western Psychological Association, San Francisco, California, April, 1971.
4   Harris, M. B. Self-directed program for weight control—A pilot study. *J. Abnorm. Psychol.* **74**, 263–270, 1969; Bruner, C. G. A comparison of a self-control and a contract procedure for weight control. *Behav. Res. Ther.* **9**, 347-354, 1971.
5. Wollersheim, J. P. Effectiveness of group therapy based upon learning principles in the treatment of overweight women. *J. Abnorm. Psychol.* **76**, 462–474, 1970.
6. Further details of the research studies, an annotated bibliography on obesity, and a therapist manual with a behavioral contract and forms are available from D. Balfour Jeffrey, Department of Psychology, University of Utah, Salt Lake City, Utah 84112.
7. Jeffrey, D. B. Christensen, E. R. and Pappas J. P. A case study report of a behavior modification weight group: Treatment and follow-up. Paper presented at the meeting of the Rocky Mountain Psychological Association, Albuquerque, New Mexico, 1972.
8. Jeffrey, D. B. and Christensen, E. R. The relative efficacy of behavior therapy, willpower, and no treatment control procedures on the modification of obesity. In A. Stunkard (Chm.), *Behavior therapy approaches to the treatment of obesity: Recent trends and developments.* Symposium presented at the meeting of the Association for the Advancement of Behavior Therapy, New York, October, 1972.
9. Stuart, *op. cit*; Mann, *op. cit*; Harris, *op. cit*; Wollersheim, *op. cit*; Jeffrey, Christensen, Pappas, *op. cit*; *Ibid.*

PART VI

SELF-CONTROL TECHNIQUES

Introduction[1]

D. BALFOUR JEFFREY
Emory University

The growing interest in self-control[2] seems to be based on humanistic concerns, cultural beliefs, and a desire to improve the efficacy and efficiency of available treatment methods. Behavioral self-control approaches compliment humanistic concerns because they help the individual to master his environment and to change himself if he so desires. Researchers in behavioral self-control do not view the individual as a passive recipient of environmental forces. Instead, as Bandura (1969) suggests, the relationship between the individual and his environment is a continuous reciprocal influence process. This is another way of saying that people affect their environment and in turn are affected by it. This interdependence is continuous and needs to be taken into account in behavioral applications.

Culturally, self-control approaches are generally acceptable to the public because of Western society's strong belief in the individual plus the fact that they require the individual's active and voluntary participation in his own treatment. Researchers also believe that self control approaches enable the individual to maintain his behavioral changes in the absence of therapist influences better than other treatment approaches.

Finally, some researchers feel that self-control approaches are more efficient than other interventions since the individual conducts much of the treatment himself, thus saving the therapist time. The first two beliefs are attitudes about psychology and society that are difficult to fault or disprove. Only the last two assumptions about efficacy and efficiency are empirical; unfortunately, there is a paucity of data to support either of them at this time.

---

[1] This introduction was written especially for this book. Special thanks are extended to Roger C. Katz for his comments on an earlier draft.

[2] There is some confusion in the use of the terms self-control, self-regulation, self-management, and self-directed behavior. In this introduction, these terms are used synonymously to denote any response made by an individual to change or maintain his own behavior. For a detailed discussion of the definitions and techniques of self-control, see Goldiamond (1965), Goldfried and Merbaum (1973), Jeffrey (1974), and Thoresen and Mahoney (1974).

SELF-CONTROL TECHNIQUES

In order to examine self-control research, and in particular, research related to obesity management, it may be helpful to review various control techniques that are currently being used. First, there is a general class of self-managed antecedent stimulus control techniques — that is, techniques by which the individual learns to engage in specific behaviors that precede the target behavior. These consist of (a) self-monitoring of eating, physical activity, and body weight; (b) self-initiated goal-setting for eating, exercising, and weight loss; and (c) self-initiated environmental planning. The last involves having the individual rearrange environmental situations that lead to high food consumption or low energy expenditure. These techniques are often referred to as stimulus control techniques.

A second class of self-control techniques consists of self-initiated consequent control, or reinforcement control. These techniques include (a) self-reinforcement for food and exercise management; (b) self-punishment for the lack of weight management; and (c) self-initiated environmental reinforcement. The last involves having the individual prompt significant people in his environment to reinforce him for his weight-management efforts. With a definition, assumptions, and techniques of self-control in mind, let us review this section's studies on obesity management by behavioral self-control.

SELF-CONTROL STUDIES

The first three articles in this section are classics in the field (Ferster, Nurnberger, and Levitt, 1962; Stuart, 1967; Stuart, 1971). The Ferster, Nurnberger, and Levitt (1962) article is the first study in which a model of self-control of overeating is presented. Perhaps the most important contribution of this conceptual paper is its emphasis on stimulus control. The authors recommend a detailed analysis of antecedent discriminative stimuli for eating after which these stimuli are rearranged to lessen the temptation to eat. In light of Schachter's (1971) research that obese people are more responsive to external environmental stimuli than normal-weight people, this early work on stimulus control has great importance. Ferster *et al.* also discuss shaping and maintaining self-control responses. They write, "Self-control is a very complex repertoire of performance which cannot be developed all at once" and suggest that self-control must be developed in slow steps over long periods of time. These early observations are very astute in light of recent studies (Hall *et al.*, 1974) that suggest short-term training periods in self-control may not be sufficient for establishing and maintaining self-control behavior related to obesity. Ferster *et al.* also recommend that weight reduction proceed slowly to allow for proper development of self-control responses. This gradual approach to weight reduction is also recommended by Stuart (1967). However, it should be noted that Ferster *et al.*'s recommendations for gradual weight loss, which have been adopted in almost all behavioral studies, do not have an empirical basis. Studies which compare rapid versus gradual behavioral treatment of weight loss are still lacking. In fact, a review by Stunkard and Rush (1974) suggests that an initial rapid weight loss followed by gradual weight loss may be more preferable than a sustained gradual weight loss. Unfortunately no data are presented by Ferster *et al.* to substantiate their ideas about self-control, although the data have been reported elsewhere (cited in Penick *et al.*, 1971) that the modal weight loss for their ten subjects was 10 lb, with a range of 5 to 20 lb.

Stuart's (1967) study, our second article, is important because of its adaption of Ferster *et al.*'s stimulus control procedures, its clinical refinements, and its encouraging results. Stuart reports impressive weight losses in eight of ten women over a combined treatment and follow-up period of one year. However, although the program was extremely successful in producing weight losses, it is not clear whether the patients reached their desired weight goals, and no data are given indicating whether they maintained their weight loss after formal intervention had ceased. Stuart's (1971) subsequent study, our third article, is a more refined version of his initial treatment model, and adds the important dimensions of exercise and nutrition management. An excellent expanded version of this article can be found in a book by Stuart and Davis (1972). Although Stuart (1971) refers to his intervention model as situation control rather than self-control, his treatment does, to a large extent, require the *individual* to initiate behaviors which will change his environment and thus modify his eating. In view of the general definition and techniques of self-control presented earlier, Stuart's (1971) study can be considered a self-control approach.

The next five articles (Wollersheim, 1970; Hagen, 1974; Harris, 1969; Harris and Hallbauer, 1973; Penick *et al.*, 1971) are examples of experimental therapy outcome studies which have compared a variety of self-control and other behavioral techniques with no-treatment, attention-placebo, and traditional obesity treatment control groups. Wollersheim's (1970) article is an excellent psychotherapy outcome study in terms of its experimental design, detailed procedures, and exhaustive data analysis. Motivated overweight female college students were randomly assigned to one of four experimental conditions: (a) behavior therapy consisting of reinforcement and stimulus control procedures; (b) an analogue of traditional insight psychotherapy; (c) positive expectation or social pressure to lose weight; or (d) a no-treatment control group. At post-treatment and follow-up the behavior therapy group was superior in both weight reduction and a decrease in reported frequencies of eating behaviors.

Hagen (1974), in a sequel to Wollersheim's study, investigated whether written presentation of principles previously found effective produced significant weight reduction without face-to-face encounters between client and therapist or therapy group. Female college students were randomly assigned to a (a) behavior therapy group (which was the same as Wollersheim's behavior therapy group), (b) "manual only" group (which had the same lessons as the behavior therapy group but in which all the lessons were sent and returned by mail), (c) behavior therapy plus manual group, or (d) no-treatment control group. All treatment conditions produced significantly more weight loss than the control group, with the "manual only" group doing as well as the other two treatment groups. However, a recent long-term follow-up by Hagen (personal communication), revealed that none of his groups maintained their weight losses.

Harris (1969) compared a no-treatment control group to a self-control group consisting of stimulus control and self-reinforcement. Individuals who participated in the program lost more weight than the controls. In a subsequent study, Harris and Hallbauer (1973) experimentally investigated Stuart's (1971) recommendation to include exercise management as part of treatment. They compared a self-control group with a self-control plus exercise management group and an attention placebo treatment group. The results indicated that all three groups lost weight during the 12-week program, with no significant differences between them. A 7-month follow-up showed that individuals in the two self-control groups lost more weight than the control group, and the self-control plus exercise group lost more weight than the self-control only group.

Penick et al. (1971), in an intensive day-care program for the treatment of obesity, compared a behavior modification group with a traditional psychotherapy group. The behavior modification procedures consisted of self-initiated stimulus control and external reinforcement. Both groups received training in nutrition and exercise. The behavior modification group did better during treatment than the traditional psychotherapy group. Furthermore, the subjects in both groups continued to lose weight at a 6-month follow-up.

The next set of five experimental studies (Hall, 1972; Mahoney, Moura, and Wade, 1973; Mahoney, 1974; Jeffrey, 1974a; Romanczyk et al., 1973) compares the relative efficacy of external and self-control techniques.

In the first study, Hall (1972) compares self-management environmental planning with therapist control. The former treatment consisted primarily of Ferster et al.'s stimulus control procedures and the latter primarily of the experimenter paying each subject for weekly weight losses. Both treatments were successful in producing weight losses; however, the external reinforcement procedure resulted in losses of a greater magnitude for most subjects than did the self-managed environmental planning.

The article by Mahoney, Moura and Wade (1973) compares the relative efficacy of self-reward, self-punishment, self-monitoring, and information-only. All subjects were given information of effective stimulus control techniques for weight loss. After 4 weeks of treatment, self-reward subjects had lost significantly more weight than either the self-monitoring or self-punishment groups. These findings were interpreted as providing a preliminary indication that self-reward strategies may be superior to self-punitive and self-recording strategies. At 4-month follow-up, the self-reward subjects continued to show greater improvement than either self-punishment or the control subjects. However, since there was about a 60% drop-out rate at follow-up, it is very difficult to interpret the follow-up data. In a subsequent study, Mahoney (1974) compares self-reward for eating-habit improvement, self-reward for weight loss, self-monitoring, and a delayed-treatment control. The results indicated that all three treatment groups lost weight. However, the self-reward conditions were most effective, with self-reward for eating-habit improvement producing the greatest weight loss. An important aspect of this study is that self-reward contingent on eating-habit improvement resulted in better weight loss than self-reward contingent on weight loss.

Jeffrey (1974a) conducted a study in partial collaboration with Mahoney (1974). Taking Kanfer's (1971) model of self-regulation as a theoretical basis, self-monitoring and standard setting were held constant for each group, with only the locus of reinforcement manipulated. The external-control group consisted of therapist reinforcement and an explicit attribution set that the therapist was responsible for the weight loss, while the self-control group consisted of self-reinforcement and an explicit attribution set that the subject was responsible for his own weight management. Jeffrey found that self-control subjects did as well as the external-control subjects during treatment, and maintained better during follow-up. Although these findings appear contradictory with Hall's (1972) results, procedural differences exist between the two studies which could account for the discrepancies in outcomes. For example, Hall's self-control treatment consisted primarily of stimulus control, while Jeffrey used stimulus control, self-monitoring, and self-reinforcement for both eating habit and weight-reduction improvement together with an explicit self-attribution set. The findings of these studies suggest that a combination of self-managed antecedent stimulus control and consequent reinforcement control may be more powerful than either used separately.

Romanczyk *et al.* (1973) conducted an excellent component analysis of self-monitoring of weight, self-monitoring of caloric intake, aversion imagery, relaxation therapy, and combined self-control procedures. In general, their results indicate that all of the self-management procedures were more effective than no-treatment control or self-monitoring for weight only. In a second study, reported in the same article, they found that self-monitoring for caloric intake was effective; however, the use of combined self-control procedures resulted in greater weight losses which were sustained during a 12-week follow-up. The authors concluded that the enduring weight losses suggest that subjects learned behavioral skills which they were able to implement on a continuing basis. Hopefully, this interpretation is correct. However, these researchers, as many researchers in this section, have the same problems of analyzing and interpreting follow-up data when there are high drop-out rates (over 30% at posttreatment and over 60% at follow-up for the Romancyzk *et al.*, 1973, study). A plausible rival hypothesis is that the sustained weight loss was simply due to the fact that the seventeen of twenty-eight patients who dropped out between pretreatment and follow-up had not lost or had even gained weight. If the drop-out data had been included in the analysis, the posttreatment and follow-up data might not have been so impressive. The problem of drop-outs is a difficult one which needs further attention.

All of the previous studies have involved professionally trained behavior therapists who administered treatment to a limited number of people. Our next study (Levitz and Stunkard, 1974) extends self-control techniques to a larger audience of therapists and patients. Levitz and Stunkard (1974) applied their behavioral treatment programs with a self-help group called TOPS — Take Off Pounds Sensibly. The results indicated that professional therapists could implement a behavioral program in a community based self-help group. Another study (McReynolds *et al.*, 1976) trained nutritionists in self-management techniques and found that with a minimum of training and continued supervision, nutritionists could successfully implement several types of self-control programs with overweight women.

The final two articles (Hall, 1973; Hall *et al.*, 1974) deal with the issue of sustaining and maintaining weight loss. All of the self-control studies and essentially all the other studies in this book have demonstrated successful weight loss during treatment. However, *no* study has demonstrated continued weight loss up until the individual reaches his desired weight goal. Most of the studies which reported short-term follow-ups indicate that while weight gain did not necessarily occur, there was no continued weight loss either. These last two studies specifically deal with the issue of long-term maintenance of weight loss.

Hall's (1973) 2-year follow-up of her earlier study (Hall, 1972) indicates that neither her external nor self-control groups maintained weight loss. And finally, Hall *et al.* (1974) indicate that despite short-term treatment and follow-up success of two self-managed treatments, long-term weight losses were not maintained.

These findings are in disagreement with Harris and Hallbauer's (1973) successful 7-month follow-up. However, the negative findings of Hall's studies question the "proven" efficacy of behavioral modification for obesity; they also question a cardinal assumption that self-control approaches will lead to better maintenance than other treatment approaches. Furthermore, no existing studies have included efficiency measures to test the hypothesis that self-control treatments are now more efficient than other treatments.

TREATMENT TRENDS

The studies included in this section point to the following conclusions about the effects of various antecedent stimulus control and reinforcement control approaches to weight management:

1. Self-monitoring of weight appears to have temporary effects on weight

reduction (Stuart, 1971). However, self-monitoring of eating habits does appear to have some therapeutic effects (Romanczyk *et al.*, 1973). Probably the most important value of self-monitoring is the detailed information it provides for the patient and therapist about the antecedent and consequent stimuli controlling the patient's eating and exercise habits. This information is essential for planning comprehensive treatment.

2. A combined self-control intervention seems to be as effective as an external-control intervention in producing weight losses during treatment and seems to be more effective in promoting maintenance during short-term follow-up. Furthermore, a refundable contingency results in fewer drop-outs and absentees than a nonrefundable contingency. Finally, a self-control refundable contingency results in less inappropriate reinforcement than a self-control nonrefundable contingency (Jeffrey, 1974a).

3. It makes theoretical and empirical sense to place the stimulus control and reinforcement contingencies on the target behaviors of eating and exercise improvement rather than on weight loss (Mahoney, 1974). Most researchers, however, still focus on a weight loss rather than on relevant eating and exercise behaviors, of which weight loss is a function (Stuart, 1973). Clearly future research needs to emphasize the assessment and modification of exercise habits. The initial study by Harris and Hallbauer (1973) suggests very promising results.

4. Although stimulus control and reinforcement approaches facilitate weight loss, most researchers typically do not systematically combine them. It would seem that a combination of the two would lead to more powerful results (Stuart, 1973).

5. Individuals vary considerably in their responsiveness to behavioral weight-control procedures (Penick *et al.*, 1971). Possible sources of variation may be that the techniques themselves vary in effectiveness, or individuals vary in their abilities to implement behavioral techniques, or therapists vary in the emphasis they place on implementing the different techniques. Research is clearly needed to evaluate treatment, subject, and therapist factors in order to better understand this response variability.

6. Although frequent weigh-ins and therapist or group support may enhance self-control efforts, these factors by themselves appear to be insufficient for successful weight management (Wollersheim, 1970; Hagen, 1974).

7. When the patient is introduced to the program it should be clearly explained that he will need to make a lifelong commitment to managing his weight and that it will take a great deal of effort in the beginning to permanently modify his eating and exercise habits. The therapist and patient should undertake a thorough assessment to see if the patient is ready to begin such a program (Jeffrey, 1976). If he is not ready, then it is probably best to tell the patient not to begin until he is ready to commit himself to a long-term program. In addition to an individual readiness assessment, there also needs to be an environmental readiness assessment. Careful evaluation of the patient's family, social, and work

L

environment needs to be undertaken to see if the patient can elicit support in an effort to facilitate weight management. If it appears that the immediate environment will not be supportive of sustained weight loss, then the first phase of the treatment needs to focus on this.

All self-control studies in this section and other studies in this book have demonstrated short-term weight loss by behavioral methods. However, none of these studies continued treatment until the patient reached his desired weight goal. This in part may account for the lack of maintenance because the patient has not had the chance to reach his weight goal and stabilize his new eating and exercise habits before treatment is completed. It seems time for therapists and researchers alike to begin to continue treatment until the patient's desired weight goal is attained.

In closing, present research indicates that weight losses can be achieved with behavior modification procedures. However, this research also indicates that future research needs to systematically attempt to program maintenance of weight loss. Therapist-initiated and self-initiated antecedent stimulus control and consequent reinforcement control seem to offer the most promising approaches to weight management. In outpatient settings, a combination of self- and therapist-control approaches will probably lead to the most powerful treatments of obesity. Finally, behavior modification can be considered an advancement in the management of obesity, however it should not be considered a panacea or an easy solution to this complex and difficult health problem.

References

Bandura, A. *Principles of behavior modification*, New York: Holt, Rinehart & Winston, 1969.

Ferster, C. B., Nurnberger, J. I., and Levitt, E. E. The control of eating. *Journal of Mathetics*, 1962, 1, 87–109.

Goldiamond, I. Self-control procedures in personal behavior problems. *Psychological Reports*, 1965, 17, 851–868.

Goldfried, M. R. and Merbaum, M. (Eds.), *Behavior change through self-control*. New York: Holt, Rinehart & Winston, 1973.

Hagen, R. L. Group therapy versus bibliotherapy in weight reduction. *Behavior Therapy*, 1974, 5, 222–234.

Hall, S. M. Self-control and therapist control in the behavioral treatment of overweight women. *Behaviour Research and Therapy*, 1972, 10, 59–68.

Hall, S. M. Behavioral treatment of obesity: A two-year follow-up. *Behaviour Research and Therapy*, 1973, 11, 647–648.

Hall, S. M., Hall, R. G., Hanson, R. W., and Borden, B. L. Permanence of two self-managed treatments of overweight in university and community populations. *Journal of Consulting and Clinical Psychology*, 1974, 42, 781–786.

Harris, M. B. Self-directed program for weight control: A pilot study. *Journal of Abnormal Psychology*, 1969, 74, 263–270.

Harris, M. B. and Hallbauer, E. S. Self-directed weight control through eating and exercise. *Behaviour Research and Therapy*, 1973, 11, 523–529.

Jeffrey, D. B. A comparison of the effects of external control and self-control on the modification and maintenance of weight. *Journal of Abnormal Psychology*, 1974, 83, 404–410 (a).

Jeffrey, D. B. Self-control: Methodological issues and research trends. In M. J. Mahoney and C. E. Thoresen (Eds.), *Self-control: Power to the person.* Belmont, California: Brooks/Cole, 1974 (b).

Jeffrey, D. B. Behavioral management of obesity: Learning principles and a comprehensive intervention model. In E. Craighead, A. E. Kazdin, and M. J. Mahoney (Eds.), *Behavior modification: Principles, issues and applications.* New York: Houghton Mifflin, 1976.

Kanfer, F. D. The maintenance of behavior by self-generated stimuli and reinforcement. In A. Jacobs and L. B. Sachs (Eds.), *Psychology of private events.* New York: Academic Press, 1971.

Levitz, L. S. and Stunkard, A. J. A therapeutic coalition for obesity: Behavior modification and patient self-help. *American Journal of Psychiatry,* 1974, **131,** 423–427.

Mahoney, M. J. Self-reward and self-monitoring techniques for weight control. *Behavior Therapy,* 1974, **5,** 48–57.

Mahoney, M. J., Moura, N., and Wade, T. The relative efficacy of self-reward, self-punishment, and self-monitoring techniques for weight loss. *Journal of Consulting and Clinical Psychology,* 1973, **40,** 404–407.

McReynolds, W. T., Lutz, R. N., Paulsen, B., and Kohrs, M. B. Weight loss resulting from two behavior modification procedures with nutritionists as therapists. *Behavior Therapy,* 1976, **7,** 283–291.

Penick, S. B., Filion, R., Fox, S., and Stunkard, A. J. Behavior modification in the treatment of obesity. *Psychosomatic Medicine,* 1971, **33,** 49–55.

Romanczyk, R. G., Tracey, D. A., Wilson, G. T., and Thorpe, G. L. Behavioral techniques in the treatment of obesity: A comparative analysis. *Behaviour Research and Therapy,* 1973, **11,** 629–640.

Schachter, S. Some extraordinary facts about obese humans and rats. *American Psychologist,* 1971, **26,** 129–144.

Stuart, R. B. Behavioral control of overeating. *Behaviour Research and Therapy,* 1967, **5,** 357–365.

Stuart, R. B. A three-dimensional program for the treatment of obesity. *Behaviour Research and Therapy,* 1971, **9,** 177–186.

Stuart, R. B. Behavioral control of overeating: A status report. Paper presented at the Fogarty International Center Conference on Obesity. Bethesda, Maryland, October 1973.

Stuart, R. B. and Davis, B. *Slim chance in a fat world: Behavioral control of obesity.* Champaign, Illinois: Research Press, 1972.

Stunkard, A. J. and Rush, J. Dieting and depression re-examined: A critical review of reports of untoward responses during weight reduction for obesity. *Annals of Internal Medicine,* 1974, **81** 526–533.

Thoresen, C. E. and Mahoney, M. J. *Behavioral self-control,* New York: Holt, Rinehart & Winston, 1974.

Wollersheim, J. P. Effectiveness of group therapy based upon learning principles in the treatment of overweight women. *Journal of Abnormal Psychology,* 1970, **76,** 462–474.

CHAPTER 33

The Control of Eating

CHARLES B. FERSTER, JOHN I. NURNBERGER and EUGENE E. LEVITT
Indiana University Medical Center

Although many investigators have described patterns of eating behavior and reported a wide range of factors related to obesity,[1,2,5,9,10,11], specific techniques for changing an individual's eating behavior are given little or no attention in published reports, and programs of weight control based on behavioral principles are virtually non-existent. This report is an account of the application of some elementary general principles of reinforcement theory[7] to the analysis of the behavior of the human eater. This theoretical framework of reinforcement was used to analyze actual performances in eating, and particularly self-control of eating. Supplementing the account of this system are descriptions of experimentally developed techniques which should illustrate practical applications of the theoretical principles of self-control.[1]

The theoretical analysis begins with the simple observation that the act of putting food in one's mouth is reinforced and strongly maintained by its immediate consequences: the local effects in the gastro-intestinal system. But excessive eating results in increased body-fat and this is aversive to the individual. The problem is therefore to gain control of the factors which determine how often and how much one eats. An individual will manipulate these variables if the control of eating is reinforcing to him — if he escapes from or avoids the *ultimate aversive consequences of eating* (UAC). Unfortunately for the overeater, the long-term or ultimate aversive consequences of obesity are so postponed as to be ineffective compared with the immediate reinforcement of food in the mouth. Alcoholism is a similar example in which hangover symptoms and the full impact of asocial activity are not suffered until considerable time has elapsed. Realization of self-control, then, demands an arrangement that will bring the influencing conditions into closer association with the reduction of eating behavior.

Reprinted with permission from the *Journal of Mathetics*, 1962, 1, *87–109*.

[1] The experiments are still underway and will be reported separately by the second and third authors.

The analysis and development of self-control in eating involves four steps:

1. *Determining what variables influence eating.* Almost every known behavioral process is relevant to this. Among these are control of eating by stimuli, effect of food deprivation, chaining, avoidance and escape, prepotent and competing behaviors, conditioned alimentary reflexes, and positive reinforcement.[2]
2. *Determining how these variables can be manipulated.* Specification of performances within the repertoire by which the individual can manipulate these variables. One example would be the choice of foods which are weak reinforcers, yet rewarding enough to maintain the behavior of eating them at some low level.
3. *Identifying the unwanted effects (UAC) of overeating.* Avoidance of these is the basic motive for developing the required self-control.
4. *Arranging a method of developing required self-control.* Some of the required performances may call for so drastic a change of behavior that it may be necessary to produce the required repertory in stages by reinforcing successive approximations.

Self-control requires for our purposes a more precise definition than is conveyed by the term "will-power". It refers to some specific performances which will lower the disposition to emit the behavior to be controlled. These performances involve the manipulation of conditions influencing this behavior. A convenient datum for our analysis is the *frequency* of the behavior's occurrence. The strength, durability or persistence of the behavior is measured by its frequency. Frequency has the measurement advantage of being a continuous variable. Similarly, the disposition to eat can vary from small to large. The various conditions which the individual himself can manipulate to lessen the frequency of the controlled behavior will be presented in detail in the next section, *Avenues of Self-control.* The technical problem of generating the self-control performance and maintaining it in strength will be dealt with in the section *Shaping and Maintaining the self-control Performance.*

Avenues of Self-control

THE ULTIMATE AVERSIVE CONSEQUENCES

Avoidance of the ultimate aversive consequences (UAC) of uncontrolled eating is essential in developing performances with which a person may regulate his eating behavior. Self-control is needed because of the time lapse between the act of eating and its UAC. To overcome this time lapse, techniques were sought which would derive a conditioned stimulus from the UAC and apply it at the time the disposition to eat was strong. This is based on the principle that almost any event may become aversive when paired with a known aversive event. Such a conditioned stimulus may be the person's own verbal behavior, if specific training procedures are applied. It is not enough for the subject to *know* what the aversive effect of overeating is, for such knowledge by itself leads only to verbal responses weaker than the food-maintained behavior and may not lessen the strong disposition to eat. Therefore an extensive repertoire must be established so that the subject has under his control large amounts of verbal behavior dealing with the consequences of eating. The continued intensive pairing of facts about the UAC with various kinds of eating performance will make the performances themselves conditioned aversive stimuli. Once a given performance such as eating a piece of pie acquires conditioned aversive properties, any approach to it will produce aversive stimuli. These stimuli will reinforce any self-control because the self-control terminates the aversive stimulus and prevents the uncontrolled act. By such a process, certain foods like pies, cakes, cokes, doughnuts or candy may become conditioned aversive stimuli, at least until other avenues of control become available.

Before the unwelcome consequences of overeating can be used in developing self-control, they must be identified and developed for the individual. It cannot be assumed that an obese person already has a repertoire about the UAC of eating. In the application of the principles to human subjects being studied, the development of the UAC was one of the major parts of the practical program. However, developing a repertoire by which the subjects could create an aversive state of affairs for themselves presents serious technical problems. First, to establish this repertoire, the actual aversive events must be identified for the subject in terms that are meaningful for his daily life. Second, the subject must learn an active verbal repertoire with which he can translate caloric intake into ultimate body fat.

We first disclosed, in great detail, the consequences of uncontrolled eating for each individual. After each subject described anecdotes about UAC in group sessions, we helped each one to develop a fluent verbal repertoire about the relevant aversive consequences. We found that simply *recognizing* the various aversive consequences did not give these subjects an active verbal repertoire which could be invoked immediately and whenever needed. To develop an active repertoire about the UAC, we arranged rehearsals, frequent repetitions, and written examinations. In general, the subjects were unaware of their inability to verbalize the relevant aversive consequences, and were surprised by the poor results of the early written and oral examinations. Verbal descriptions of aversive consequences the subjects had actually experienced were far more compelling than reports of future and statistically probable consequences, such as diabetes, heart disease, high blood pressure, or gall bladder disorder. In other words, descriptions of actual or imagined social rejection, sarcastic treatment, extreme personal sensitivity over excess weight, demeaning inferences concerning professional incompetence or carelessness, or critical references to bodily contours or proportions were much more potent. All of our subjects found their constant and unsuccessful preoccupation with dieting aversive, and any ability to control their own habits highly rewarding.

All of the exercises in this area were designed to develop a strong and vivid repertoire that could be introduced promptly in a wide variety of situations intimately associated with eating and despite a strong inclination to eat. The actual aversive effects of being overweight are largely individual matters which differ widely from person to person. We therefore used group discussions as an aid for each person to discover how her body weight affected her life. The discussion was guided toward explicit consequences and anecdotes rather than general statements such as "I want to lose weight because I will feel better". We found that after only four or more group sessions, subjects shifted from vague statements such as "I'll look better in clothes" to specific ones such as "My husband made a sarcastic remark about an obese woman who crossed the street as we were driving by". Perhaps, the verbalization of the UAC was too aversive before we had demonstrated that self-control was possible.

Amplifying the aversive consequences of overeating. To establish the bad effects of eating more than one's daily requirements, it is necessary that the individual know the metabolic relationships between different kinds of food, general level of activity, and gain or loss of weight. Phrases like "Everything I eat turns to fat" illustrate that the required repertoire is frequently absent. Thorough training should be given in the caloric properties of all of the kinds of foods which the individual will encounter. The aversive effects of eating certain undesirable foodstuffs can be amplified by generating verbal repertories which describe the full consequences of eating them. For example, the subject should be made to recognize that a 400-calorie piece of pie is the caloric equivalent of a large baked potato with butter plus a medium-size steak. The pie is equivalent to one-tenth of a pound of weight gained, and so forth. Again, *knowing* these facts is not at issue. The issue is that a strong-enough repertoire be established, and with enough intraverbal connections, that the UAC behavior will occur with a high probability in a wide enough variety of situations.

An important exercise early in the weight-control program is the identification of the individual's actual food intake. The subject's casual summaries of his daily food intake are likely to be grossly inaccurate. His ability to recognize his actual food intake is improved by an interview technique in which the interviewer probes and prompts him: "What did you have for breakfast?" "How many pieces of toast?" "How many pieces of bread?" "What did you do between ten and eleven in the morning?" "Were you at a snack bar or a restaurant at any point during the day?" "Were you offered any candy at any point?" and so forth.

With the pilot subjects, we leaned most heavily on a written protocol which we used as a basis for individual interviews about their diets. Each subject kept a complete written account of everything she had eaten, along with calculations of fat, carbohydrate, protein, and numbers of calories. A large part of the early sessions was devoted to problems in recording food intake, such as difficulties in estimating mixed foods like gravies, stews, or sauces.

For the first 4 weeks of the program, when some simpler kinds of self-control were developed, the subjects' caloric intake was set to maintain a constant weight. We over-estimated the maintenance levels, and all subjects gained weight during this month. However, the weight increase proved the relationship between caloric intake and weight change in a situation where the caloric intake was carefully defined. In spite of the weight gain, however, some measure of self-control emerged, particularly in changes in the temporal pattern and regularity of eating.

Deprivation

The effect of food deprivation may be observed in a pigeon experiment in which the frequency of a pigeon's key pecking, maintained by producing food, is measured as a function of changes in the level of food deprivation. Changes in the level of food deprivation produce continuous changes in the bird's performance over an extremely wide range if we can measure the frequency of the bird's pecking. This frequency of pecking is intuitively close to notions like the bird's disposition to eat, probability of action, or motivation. When a wide range of frequency response can be measured sensitively, the level of deprivation affects the bird's performance continuously, from the free-feeding body weight to as low as 65 or 70 per cent of normal body weight. Food deprivation of the order of 6 to 24 hours constitutes a very small part of the effective range. The magnitude of food deprivation therefore continues to increase the organism's disposition to emit responses, reinforced by food, long after no further changes occur in gastrointestinal reactions (e.g., hunger pangs) and other conditioned effects of food in the mouth. The hunger pangs, which are ordinarily taken as symptoms of hunger (from which the effect of food deprivation is inferred), are more closely related to the conditioned stimuli accompanying past reinforcements of eating than to the level of food deprivation. The conditioned reflexes involving the gastrointestinal system occur at relatively low levels of deprivation compared with the effective range of food deprivation in respect to the changes in frequency of operant behavior. There may be a similar lack of correspondence between the tendency to verbalize, introspectively, reports of hunger and the actual disposition to eat. For purposes of developing self-control, the actual performances resulting in food in the mouth are more relevant than the introspective reports of "hunger".

Controlling the rate at which the subject loses weight proves to be a major technique of self-control. For any degree of establishment of a self-control repertoire, there is probably some level of food deprivation which will cause the subject to eat in spite of the self-control behavior. Therefore, a major principle of self-control would be to pace the rate of the subject's weight loss so that the effect of the weight loss on the disposition to eat would be less than the given stage of development of self-control. Many avenues of self-control may be learned without causing any weight loss. Placing the eating behavior under the control of specific stimuli or breaking up the chain of responses usually present in the compulsive eater are examples of this. The former will be discussed below. Breaking up a chain causes the eating performance to become a series of discrete acts which are more easily interrupted than a continuous performance in which each chewing response or each swallow occasions placing the next bit of food on the fork.

If the self-control performances which may be developed are to be useful, they must be maintained by conditions which will be present continuously, even after the weight-control therapy procedures are discontinued. Many unsuccessful crash-diet programs illustrate the way in which too rapid a loss of weight produces a level of deprivation and a disposition to eat exceeding the existing self-control. The usual diet involves some program which taps the motivation of the dieter temporarily. For example, slight aversive pressure from the husband or family doctor may produce a rapid loss in weight, perhaps on the order of 3 to 5 pounds a week. The effect of the rapid weight loss is a large increase in the disposition to eat which then overcomes the subject's temporary motive.

Limiting the diet to one specific food, such as protein, probably will produce a heightened disposition to eat other food stuffs regardless of the general weight level. These are the traditional specific hungers. An all-protein diet, for example, even if taken without limit of calories, would probably generate an enormous disposition to eat carbohydrates, sugars, and fats. Therefore, a balanced diet should be maintained and a weight loss brought about by a uniform reduction in amount rather than kind of food.

Although the major effects of food deprivation appear when weight losses are of the order of pounds, the time elapsed since eating would have local effects on the disposition to eat. Local satiation effects may best be used as a limited avenue of self-control by arranging the eating schedules so that the subject ingests a meal or a significant amount of food just before a situation in which the disposition to eat might be unusually strong. An example is a social situation in which eating has frequently occurred in the past or when preferred foods are present. The housewife who eats continuously while preparing dinner can control the disposition to nibble the foods being prepared by shifting the preparation of the dinner meal to the period of time immediately following lunch, when her disposition to eat is lower because she has just eaten.

In the application of the self-control principles to actual exercises, we specified a weight loss of 1 pound per week and insisted that our subjects adhere to this rate of weight loss even though each of them wanted to cut her diet more stringently in order to lose weight at a greater rate. Different rates of weight loss might possibly be arranged at different stages of development of self-control after more is known about the effectiveness of different avenues of self-control and about the relative effects of weight loss depending upon the initial level.

The continued ingestion of food during a meal provided another variation in level of food deprivation which was used to provide a gradual transition to the final self-control performances. Exercises, such as brief interruptions in eating, were first carried out toward the end of the meal when some satiation had occurred. After the subjects began to learn how to use auxiliary techniques to stop eating and their existing eating patterns began to break down, the exercises were moved progressively toward the early part of the meal, when their levels of deprivation were higher so that the exercises had to be more difficult.

SELF-CONTROL BY MANIPULATING STIMULI

The characteristic circumstances when an individual eats will subsequently control his disposition to eat. The process is illustrated by the pigeon whose key pecking produces food only when the key is green and not when it is red. The frequency with which the pigeon pecks the key (reinforced by food) will later depend upon which color is present. Thus, changing the color of the key can arbitrarily increase or decrease the frequency of pecking independently of the level of food deprivation. A frequent factor in the lack of self-control in the obese person may be the large variety of circumstances in which eating occurs. In contrast, a much narrower range of stimuli is present during the more infrequent eating periods of the controlled person. Therefore, the disposition to eat possibly could be decreased by narrowing the range of stimuli which are the occasions for the reinforcement by food. By proper choice of the actual stimuli controlling the eating behavior, it should also be possible to increase the individual's control over these stimuli. There are circumstances when even the pathologically compulsive eater will have a considerably lower disposition to eat for periods of time simply because the environment is novel enough so that eating has never occurred then. Consider, for example, walking in an isolated forest area.

The first step in the development of self-control in this category is to narrow the range of existing stimuli which control eating. The overweight individual eats under a large variety of circumstances. Thus, the problem of self-control is made difficult by the large number of daily occasions which bring the tendency to eat to maximal levels because in the past they have been the occasions when eating has occurred. Two kinds of behavior need to be brought under stimulus control. The first is the elicited reflex effects of food, such as salivation, gastric secretion, and other responses of the gastrointestinal tract. The other involves operant behavior, or the behavior involving the striated musculature of the organism — walking, talking, reaching, cooking, and so forth. In the so-called voluntary behaviors, the major datum is the frequency of the behavior rather than the magnitude of an elicited reflex, as with the smooth-muscle response of the digestive system. Although these two types of behavioral control are inevitably tied together, their properties are different and they must be distinguished both dynamically and statically. In order to break down the control of eating by the stimuli which have been the characteristic occasions on which eating has been reinforced in the past, the stimuli must occur without the subsequent reinforcement by the food. The process is a direct extrapolation from the extinction of a Pavlovian conditioned response. If the dog is to discontinue salivation on the occasion of the bell, the bell must be presented repeatedly in the situation in which the food no longer follows. The amount of saliva the bell elicits then declines continuously until it reaches near-zero. Similarly, the stimuli characteristic of the preparation of a meal will cease to control large amounts of gastric activity if these stimuli can be made to occur without being followed by food in the mouth. Initially, the stimuli will elicit large amounts of gastric activity; but with continued exposure to these stimuli, the amount of activity will decline continuously until low levels are reached.

Delimiting existing stimulus control of eating may take considerable time because (1) the loss of control by a stimulus is a gradual process, requiring repeated exposure to the relevant stimuli; and (2) it may be a long time before the individual encounters all of the situations in which he has eaten in the past. The sudden temptation of the ex-smoker to light a cigarette when he meets an old friend is an example of the latter kind of control.

Self-control developed under procedures involving very special situations and foods (for example, liquid diets, all-protein diets, or hard-boiled eggs and celery) will be difficult to maintain when the diet circumstances return to normal. The very abrupt shift in eating patterns, kinds of food eaten, and characteristic circumstances surrounding eating will weaken the self-control performances as well as strengthen eating behaviors which were previously in the person's repertoire under the control of the more normal environment. Hence, self-control performances must be developed under circumstances and with foods which are to be the individual's final eating pattern.

TEMPORAL CONTROL OF EATING

The time of day is an important event controlling eating. With the individual who characteristically eats at regular intervals, gastric activity comes to precede these occasions very closely, and is at low levels elsewhere regardless of levels of deprivation. The same can be said for operant behavior associated with eating, although the order of magnitude of some of the parameters may be difficult. After the conditioned responses associated with eating are brought closely under the control of a strict temporal pattern, feelings of hunger should disappear except just before meal-time. However, many individuals have no such routine patterns of eating, so that the temporal pattern of eating does not limit the amount of gastro-intestinal activity. The obese person frequently eats in the absence of any gastric activity. A technique of self-control in this category would rigidly specify a temporal pattern of eating and find conditions for adhering to it. As with gastro-intestinal reflexes, this general disposition to engage in operant behaviors reinforced by the ingestion of food can be brought under the control of a temporal pattern of eating, with a resulting lower disposition to eat during the intervals between regular meals. In the early stages of learning self-control, the development of a rigid temporal pattern perhaps should be carried out under conditions in which no weight loss is to be expected and the amount of food, ingested at specified meals, is large enough to minimize the disposition to eat on other occasions. The subsequent maintenance of this temporal pattern of eating when the subject begins to lose weight will depend upon the concurrent action of other categories of self-control performances. The control of eating by temporal factors can also be developed for situations other than the normal routine meals, as, for example, at social gatherings and parties. Because the availability of food is predictable here, early stages of self-control can include arranging a specific time when the eating will occur rather than indeterminate consumption of whatever foods happen to be available.

THE EATING SITUATION

As with the temporal properties of eating, the actual characteristics of the eating situation may be used to control the disposition to eat. However, the stimuli here are clearer and probably exert control of an even larger order of magnitude than that of the temporal pattern. This application of the principle of stimulus control is the same as in the temporal contingency: to arrange that eating occurs on limited and narrowly circumscribed occasions and never otherwise. To simplify the development of the stimulus control, eating situations should be associated with stimuli which occur infrequently in the individual's normal activities. For example, an eating place in the home should be chosen so that it is maximally removed from the routine activities of the day. Nor should eating occur together with any other kind of activity such as reading. If reading occurs frequently enough while the subject is eating, then reading will increase the disposition to eat because it has been an occasion on which eating has been reinforced.

EMPHASIZING THE STIMULUS CONTROL

The occasions characterizing eating can be emphasized by deliberately arranging very obvious stimuli. For example, the subject always eats sitting down at a table which has a napkin, a place setting, and a purple table cloth. The latter makes the situation even more distinctive. In the extreme case, a specific item of clothing might be worn whenever the subject eats. Narrowing the range provides another form of stimulus control. By eating only specific foods in specific places, the disposition to eat when other foods are available will be minimized. This factor will also be discussed under chaining; but the aspect emphasized here is the effect of the foods eaten as one of the elements in the occasion associated with eating. If a subject has eliminated ice cream, candy, and cake from his diet, the sweet shop will have little control over his behavior.

In the actual procedures with subjects, stimulus control was the first avenue of self-control developed. The subjects learned to keep daily diet protocols during the first few meetings and to determine the number of calories necessary to maintain their weight. We restricted eating to three meals a day, eliminated concentrated fats and sugars from the diet, and attempted to bring about an increase in the amount of food taken in at meals, particularly at breakfast, to bring about a normal pattern of eating without any expected weight loss. For individuals having difficulty in restricting their eating to meals, we arranged a specific and routine extra feeding, as, for example, a glass of milk and a few crackers at bedtime. The extra feeding was to be taken routinely, however, so it did not become a reinforcer for increasing the probability of eating on a wide variety of occasions. No weight loss was attempted until the subjects were successful in eating a normal range of food at meals without any eating at other times. We attempted to create an eating pattern which could be carried out without interruption after the weight-control program was terminated. Our major problems were insufficient protein or excess fat in the diet. None of the subjects ate excessive amounts of carbohydrate except perhaps as candy. However, all subjects had trouble eating a full meal. It was paradoxical that women who joined the program because they could not limit their eating had difficulty in ingesting a maintenance diet at mealtimes. One complained of nausea, another of chest pains, and a third of discomfort from overeating. All of the complaints disappeared in a week, however.

CHAINING

Eating is a rough designation for a chain of behavioral sequences culminating in swallowing and the subsequent gastrointestinal reflexes. An illustrative sequence might be as follows: Dressing makes possible leaving the house; leaving the house leads to walking to the store; entering the store is followed by the selection of foods, a basket of food is the occasion for paying the clerk and leaving the store; a bag of groceries at home leads to storing the food; stored food is the occasion for cooking or otherwise preparing the food; the prepared food is the occasion for setting the table and sitting down; the sight of food is the occasion for cutting it with a fork or knife; the dissected food leads to placing food in the mouth; food in the mouth is followed by chewing; and chewing is followed by swallowing. The sequence differs from individual to individual and from time to time, but any selected elements illustrate the process.

Because the frequency of occurrence of the final member of the chain depends on the nature of the earlier members of the seating sequence, some degree of self-control can be arranged by dealing with the dynamic properties of the eating sequence. The length of the chain of responses leading to swallowing will markedly influence the frequency with which the eating sequence is carried out. The longer the sequence of behaviors in the chain and the more behavior sequences in each member of the chain, the weaker will be the disposition to start the chain. This property of chaining suggests a technique of control which could be useful if used in conjunction with the other avenues of control. By arranging that all of the foods available or accessible require a certain amount of preparation or locomotion, the tendency to eat can be reduced simply because the chain of responses leading to swallowing was lengthened. Keeping food out of areas normally entered, shopping on a day-to-day basis (at a time when the disposition to eat is low), buying foods which are not edible without cooking or other preparation, and placing food in less accessible places are some techniques for weakening the disposition to eat by lengthening a chain. As in some of the avenues of control, this technique would be inadequate under extreme levels of deprivation without additional support from other types of control. The chain must not be lengthened too much, or it might become so weakened that prepotent eating behaviors would occur or the chain shortcircuited.

The actual form of the eating chain in the latter members just before swallowing may be rearranged to reduce the rate of eating. The behavior of swallowing is so strongly reinforced that it could occur very soon after food enters the mouth, without very much chewing. Similarly, the behavior of placing food in the mouth (reinforced by the taste of food) has high strength and occurs as soon as the mouth empties. Many eaters carry out this sequence at a very high rate by reaching for additional food just as soon as food is placed in the mouth and by swallowing while the fork is in transit to the mouth. This analysis is confirmed by the high rate with which many obese people eat compared with that of normal obese eaters.

To reduce the rate of eating and to make it possible for the subject to stop eating at any point, we designed simple exercises to break the chain, particularly the near-final members, so that the occasion for placing food on the fork is swallowing rather than chewing. The new sequence was: food on the fork only after other food is swallowed and the mouth is empty. These exercises depended on ancillary techniques of control already developed by other techniques of self-control. At the start, the interruptions were only a few seconds; then, they were gradually increased to several minutes. The ability to stop eating at *any* point represents the final effect of nearly all of the other avenues of control; nevertheless, it constitutes a separate technique of control demanding special exercises. In later, more difficult exercises, the subject holds food on a fork for various periods of time without eating. Similarly, chewing is prolonged before swallowing for increasing periods. These exercises are carried out initially at the end of a meal, when the deprivation level is low.

The type of food eaten is of major importance in how reinforcing it would be, and hence how long a chain of responses can be maintained by the food reinforcement. The disposition to eat could be somewhat regulated by a selection of foods in the individual's diet that are sufficiently reinforcing (appetizing, caloric, etc.) to be eaten, but minimally reinforcing so as to minimize the resulting disposition to eat. A certain balance must be achieved; if the foods chosen are so unappetizing or unappealing that their reinforcing effect is negligible, the subject will simply switch to other foods. Also relevant here are the dynamic effects of food deprivation. Foods which are maximally reinforcing should be eaten when the individual is less deprived, and minimally reinforcing foods should be eaten under stronger conditions of deprivation. In other words, the effect of the highly reinforcing foodstuffs on the disposition to eat would be minimized by a lower level of deprivation so that the subject can stop eating more easily. In special cases, the food intake could be increased temporarily in order to minimize the highly reinforcing effect of certain foods. For example, if an individual who is highly reinforced by caloric pastries knows she will be in a situation where such pastries are being served, she could lessen the probability of eating them by increasing her food intake during the preceding meal or by a glass of milk before entering the situation.

PREPOTENT REPERTOIRES

One way to lessen the disposition to eat is to supplant it by establishing other activities incompatible with eating. In an extreme case, an apparently large disposition to eat is often due to a behavioral repertoire in which eating appears strong because the rest of the repertoire is weak. Some degree of self-control should be possible if some activity could be maintained at a potentially high strength and circumstances arranged so that the subject could engage in this activity whenever the disposition to eat was strong. An example of such an activity might be telephoning a friend just after breakfast instead of indulging in the customary between-meal nibbling. The use of prepotent repertoires as a technique of control implies a certain amount of control over the prepotent repertoire. In order for these substitutive repertoires to be effective, special attention must be given to methods for strengthening them, particularly when they are needed. For example, instead of reading the newspaper as soon as it arrives, it could be put aside until some time when the peak tendency to eat occurs. Similarly, the telephoning of friends could be postponed in order to keep this behavior at high strength. Such activities occur initially because of independent reinforcement. Another kind of prepotent repertoire may be established by starting some strongly reinforced activity whose reinforcement occurs only if the behavior occurs uninterrupted for a period of time. Examples are washing a floor, going to a movie, taking a bus ride, reading a short story, or going for a walk. Such performances will be prepotent over eating because of the temporary aversive consequences resulting from their interruption. In many cases, the prepotent repertoires physically remove the individual from the place where eating can occur.

The effective use of prepotent repertoires depends upon the development of other avenues of control. Probably no one of these "prepotent" performances would be effective by itself if the disposition to eat were strong. For example, the individual going for a walk could simply stop at a restaurant to eat. Nevertheless, there is still a net advantage, because the supplementary types of self-control needed are relatively easy. For example, compare the disposition to stop at a restaurant during a walk with the disposition to eat in the normal situations when eating usually occurs. If the individual usually eats at home, the tendency to stop at a restaurant and eat will be considerably less than the tendency to eat at home. No explicit training was required in the pilot experiment to establish self-control by the use of prepotent repertoires; but all of the subjects used them during several phases of the experiment.

Prepotent repertoires may be affected by emotional factors. For example, many persons eat when depressed, affronted, thwarted, or frustrated. In the terms of the functional analysis of eating used here, emotional factors may weaken behaviors other than eating so that eating becomes relatively stronger. Putting food in one's mouth remains a highly reinforcing activity even if the remainder of the individual's repertoire is severely depressed. Eating then occurs because it is less disrupted by the emotional variables depressing the rest of the individual's repertoire.

Eating may interact with emotional factors in more subtle, but nonetheless important, ways, as a mechanism by which a person might escape or avoid emitting verbal behavior which is highly aversive, e.g., thinking about impending circumstances which are highly aversive. Because of its very strong and immediate reinforcement, eating will be prepotent over thinking about anxiety-evoking occurrences. Thus, eating comes to acquire two sources of strength: the immediate reinforcement from food in the mouth, and the reinforcement from postponing or avoiding the aversive consequences of emitting the verbal behavior which the eating supplants. Emotional disturbances will also disrupt the performances by which the individual controls himself, as will any general depression or disturbance of the individual's over-all repertoire. Self-control performances will be especially liable to disruption early in their development, before they become strong and maintained.

The manipulation of factors to minimize the effects of emotional disturbances is a separate topic, involving self-control of variables different from those in eating and thus requiring a separate analysis. The main avenue of control in eating lies in increasing the strength and durability of the self-control performances so that they will remain intact during emotional disturbances. For example, a person who has acquired an active and extensive verbal repertoire about all of the personal aversive consequences of being overweight will be able to emit these behaviors even during some general depression of his behavioral repertoire. The behavior about the ultimate aversive consequences of eating will be even more durable during possibly disrupting situations if it has already been effective in producing self-control, that is, if the behavior about the UAC has been reinforced effectively by suppression of the disposition to eat.

If existing levels of self-control are certain to break down because of an emotional disturbance, the individual should be trained to plan a controlled increase in food intake. The advantage of explicitly increasing the level of food intake would be that the food would be eaten under controlled conditions, so that stimulus control and other factors of self-control already developed would be maintained, and the effects of absence of progress in self-control would be minimized. Overeating under planned conditions would probably weaken the already developed self-control repertoires less than unplanned or uncontrolled eating.

In many situations, the general depression of an individual's repertoire occurs only for a limited time. Here, the necessary self-control performances would be a manipulation of the physical environment so that food is not available then, or would be the creation of a prepotent environment. The depressed individual who wishes to control his eating goes to a movie, takes a ride on a bus, or goes for a walk. These activities give time for the emotional states to disappear and simultaneously provide an environment in which eating has not been reinforced very frequently in the individual's past experience. Of course, applications of these techniques of control depend upon the prior achievement of a certain amount of self-control, and probably are some of the most difficult areas of self-control to acquire. Such items would not be attempted at an early stage of the self-control program.

Shaping and Maintaining the Self-control Performance

Self-control is a very complex repertoire of performance which cannot be developed all at once. If self-control consists of items of behavior with the same dynamic properties as those of the rest of human behavior, the self-control performance, as a complicated repertoire, must be developed in slow steps. These would begin with some performance already in the individual's repertoire and proceed in successive stages to more complicated performances. With each gain in self-control, the individual has a repertoire from which a new degree of complex behavior may emerge. Simply "telling" the subject the nature of the performances required for the development of self-control is not a sufficient condition for their development. The situation is analogous to that of a complicated motor or intellectual activity. One cannot explain to the novice how to differentiate an equation in calculus without first establishing a repertoire in algebra. Similarly, as most golfers have learned, no amount of verbal instruction will take the place of slow development of behavior reinforced by its effect on the golf ball. The actual disposition to emit the self-control behavior builds up because it was emitted successfully to reduce the long-term aversive effects of the behavior to be controlled. What is required here is to begin with some performance very close to one in the individual's repertoire, and to arrange circumstances so that those performances have at least some effect on the disposition to eat. The early reinforcement of this initial repertoire by a discernible movement in self-control provides the basis for the subject's continued attendance to the self-control program.

In the development of self-control, the concern is not simply the presence or absence of a self-control performance. A group of behaviors must be built constituting a repertoire that will occur with a sufficient degree of certainty to be maximally effective.

Just as the disposition to eat can vary from near-zero to large values, the behaviors involved in self-control can also be weak or strong. Whether the individual "knows" what the potential techniques of self-control are, or even can emit them, is not so important as the durability of the self-control repertoire. A set of performances is needed which will occur with high enough probability despite competition from the individual's other repertoires. The maintaining event for the self-control performance is the reduction in the disposition to eat. The effect of the reinforcement is not an all-or-none matter, and the reinforcing effect of gains in self-control repertoires can be variously small, large, or even intermittent. Uncontrolled eating should not be viewed as a failure in control, but simply as the absence of progress. If the positive aspects of the program are emphasized, as well as the development of specific performances to control the disposition to eat, each small increment in the ability of the subject to control himself will reinforce further participation in the self-control program. A failure of a self-control performance to prevent eating defines an intermittent schedule of reinforcement of the self-control behavior. It may still continue to maintain the performances, just as any other act that is intermittently reinforced.

Some types of self-control require that old performances disappear rather than a specific repertoire, as, for example, the development of stimulus control, be built. The development of this kind of self-control is largely a function of the number of exposures, without eating, in situations when the individual has eaten in the past. Verbal behavior has only limited relevance here, since it can be little more than a report of what is taking place. Recognizing that the preparations for dinner are increasing the disposition to salivate and eat is of little use in controlling these effects. Extinguishing the effects of these stimuli is an orderly process requiring only exposure to the stimuli and passage of time. However, knowledge of the process might be of use in conjunction with the various avenues of self-control, particularly in respect to emphasizing the stimuli involved. Once the subject recognizes that the extinction of the stimulus control is a slow process, even minor decrements in the extent of the control by the stimuli will provide reinforcements for maintaining the self-control, as, for example, when several days are required for extinction. In the absence of knowledge of the order of magnitude of the course of the process, weakly maintained self-control behaviors might extinguish. In the actual self-control program, noting reductions in the strength of eating behavior during its extinction provides interim reinforcement for the self-control performances.

Discussion

Traditionally, the development of self-control has been in a framework of classical psychoanalytic and dynamic psychotherapeutic approaches to human behavior. These approaches view self-control in terms of its developmental and dynamic origins and the inner-directed, private forces which sustain, direct, or distort its external manifestations. Prior life experiences are considered in detail through interviewing and related techniques, including analyses of current actions and attitudes (transference and counter-transference). The focus is on the past to assist the individual in discovering those formative experiences and relationships which have functioned to establish current attitudes and current modes of alleviating anxiety and guilt. A major structural goal of this system is the development of effective insight with increased intellectual freedom and more realistic self-appraisal. A major symptomatic goal is the ultimate reduction of anxiety and guilt, with a resultant diminished need to exploit heroic or uneconomic measures in the control of either or both. A fundamental assumption here is that the human being who becomes sufficiently aware of his personal developmental behavioral determinants and who is sufficiently relieved of neurotic anxiety of guilt, will, by virtue of this achievement, progressively lose his dependence on irrational and restrictive defenses. A corollary is that a healthy behavioral repertoire is potentially available at any time the individual gains relief from the guilt and anxiety of his deviant developmental history. These assumptions are not at all unreasonable for many problems encountered by the clinician, and sometimes appear to be convincingly supported by satisfactory therapeutic outcome. However, there are outstanding exceptions, characterized by certain common behavioral elements. Among these are (1) elaborately ritualized performances; (2) long-standing maintenance of such patterns; and (3) large amounts of strongly maintained and sustained activity. These are the symptoms present in many alcoholic individuals, in all obsessive-compulsive neurotics, in many patients with neurotic depressive reactions, in drug addicts, in a variety of schizophrenic patients, and in many individuals with eating disturbances (obese as well as anorexic). Successful and sustained therapeutic improvement is exceptional for all, including the obese,[8] however prolonged and insightful the therapeutic experience may be. The kind of functional analysis of behavior proposed here may provide a conception of human behavior as an alternative to the classical psychoanalytically oriented systems.

The terms in such an analysis are the actual performances of the patient and their exact effects on his environment. The frequency of occurrence of the performance is studied as a function of its effect on the environment, and every attempt is made to observe and deal with the relevant performances rather than with inferred processes. The specificity of the analysis does not mean that the patient must have an intact repertoire by which he deals with the world, and attention can be focused on creating whatever repertoire is necessary. Most of the present report is a presentation of certain practical techniques which can be applied to the problem of uncontrolled eating. The preliminary results of this pilot program are not included as a record of even mediocre success, but rather as a description of the medium within which the specific techniques of control were imparted. A much longer follow-up period and a larger number of cases are necessary to develop a successful program as well as test it. Nor can we now designate these aspects of the program which were effective or ineffective. This report is intended to provide a theoretical and practical model for more structured programs of self-control in eating. We have shown eating habits can be changed in a short-term, small-group-therapy program by the use of the basic principles outlined here. Whether or not the weight losses reported during the first 15 sessions are primarily due to the application of the principles outlined can be determined only by appropriately controlled study experiments. We are not concerned whether one or another program can effect weight loss, since many pharmacologic individual-and group-therapy programs lead to temporary loss of weight, as is generally known. The central issue is the development of self-control in eating which will endure and become an available part of the individual's future repertoire. Most conventional programs do not focus on the eating patterns available to the subject after he has lost weight, nor do they present recognizable techniques for developing such future control. Possible exceptions are in individual programs of psychotherapy which are directed toward an exploration and resolution of the unconscious determinants of eating behavior, and in certain of the conditioned-reflex techniques. Yet, even in these programs, this question remains: Do proper eating habits exist after the individual is free of the relevant disability? The program outlined here has the special advantage of focusing directly and specifically on future eating behavior and of presenting even more specific techniques for bringing this behavior under control. Application of the basic principles requires no special instrumental or technical training and is relatively economical. Slow and controlled weight loss under relatively high-caloric intake levels minimizes medical and psychological problems.

We cannot state whether the program we carried out is suitable for severely obese individuals (particularly those who have medical or psychiatric complications). Nor can we specify how the technical principles and procedures can be applied to subjects of low educational level or of limited intelligence. A major problem here would undoubtedly be the difficulty of daily and accurate caloric-intake records. Some of these fundamental questions are subjects for future study.

References

1. BRUCH, H. *The importance of overweight*. New York: W. W. Norton, 1957.
2. CAPPON, D. Obesity. *Canadian Medical Association Journal*, 1958, 78, 568–573.
3. FERSTER, C. B. Reinforcement and punishment in the control of human behavior by social agencies. *Psychiatric Research Report*, 1958, 10, 101–118.
4. FERSTER, C. B. and SKINNER, B. F. *Schedules of reinforcement*. New York: Appleton–Century–Crofts, 1957.
5. GALVIN, E. P. and McGAVACK, T. H. *Obesity, its cause, classification and care*. New York: Hoeber-Harper, 1957.
6. SKINNER, B. F. *The behavior of organisms*. New York: D. Appleton Century Co., 1938.
7. SKINNER, B. F. *Science and human behavior*. New York: Macmillan, 1958.
8. SKINNER, B. F. *Cumulative record*. New York: Appleton–Century–Crofts, 1959.
9. STUNKARD, A. The results of treatment for obesity. *Archives of Internal Medicine*, 1959, 103, 79–85.
10. STUNKARD, A. Eating patterns and obesity. *Psychiatric Quarterly*, 1959, 33, 284–295.
11. STUNKARD, A. Obesity and the denial of hunger. *Psychosomatic Medicine*, 1959, 21, 281–289.

CHAPTER 34

Behavioral Control of Overeating

RICHARD B. STUART

School of Social Work, University of Michigan

Summary— A behavioral treatment for overeating, utilizing operant and respondent conditioning techniques is described. To date, all eight patients with whom this treatment has been employed have been successfully treated and no negative secondary reactions have been observed.

Obesity is well recognized as a major health hazard. Only two common characteristics have been observed in obese persons: a tendency to overeat and a tendency to underexercise (U.S. Public Health Service, undated). While obesity has been ascribed to various causes (Bychowski, 1950; Hamburger, 1951; Deri, 1955; Stunkard, 1959; Mendelson, 1966), the treatment of overeating has been successful when it is based solely upon a functional analysis of the maladaptive response (Ferster *et al* 1962). The present paper presents Ferster's approach in somewhat modified form and reports upon the clinical results to date.

Self-control

Man clearly controls his own behavior so as to achieve his own objects. The source of this control is commonly ascribed to central adaptive mechanisms ranging from the ego to the conscience. From a behavioral point of view, self-control is an inference drawn from the functional relationships among observable responses (Bijou and Baer, 1961). The behavioral processes involved in a person's control of himself are the same as those one would use in controlling the behavior of others (Skinner, 1953).

The first step in self-control is a precise analysis of the response to be controlled and its antecedent and consequent conditions. An analysis of overeating would naturally include a precise description of the topography of the response, the conditions under which it occurs, and its consequences. The second step is the identification of behavior which facilitates eating a proper amount of food (including behavior which interferes with overeating). The third step is the identification of positive or negative reinforcers which control these behavior patterns. A reinforcer can be identified for every response, using Premack's principle ("Of any two responses, the more probable response will

Reprinted with permission from *Behaviour Research and Therapy*, 1967, 5, 357–365.

reinforce the less probable one", Premack, 1965). Thus a reinforcer is always available for any desired response, independent of the topography of that response. The fourth step requires the application of the reinforcement to alter the probability of the preselected response (Homme, 1965). The outcome of self-control can be termed "contingency management" and is designed to increase the frequency of desired overt responses while decreasing the frequency of undesired responses.

Structure of Treatment

Treatment sessions are scheduled three times per week, usually last for approximately 30 min, and extend over a 4- to 5-week period. Subsequent sessions occur as needed, but usually at intervals of 2 weeks for the next 12 weeks. "Maintenance" sessions are scheduled as needed, while follow-up sessions occur on a planned monthly basis. The logic of scheduling frequent sessions at the start of treatment is that it is assumed that learning can occur most efficiently when teaching occurs in massed trials. As sessions become less frequent, more relevant experience is accumulated than can be fully discussed, and too much irrelevant or competing experience is accumulated. Massed sessions at the start also increase the opportunity for monitoring the patient's performance, which helps to make success more likely. It is essential that the patient encounter immediate success, for "if the self-contingency manager does not get reinforced for self-management, extinction will occur" (Homme, 1965).

Initial Interview

The initial interview combines the processes of behavioral assessment with the establishment of a working therapeutic contract. All techniques utilized in each session are explained to the patient, along with a discussion of their rationale. In this way, the patient is able to focus his attention upon a particular routine and can work with the therapist in finding ways of achieving greater success. He is also trained in a new method of describing his own behavior. "Rather than telling him to modify them (something which he may have already told himself), he is trained in the experimental analysis of behavior, and also in the variables which maintain it, or which he can recruit to modify it" (Goldiamond, 1965). No diagnostic formulations are entertained unless they are relevant to the current therapeutic contract, and all such formulations are communicated to the patient. A record is kept of all phases of the treatment, and this record is reviewed by the patient periodically. In addition to an anecdotal record of the treatment maintained by the therapist, two daily records are kept by the patient throughout therapy.

1. FOOD DATA SHEETS

These records account the time, nature, quantity and circumstance of all food and drink intake. Time is important as a means of determining the pattern of between-meal eating as well as the duration of scheduled meals. The nature and quantity of food consumed is important because of its obvious bearing upon weight gain. This entry includes the mode of preparation, e.g. broiled, fried, etc., often as much a source of unnecessary weight gain as the nature of the food-stuffs themselves. Describing the precise weight or volume of foods is useful not only as a monitoring procedure, but because it requires a slight interruption in the normal chain of eating responses. Finally, knowledge of the circumstances under which eating occurs provides clues to the ways in which it can be controlled, through identification of the current controlling conditions. Such factors as tension, solitude, cleaning up, reading or watching television are commonly associated with excessive eating. When this is known, it is possible to take steps to change the responses to these stimuli.

2. WEIGHT RANGE SHEETS

The patient's weight range is important because it consists of a running record of fluctuations in gross body weight. Weight is to be recorded before breakfast, after breakfast, after lunch, and before bedtime. There is a natural reduction of weight during the night as energy is expended in maintaining body functions such as breathing, temperature regulation and heartbeat, while food and liquid consumption are almost nil. This weight is gradually regained during the day as caloric intake exceeds caloric expenditure. Obesity occurs because the amount of food consumed is in excess over that which is needed for energy. This gross weight is the target of the therapeutic program. Having the patient weigh himself four times daily serves as four daily reminders of the therapeutic program. In addition, the patient is provided with direct evidence of the effect of food and drink intake upon his weight. This serves as a periodic, mildly aversive stimulus associated with overeating.

Additional data is gathered in two areas. First, the patient is asked to list high probability behavior patterns, free operant responses which occur with high frequency and which, by implication, are positively reinforcing. For some patients, activities such as reading, talking to friends, watching television or reading the newspaper are readily available. For other patients, those suffering from a "behavioral depression", eating may be the only readily available high probability behavior. It may be necessary to help the patient to cultivate a reservoir of positively reinforcing responses. For example, two patients were helped to develop intense interests in caged birds and growing African violets. While these responses are not to be used until the fifth step in the treatment, it is essential to gather the necessary information at the beginning to allow time for the development of new interests. A second type of data, with the same eventual application, deals with the patient's most urgent, weight-related fears. For some patients, these fears concern ultimate physical consequences of overeating, such as cardiovascular disease or death from infection because surgery is impossible. For other patients, these fears concern social consequences, such as the loss of a mate or the total cessation of sexual experiences.

A weight-loss goal of from 1 or 2 lb/week is set during the initial interview. Greater loss of weight poses certain physiological hazards and creates the risk of food deprivation, while loss of less than 1 lb/week is not sufficiently reinforcing and is relatively ineffective. Finally, treatment recommendations are made in the first as well as all subsequent sessions, as needed.

Behavioral curriculum—Step One. Behavioral therapy, as an active therapy, emphasizes patient activity as a means of goal attainment. The first step in treatment, following introduction of the recording procedures, requires the patient to interrupt his meal for a pre-determined period of time, usually 2 or 3 min which is gradually increased to 5 min. He is instructed to put down his utensils and merely sit in his place at the table for a specified period of time.

Rationale. The logic of this maneuver is that the patient is given an early experience of control over one aspect of his eating, however small, and learns that eating is a response which can be broken down into components which can be successively mastered. The reinforcement for success is immediate, and consists of the knowledge that the patient has taken his first step toward overcoming his compulsion. It is important that the patient be successful in his first step, and he is instructed to telephone the therapist if he encounters any difficulty. In such instances, the interval would be reduced to the point at which the patient can meet with success. The therapist is available by telephone at all times, in order to guard against any failure by the patient which might adversely affect his expectation of success.

Second Interview

Each interview following the first has the same general format: The Food Data and Weight Range Sheets are discussed; the patient's progress with the behavioral curriculum is discussed with abundant praise for success; and new steps are planned and put into operation with the patient's full participation. Patients are asked to anticipate any forthcoming stressful events in their lives, and this is followed by planning how to minimize the possibility of compensatory overeating.

As the Food Data Sheets are reviewed, the patient is asked if he sees any obvious changes which might be made. There are often suggestions for changing the mode of food preparation or for the substitution of a less-fattening substance for a particularly harmful one, such as sherbet in place of ice-cream.

Changes are rarely suggested by the therapist, as *self-dosing* is an important prerequisite for complete self-control. At times, patients have been cautioned to be more temperate in their deletion of foods so as to reduce the possibility of deprivation.

Behavioral curriculum—Step Two. The patient is instructed to remove food from all places in the house, other than the kitchen. He is also instructed to keep in the house only those foods which require preparation, other than salad greens and the like, and he is instructed to prepare only one portion at a time.

Rationale. Much compulsive eating is "automatic", in the sense that the patient may be unaware of the fact that he is eating. If a series of actions is required prior to eating, the patient is forced to become aware of his behavior. Therefore, a trip to the kitchen and the task of food preparation are both reminders that eating is about to occur. This may be an effective deterrent. If not, the need for preparation of individual portions may serve as an effort which outweighs the reward of eating.

Behavioral curriculum—Step Three. The patient is instructed to make eating a "pure experience", that is, he is instructed to pair eating with no other activity, such as reading, listening to the radio, watching television or talking on the telephone or with friends.

Rationale. If the patient reads while he eats, he is most likely to want to eat while he reads, etc. If eating can be held separate from other behavior, it will not continue as a conditioned response to the occurrence of this other behavior.

Confinement of the food to the kitchen and the elimination of other responses associated with eating are means of promoting stimulus control of the response. These are stimuli which set the occasion for eating. Additional steps, such as controlling the interval during eating, are designed to promote control of the proprioceptive or mediating stimuli inherent in the complex response of eating.

It should be noted that despite the rigors of steps two and three, no direct limitation of the type or quantity of food has been suggested. The goal of these steps is not the immediate reduction of food intake. Instead, it is to so manipulate the eating response as to make it more readily self-controlled, first by bringing it to awareness and then by disrupting its chaining to other behavioral responses.

Third Interview

No new steps are suggested in the third interview, to avoid "overloading" the patient with behavioral prescriptions. Instead, following a review of his experiences, the patient's help is elicited in refining the steps which have been taken.

Fourth Interview

The first week of treatment will have been accomplished by this time. The Weight Record is therefore reviewed, and the first entry is made on a chart recording weekly weight changes. This chart is retained by the patient and serves as a reminder of progress. It should be noted that weight loss may be greater during the first 2 weeks of treatment than it will be subsequently. This is probably related to the "honeymoon effect" of treatment and to the fact that the patient has a greater amount of voluble fat which is convertible to energy during this time. Accordingly, the patient is forewarned to anticipate a more gradual weight loss of between 1 and 2 lb weekly.

Behavioral curriculum—Step Four. Obese patients have been observed to eat very rapidly whenever they eat, so that large quantities of food are consumed in very brief periods. To slow the process of ingestion, the patient is instructed to put a small amount of food in his mouth, and to replace his utensils on the table until he has swallowed.

Rationale. This step is aimed directly at manipulation of the eating response, and success with this step is tantamount to direct control over the response. In addition to its control value, this step also helps the patient to derive more enjoyment from his food so that he can replace quantity with quality in his eating. Rapid eating not only leads to indigestion, but it also obviates the possibility for full enjoyment of the taste and aroma of food. By eating more slowly, the patient can improve his digestion and learn to savor his food. He may eventually achieve a normal state of satiation with less food intake. This step is easily followed at all meals, including those eaten socially, and has the added value of making the patient a more tolerable eating companion.

Fifth Interview

Following all of the normal interview procedures, the therapist enlists the patient's aid in identifying "danger periods" of between-meal eating. These are times of high arousal when "the probability of the most practiced response appearing is increased" (Pyke *et al.*, 1966). As eating is the most practiced response, it is highly likely to occur at these times. Training the patient in controlling eating under high arousal circumstances is tantamount to training him in temporal control of eating.

Behavioral curriculum—Step Five. The patient is instructed to engage in one of the previously identified high probability behaviors at times when he would normally eat. This is analogous to a procedure developed for the control of smoking: "If a response other than smoking can be conditioned to stimuli which ordinarily lead to smoking and the link between these stimuli and the response of smoking weakened, then it should become easier for the individual smoker to cut down his consumption or to quit entirely. That is, the smoker now has at his disposal an alternative response to smoking" (Pyke *et al.*, 1966). The patient is instructed to read the newspaper or to call a friendly neighbor at exactly 10:00 a.m. if eating occurs consistently at this hour. Similar alternative responses are planned for other times of the day which have been identified as periods of high arousal. Before embarking upon the substitute behavior, the patient is instructed to repeat the phrase: "I can control my eating by engaging in other activities which I enjoy."

Rationale. Between-meal eating is understood to be an important source of positive reinforcement for patients who overeat. They cannot be expected to forego this reinforcement without a substitute. The substitute has inherent reinforcing value (it is a high probability behavior) and it implies the occurrence of self-control which is reinforcing. Specifically, the patient learns a new response to stimuli which previously set the occasion for eating. In order to set the occasion for the emission of the alternate response, the patient is trained to verbalize the rationale for the procedure. Since this behavior is in the service of the patient's goal attainment, following the prescription adds a measure of reinforcement for the new behavior.

Sixth Interview

This session, like the fourth, is used to consolidate gains made to date. There is considerable discussion of ways of refining behavioral steps so as to maximize their effectiveness. By this time, patients are often active in planning their own curricula and have been ingenious in devising procedures of great value to themselves. For most patients, the behavioral curriculum is complete at this point, with subsequent sessions being devoted to refinement of the program, and with patient decisions about dietary changes. At the request of one patient, the service of a dietitian was contracted for an hour in which professional advice was obtained in careful food selection. This service is of help, but not essential.

Seventh Through Twelfth Interviews

These sessions further refine the curriculum and reinforce progress. Two patients who encountered difficulty with the control of between-meal eating were offered one additional therapeutic step.

Behavioral curriculum—Step Six. Joseph Cautela (1966) has described the process of "coverant sensitization" in which the patient is trained to relax, then to imagine that he is about to indulge in a compulsion, then to imagine the occurrence of an aversive event.* One patient found considerable difficulty in

*In the original work done with the patients discussed in this report, patients were told to imagine that they were actually tasting the forbidden food before then being told to imagine the aversive condition. In a personal communication, Dr. Cautela correctly labeled this a punishment procedure. It lacks the forward conditioning advantage of an escape or avoidance conditioning procedure in which the aversive condition is applied *before* commission of the compulsive act.

controlling the eating of a particular kind of cookie at specific times during the day. She was first trained in vivid imagery and then instructed to imagine eating her favorite cookie (taking it from the package, bringing it to her lips, hearing her teeth crunch as the cookie crumbles, tasting its sweetness, etc.), and she was finally instructed to immediately switch to the detailed image of her husband in the process of seducing another woman—a great fear she had identified during the initial interview. This process proved highly successful in both instances of its use (requiring one session with one patient and two with the other) in reducing between-meal eating, without any disturbance of normal food intake. In short, it proved highly specific and powerful in its effect.

Rationale. In this treatment, the image of a forbidden object (CS) is paired with the image of an aversive stimulus (also a CS). The imagined aversive CS then forestalls the occurrence of the forbidden CS and ultimately interferes with eating. Two aspects of this procedure are of note. First, the patient demands the occurrence of a thought, or coverant (Homme, 1965). The reinforcement for the occurrence of the thought is the removal of the aversive stimulus. Second, salivation and the so-called "gustatory responses" are respondent behaviors. In this treatment, operant behavior (a thought) elicits fear which, in turn, prevents the elicitation of salivation.

Discussion

There are several differences between the approach described by Ferster and his associates and the procedure which has been presented here. Ferster's treatment is a purely operant procedure, while this treatment combines operant and respondent techniques. Ferster worked with his patients in groups, while the treatment described here is conducted entirely on an individual basis. Finally, Ferster stressed the ultimate aversive consequences of obesity, while reference to these consequences was only incidental in the treatment described here.

The treatment is aimed at building the skill of the patient in being his own contingency manager. This is a self-control procedure which is reinforced through the patient's experience of success in the control of his own behavior, the reduction of the aversive consequences of a lack of self-control, and through considerable reassurance by the therapist. More occurred in the interaction between therapist and patients than the presentation of the curriculum and a review of progress. Reassurance was given as an antecedent to each new step and praise was given for success. More tightly controlled research is needed in order to isolate the contribution of the nonspecific interaction effect to total therapeutic outcome.

There are two essential features of this approach. First, treatment is offered specifically for the problem of overeating. No effort is made to distinguish the historical antecedents of the problem and no assumptions are made about the personality of overeater. This is comparable to the treatment of anorexia described by others (Ayllon *et al.*, 1964; Bachrach *et al.*, 1965). Second, the specific format of the approach is based upon verbal behavioral assignments to be followed by the patient. These assignments can be translated into techniques of self-control because the patient receives both didactic discussion of the rationale and training in the analysis of his own behavior so that he can discern opportunities for the subsequent application of the techniques.

Treatment Results

This report covers all eight patients who received the therapy for whom 12-month follow-up data is available. Long-term data is a necessity, for the essential therapeutic problem is not the reduction of overeating but the stabilization of a reduced level of eating. Two patients began but did not complete treatment, and they have been excluded from this report. One woman became pregnant while the other, a probable psychotic, wanted another type of therapy and was dropped from this project following the second session. In general, all of these patients can be classified at the least disturbed points along the continua proposed by Mendelson (1966) and Hamburger (1951).

All of the patients are women, six of whom are married (see Table 1). Of the married patients, two have children. All are voluntary patients who were referred for private treatment. The patients initially weighed from a low of 172 to a high of 224 lb, and all were judged by the physicians to be obese.

Figure 1 presents the data covering the gross weight for each patient during the 12 months for which data is available. While the figures present an almost linear line of decrease, it should be noted that the time intervals cover 4-week periods during which fluctuations were common. In actuality, weight loss varied from as little as 6 oz to as much as 5 lb/week for individual patients. Most patients showed either diminished weight loss or slight weight gains during the weeks prior to menstruation and slightly exaggerated weight losses following

TABLE 1. Age, marital status, weight loss and number of therapeutic sessions of eight female patients receiving behavior therapy for overeating

Patient	Age	Marital status	Weight loss over 12 months	Therapeutic sessions to date
1	37	M	46	19
2	21	S	38	24
3	41	S	29	30†
4	30	M	26	28
5	24	M	35	16
6	28	M	35	21‡
7	43	M	46	30
8	30	M*	47	41

*Divorced during treatment.
†One covert sensitization session.
‡Two covert sensitization sessions.

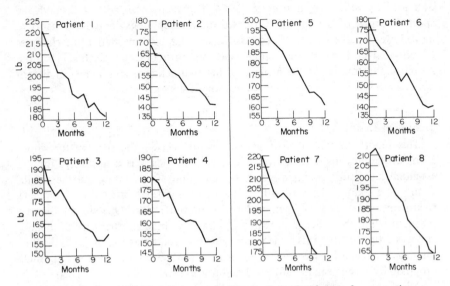

FIG 1. Weight profile of eight women undergoing behavior therapy for overeating.

menstruation. This is probably attributable to water retention associated with menstrual periods. An average overall weight loss of somewhat less than 1 lb/week was accomplished, and this is regarded as a reasonable expectation.

During the follow-up interviews at 9, 32 and 52 weeks, patients were asked to describe their current situations. Only one unusual situation was noted, one patient having obtained a divorce for which procedures were begun 1 yr prior to the start of treatment. Seven of the eight patients reported having an increased range of social activities, and three of the six married patients reported more satisfying relationships with their husbands. Three of the eight who were also compulsive smokers reported that they had self-applied the same general curriculum to smoking and either substantially reduced or eliminated smoking. While this evidence is in no sense conclusive, it suggests that "symptom substitution" has not occurred. Follow-up sessions were scheduled well in advance and undoubtedly served both as monitoring experiences and as added reinforcement for continuing the program. All patients knew of their inclusion in this clinical-research sample.

References

AYLLON, T., HAUGHTON, E. and OSMOND, H. O. (1964) Chronic anorexia: a behavior problem. *Can. psychiat. Ass. J.* 9, 147–154.
BACHRACH, A. J., ERWIN, W. J. and MOHR, J. P. (1965) The control of anorexia by operant conditioning techniques. In *Case Studies in Behavior Modification* (Eds. ULLMANN, L. P. and KRASNER, L.). Holt, Rinehart & Winston, New York.

BIJOU S. and BAER, D. (1961) *Child Development I: A Systematic and Empirical Theory,* p. 80. Appleton–Century–Crofts, New York.

BYCHOWSKI, G. (1950) On neurotic obesity. *Psychoanal. Rev.* 37, 301–319.

CAUTELA, J. R. (1966) Treatment of compulsive behavior by covert sensitization. *Psychol. Rec.* 16, 33–41.

DERI, S. K. (1955) A problem in obesity. In *Clinical Studies of Personality* (Eds. BURTON, A. and HARRIS, R. E.). Harper, New York.

FERSTER, C. B. NURNBERGER J. I. and LEVITT, E. E. (1962) The control of eating. *J. Math.* 1, 87–109.

GOLDIAMOND, I. (1965) Stuttering and fluency as manipulatable operant response classes. In *Research in Behavior Modification* (Eds. KRASNER, L. and ULLMANN, L.), p. 153. Holt, Rinehart & Winston, New York.

HAMBURGER, W. W. (1951) Emotional aspects of obesity. *Med. Clins. N. Am.* 35, 483–499.

HOMME, L. E. (1965) Perspectives in psychology: XXIV control of coverants, the operants of the mind. *Psychol. Rec.* 15, 501–511.

MENDELSON, M. (1966) Psychological aspects of obesity. *Int. J. Psychiat.* 2, 599–610.

PREMACK, D. (1965) Reinforcement theory. In *Nebraska Symposium on Motivation* (Ed. LEVINE D.), p. 132. University of Nebraska Press, Lincoln.

PYKE S., AGNEW, N. M. and KOPPERUD, J. (1966) Modification of an overlearned response through a relearning program: a pilot study on smoking. *Behav. Res. & Therapy* 4, 197–203.

SKINNER, B. F. (1953) *Science and Human Behavior.* Macmillan, New York.

STUNKARD, A. J. (1959) Eating patterns and obesity. *Psychiat. Quart.* 33, 284–295.

U.S. Public Health Service (undated) *Obesity and Health.* Public Health Service Publication Number 1485, Washington, D.C.

M

CHAPTER 35

A Three-dimensional Program for the Treatment of Obesity[1]

RICHARD B. STUART[2]

The University of Michigan, Ann Arbor, Michigan, U.S.A.

Summary— Obesity is seen as a consequence of a positive balance of energy consumed over energy expended. The reduction of obesity is accordingly sought through the reduction in the amount of food eaten coupled with an increase in the rate at which energy is expended. Both the reduction in the rate of eating and the increase in the rate of exercise are sought through management of critical aspects of the environment. Specific recommendations are made for the behavioral treatment of obesity, with the success of the treatment seeming to depend upon the effectiveness with which environmental stimuli are brought under control rather than depending upon motivational or other personal characteristics of the overeater. Pre-test data generated by the use of this procedure, coupled with the results of several recent studies appear to indicate uniquely positive results for the behavioral control of overeating.

Whether overweight is determined by gross body weight (Metropolitan Life Insurance Company, 1969) or skin-fold measurement (Seltzer and Mayer, 1965) even when differences in fat as a proportion of body weight are controlled (Durnin and Passmore, undated, p. 137), at least one in five Americans is found to be overweight (United States Public Health Service, undated). The social and economic costs of being overweight are staggering and are complicated by greatly increased vulnerability to a broad range of physical diseases, including cardiovascular and renal diseases, maturity-onset diabetes, cirrhosis of the liver,

Reprinted with permission from *Behaviour Research and Therapy*, 1971, 9, 177–186.

[1] Portions of this paper were presented at the annual meeting of the American Bariatrics Society, Washington, D.C., November 1969, and at the Fourth Annual Meeting of the Association for the Advancement of Behavior Therapy, Miami, Florida, 6 September 1970. The author wishes to express his gratitude to Barbara Davis, Judith Braver and Merrilee Oakes who contributed significantly to the development and testing of the approach which is described, and to Lynn Nilles for editorial assistance in the preparation of this manuscript. A more detailed description of the procedures may be found elsewhere (Stuart and Davis, in press).

[2] Requests for reprints should be sent to Richard B. Stuart, School of Social Work, University of Michigan, 1065 Frieze Building, Ann Arbor, Michigan 48104.

and gall bladder diseases, among many others (Mayer, 1968).[3] Despite the history of concern with obesity and the magnitude of the problem, little uncontested knowledge has been accumulated with respect to its etiology and treatment. Mayer (1968) has suggested that genetic factors may contribute to the onset of a small number of cases, while an additional small number of cases can be explained on the basis of injury to the hypothalamus, hormonal imbalance and other threats to normal metabolism. The exact role of genetic and physiological factors has, however, remained a mystery, and there has been little evidence to countermand an early observation by Newburgh and Johnston (1930) that most cases of obesity are:

> ... never directly caused by abnormal metabolism but (are) always due to food habits not adjusted to the metabolic requirement − either the ingestion of more food than is normally needed or the failure to reduce the intake in response to a lowered requirement (p. 212).

Therefore most obesities can be attributed to an excess of food intake beyond the demands of energy expenditure, and a major objective in treating obesity is a reduction in the amount of excess food consumed.

Just as there is uncertainty concerning the etiology of obesity, there is great confusion over the rule of psychological factors in overeating and its management. Some authors have contributed various useful typologies; for example, Stunkard (1959a) classified eating patterns as night eating, binge eating and eating without satiation, while Hamburger (1951) classified the triggers of excessive eating as either external or intrapsychic. Despite Suczek's (1957) observation that "single psychologic factors may not relate to either degree of obesity or ability to lose weight (p. 201)", other authors have sought to identify specific psychological mechanisms associated with obesity. For example, Conrad (1954) postulates that specific intrapsychic factors, such as efforts to prevent loss of love and to express hostility or efforts to symbolically undergo pregnancy and to ward off sexual temptations, underlie obesity. In a similar vein, while eating has been seen as a means of warding off anxiety (Kaplan and Kaplan, 1957), it has also been seen as a depressive equivalent (Simon, 1963). Furthermore, while writers have suggested that "depression, psychosis . . . suicide (Cappon, 1958, p. 573)" and other stress reactions have accompanied weight loss (Cornell Conferences on Therapy, 1958; Glucksman *et al.*, 1968), other studies have shown that: (a) the so-called "depression" associated with weight loss by some people is actually just a function of lowered energy due to reduced food consumption (Bray, 1969): (b) negative psychological reactions are frequently not found (Cauffman and Pauley, 1961; Mees and Keutzer, 1967);

---

[3]It has been argued that the relationship between obesity and such illnesses as cardiovascular diseases depends in part on the way in which fat is accumulated. For example, "People who become fat on a high carbohydrate, low fat diet are much less prone to develop atherosclerotic and thrombotic complications than those on a high fat diet (Cornell Conferences on Therapy, 1958, p. 87)."

and (c) a reduction in anxiety and depression may actually accompany weight loss (Shipman and Plesset, 1963). Despite this evidence, Bruch's (1954) admonition that treatment of overeating which does not give "psychologic factors . . . due consideration (can lead) at best to a temporary weight reduction (while being) considered dangerous from the point of view of mental health (p. 49)" is still influential in dissuading experimenters and therapists from undertaking parsimonious treatment of overeating.

While the research pertaining to physiological and psychological concomitants of obesity has led to some paradoxical conclusions, Stunkard's (1968) review of environmental factors related to obesity has demonstrated a clear-cut connection between obesity and socioeconomic status, social mobility and ethnic variables. It is interesting to note, however, that where comparative data are available, the differences ascribed to each of these factors are stronger for women than men. One explanation of this sex difference may be that the physical expenditure of energy in work may reduce the tendency toward adiposity of lower class, socially nonmobile men while the women, faced with relative inactivity, may show a more direct effect of high carbohydrate, low protein diets common at lower socioeconomic strata (Select Committee on Nutrition and Human Needs, 1970).

The literature describing the treatment of obesity is dismal and confusing. One authoritative group noted:

> . . . most obese patients will not remain in treatment. Of those who do remain in treatment, most will not lose significant poundage, and of those who do lose weight, most will regain it promptly. In a careful follow-up study only 8 per cent of obese patients seen in a nutrition clinic actually maintained a satisfactory weight loss (Cornell Conferences on Therapy, 1958, p. 87).

Failure has been reported following some of the most ambitious and sophisticated treatments (e.g. Mayer, 1968, pp. 1–2; Stunkard and McLaren-Hume, 1959), while success has been claimed for some of the more superficial "diet-clinic"-type approaches (e.g. Franklin and Rynearson, 1960). The role of drugs has been extolled by many writers, while others have cautioned that their side effects strongly contraindicate their use (American Academy of Pediatrics, 1967; Gordon, 1969; Modell, 1960). Fasting has been shown to have a profound effect upon weight loss (e.g. Bortz, 1969; Stokes, 1969), but the results have been shown to be short-lived as the patient is likely to quickly regain lost weight when he leaves the hospital setting (MacCuish et al., 1968). Claims of success have also been advanced for individual and group psychotherapy (e.g. Kornhaber, 1968; Mees and Keutzer, 1967; Stanley et al., 1970; Stunkard et al., 1970; Wagonfield and Wolowitz, 1968) and hypnosis (Hanley, 1967; Kroger, 1970), although these reports are typically not supported by controlled investigation. Finally, positive outcomes have been reported for behavior therapy techniques ranging from token reinforcement (Bernard, 1968), aversion therapy (Meyer and Crisp, 1964) and covert sensitization (Cautela, 1967) through complex contingency management procedures. Illustrative of the latter approaches are the work of Stuart (1967), which has been replicated in controlled studies by Ramsay (1968) and Penick and his associates (Penick *et al.*, 1970), and the work of Harris (1969), which included control-group comparisons in the original research.

It is probably true that behavior therapy has offered greater promise of positive results than any other type of treatment. This paper will present a rationale of and description for the treatment of overeating based upon behavioral principles.

Rationale

The treatment of obesity has typically attempted to stress the development of "self-control" by the overeater whose self-control deficit is often regarded as a personal fault. Conceding that behavior modifiers recognize first that self-control is merely the emission of one set of responses designed to alter the probability of occurrence of another set of responses (Bijou and Baer, 1961, p. 81; Ferster, 1965, p. 21; Holland and Skinner, 1961, Chapter 47; Homme, 1965, p. 504), and second, that self-controlling responses are acquired through social learning (e.g. Bandura and Kupers, 1964; Kanfer and Marston, 1963), most behaviorists still appear to regard self-control as a personal virtue and its absence a personal deficit (Stuart, 1971). For example, Cautela (1969, p. 324) is concerned with the individual's ability to manipulate the contingencies of his own behavior while Kanfer (1971) offers among other explanations for the breakdown of self-control "the patient's commitment to change", a presumed index of the patient's degree of motivation, or "the patient's prior skill in use of self-reward or self-punishment responses for changing behavior", presumed index of the patient's capacity to utilize treatment.

In any event, the relevance of the concept of self-control to the management of overeating may be questioned in the light of many recent studies. The most basic of these is the work of Stunkard (1959b) who demonstrated that in comparison with nonobese subjects obese subjects are far less likely to report hunger in association with "gastric motility". Thus the cues for hunger experiences of the obese may be tied to external events. Several ingenious studies have contributed to this possibility. First, Schachter and his associates demonstrated that obese subjects are less influenced than nonobese subjects by manipulated fear and deprivation of food (Schachter *et al.*, 1968), while they are more influenced by the time they think it is than by the actual time (Schachter and Gross, 1968). In addition it was shown that when the cues of eating are absent, as on religious fast days, obese subjects are more likely to observe dietary restrictions than nonobese subjects (Schachter, 1968). In a similar vein, Nisbett

(1968) and Hashim and Van Itallie (1965) showed that obese subjects are more influenced by the taste of food than are nonobese subjects when the duration of food deprivation is controlled. These varied studies and others suggested that the first of two requirements for the treatment of overeating must stress environmental management rather than self-control because the cues of overeating are environmental rather than intrapersonal.

The second requirement for the management of obesity must be a manipulation of the energy balance — the balance between the consumption of energy as food and the expenditure of energy through exercise. If all of the energy which is derived from the consumed food is expended in exercise, then gross body weight will remain constant. Any excess of food energy consumption over energy expenditure, however, is stored as adiposity at the rate of approximately one pound of body fat for each excessive 3500 kcal (Gordon, 1969, p. 148; Mayer, 1968, p. 158). Weight can therefore be lost through: (1) an increase in the amount of exercise, holding food intake constant; (2) a decrease in the amount of food intake, holding exercise constant; or (3) both an increase in exercise and a decrease in food intake.

It has been well demonstrated that the rising problem of obesity is associated with decreasing demands for exercise. Mayer (1968) suggested that "inactivity is the most important factor explaining the frequency of 'creeping' overweight in modern societies (p. 821)", while Durnin and Passmore (undated, p. 143) revealed that food intake is typically not adjusted to reduced exercise. Recent evidence adduced by the Agricultural Research Service (1969, pp. 22–24) demonstrated that the diets of young men in higher-income brackets include 20 per cent more kcal than the diets of those with smaller incomes and presumably more physically taxing occupations, and this is most likely to result in some measure of obesity among middle-class males. Increase in the rate of exercise can, however, have a profound effect upon body weight although the amount of exercise necessary is greater than generally expected.[4] Furthermore, given the fact that an obese person actually expends *less* energy than a nonobese person doing the same amount of work (e.g. a 250-pound man walking 1.5 mph expends 5.34 kcal per min, while a 150-pound man walking at the same rate and carrying a 100-pound load expends 5.75 kcal per min [Bloom and Eidex, 1967, p. 687]), planned programs for exercise are particularly important. In addition to aiding in the management of gross body weight, exercise programs for the

---

[4] Stuart (unpublished data) asked a group of obese women to estimate the amount of exercise required to work off the weight gain attributable to such common foods as donuts, ice-cream sodas and potato chips. Comparing their answers with the estimates based upon Konishi's (1965) figures for a 150-pound man walking at the rate of 3.5 miles per hr (29, 49 and 21 min respectively), they were found to underestimate the true work required from 200 to 300 per cent.

thin as well as the obese seem definitely to reduce the risk of certain cardiovascular diseases (Mayer, 1967).

Just as it is important systematically to increase the amount of exercise, so too is it important to reduce the amount of food or change the nature of foods eaten. Mayer (1968) recommends:

> A balanced diet, containing no less than 14 per cent of protein, no more than 30 per cent of fat (with saturated fats cut down), and the rest carbohydrates (with sucrose — ordinary sugar — cut down to a low level) . . . (p. 160).

Apart from its nutritional advantages, it is important to include a substantial amount of protein in the diet because smaller amounts of protein as opposed to carbohydrates produce satiety and because a portion of the caloric content of protein is used in its own metabolism (Gordon, 1969, p. 149), leaving a smaller proportion as a possible contributor to adiposity. Conversely, it is important to reduce the amount of carbohydrates consumed because a higher proportion of its caloric content is available for adiposity, because at least certain carbohydrates — e.g. sucrose (Yudkin, 1969) — are associated with increased incidence of certain cardiovascular diseases to which obese persons are vulnerable, and because "carbohydrate food causes the storage of unusually large amounts of water (Gordon, 1969, p. 148)" — typically a special problem faced by obese individuals.

The foregoing observations lead to several basic considerations for weight-reduction programs. First, it is essential to design an environment in which food-relevant cues are conducive to the maximal practice of prudent eating habits. This is required by the fact that overeating among obese persons appears to be under environmental control. Also, training the patient in the techniques of environmental control will probably reduce the gradual loss of therapeutic effect found in certain (e.g. Silverstone and Solomon, 1965) but not all (Penick et al., 1970) other programs. Second, it is essential to plan toward a negative energy balance. In doing this, however, it is essential to avoid exercise or dietary excesses. They are unlikely to be followed, and if they are followed each may result in iatrogenic complications. Excessive exercise might lead to overexertion or serious cardiovascular illness. Unbalanced diets might lead to physiological disease, while insufficient diets might lead to enervation and physiologically produced depression. It is therefore essential to plan gradual weight-loss programs associated with progressive changes in the energy balance, as these are both safer and more likely to meet with success (Wang and Sandoval, 1969, p. 220). The exact determination of these levels must be empirically determined for each patient, beginning with tables of recommended dietary allowance (e.g. Mayer, 1968, pp. 168—169), adjusting these for the amount of exercise, carefully monitoring weight and mood changes as time on the program progresses, and being careful to make certain that the degree of weight loss provides sufficient motivation for the patient to continue using the program.

Treatment

Translation of the above rationale into a set of specific treatment procedures sometimes requires an arbitrary selection of intervention alternatives derived from contrary or contradictory conclusions in the basic research literature. For example, while Gordon (1969) repudiated his earlier contention that a patient's eating several smaller meals each day would necessarily result in greater weight loss than his eating only the three traditional meals, others (e.g. Debry *et al.*, 1968) have shown that *with caloric intake held constant* patients who eat three meals daily may not only maintain their weight but actually gain weight, while the same patients dividing their caloric allowance into seven meals lose weight precipitously. As another example, Nisbett and Kanouse (1969) demonstrated that obese food shoppers actually buy less the more deprived of food they are while nonobese shoppers increase their food buying as a function of the extent of food deprivation. In contrast, Stuart (unpublished data) demonstrated that when a group of obese women confined their food shopping to the hours of 3:30–5:00 p.m., they purchased 20 per cent more food than when they postponed their food shopping until 6:30–8:00 p.m. Thus the therapist reading the Gordon and Nisbett studies would have his patients eat three meals and delay their food shopping until they were at least moderately deprived of food, while the therapist familiar with the work of Debry *et al.* and Stuart would do just the reverse. The therapist familiar with both must decide which recommendations to follow, framing his decision as a reversible hypothesis which can be invalidated in response to patient-produced data.

The treatment procedures which have been used in this investigation fall into three broad categories. First, an effort is made to establish firm control over the eating environment. This requires: (a) the elimination or suppression of cues associated with problematic eating while strengthening the cues associated with desirable eating patterns; (b) planned manipulation of the actual response of eating to accelerate desirable elements of the response while decelerating undesirable aspects; and (c) the manipulation of the contingencies associated with problematic and desirable eating patterns. A sample of the procedures used in the service of each of these objectives is presented in Table 1.

Second, an effort is made to establish a dietary program for each patient on an individual basis. The first step in the development of a diet is completion by the point of a self-monitoring food intake form. Because patients frequently claim to exist on unbelievably small quantities of food, only to lose weight rapidly when their diet is regulated at amounts two or three times greater than originally claimed, it is helpful to provide some social monitoring of the use of the monitoring sheets to ensure accuracy. Procedures such as those employed by Powell and Azrin (1968) have proven helpful. When validated eating records have been obtained for a 14-day period, adjustments in food intake can be planned based upon recommended caloric levels, balanced diet planning and adjustments for the level of food intake in light of the patient's exercise. In

Table 1. Sample procedures used to strengthen appropriate eating and to weaken inappropriate eating

Cue elimination	Cue suppression	Cue strengthening
1. Eat in one room only 2. Do nothing while eating 3. Make available proper foods only: (a) shop from a list; (b) shop only after full meal 4. Clear dishes directly into garbage 5. Allow children to take own sweets	1. Have company while eating 2. Prepare and serve small quantities only 3. Eat slowly 4. Save one item from meal to eat later 5. If high-calorie foods are eaten, they must require preparation	1. Keep food, weight chart 2. Use food exchange diet 3. Allow extra money for proper foods 4. Experiment with attractive preparation of diet foods 5. Keep available pictures of desired clothes, list of desirable activities

↓
Reduced strength
of undesirable responses

1. Swallow food already in mouth before adding more
2. Eat with utensils
3. Drink as little as possible during meals

↓
Provide decelerating
consequences

1. Develop means for display of caloric value of food eaten daily, weight changes
2. Arrange to have deviations from program ignored by others except for professionals
3. Arrange to have overeater re-read program when items have not been followed and to write techniques which might have succeeded

↓
Increase strength
of desirable responses

1. Introduce planned delays during meal
2. Chew food slowly, thoroughly
3. Concentrate on what is being eaten

↓
Provide accelerating consequences

1. Develop means for display of caloric value of food eaten daily, weight changes
2. Develop means of providing social feedback for all success by: (a) family; (b) friends; (c) co-workers; (d) other weight losers; and/or (e) professionals
3. Program material and/or social consequences to follow: (a) the attainment of weight loss subgoals; (b) completion of specific daily behavioral control objectives

dietary planning, "food exchange" recommendations are made (Stuart and Davis, 1971) rather than recommendations for specific food choices. In food exchange dieting, foods in each of six food categories (e.g. milk, fruit, meat, etc.) are grouped according to similar caloric levels (e.g. one egg has approximately the same caloric value as one slice of bread). Selections are made accordingly to food exchanges and this greatly increases the ease and precision of meal planning. Furthermore, when this is done as a means of increasing the probability that the diet will be followed, the unavailability of specific foods frequently leads to a termination of the entire dietary program.

Third, an effort is made to develop an individualized aerobics exercise program based upon walking in most cases (Cooper, 1968). In introducing the need for exercise, the patient is offered a choice between adherence to a punishing diet which may lead to chronic discomfort throughout the day and a more permissive diet coupled with exercise which may lead to discomfort for an hour or less per day. When an exercise program is developed, an effort is made to weave the exercise activity into the normal fabric of the patient's day to increase the likelihood that it will be followed. For example, a patient might be asked to park his car 10 blocks from the home of friends he is about to visit, to avoid elevators and walk up to his destinations, and to carry each item upstairs as needed — rather than allowing several items to accumulate — as a means of increasing the number of steps necessary.

Results

The pilot investigation reported here reflects the treatment of six overweight, married, middle-class women (171—212 pounds) between the ages of 27 and 41. Each woman requested treatment on a self-referred basis. Treatment was offered on an individual basis, but women were randomly assigned to one of two cohorts. Both groups of three patients were asked to complete the Sixteen Personality Factor Questionnaire (Cattell and Eber, 1967) and to keep a 5-week baseline of their weight and food intake. The first group was then offered treatment twice weekly (average 40 min per session) for a 15-week period, while the second group was asked to practice "self-control" of eating behavior. The self-control subjects were given the same diet planning materials and ·exercise program that the treatment group was offered. They were not, however, given instruction for the management of food in the environment. At the conclusion of the 15-week period, the treated group was asked to continue the treatment program and the second group was offered 15 weeks of the same treatment. Approximately 6 months following the termination of treatment of Group 1 and 3 months following the termination of treatment of Group 2, follow-up data were collected including weight, eating patterns and the readministration of the Cattell 16 P.F. The results including follow-up data are presented in Fig. 1. It will be seen that patients in Group 1 lost an average of 35 pounds while those in Group 2 lost an average of 21 pounds. These results are consistent with the objective set for gradual weight loss approximating one pound per week. It will also be seen that the mere collection of baseline self-monitoring data was associated with mild weight loss in both groups, although these gains were dissipated as time progressed for the second group. Finally, comparison of the pre- and post-test personality test results reveal little change other than small improvement in "ego stability" and tension (Factors C and Q4) of the 16 P.F.

The results provide suggestive evidence for the usefulness of a threefold treatment of obesity stressing environmental control of overeating, nutritional planning and regulated increase in energy expenditure. The sample size was too small to permit generalization, and the superiority of the initially treated (Group 1) over the initially untreated (Group 2) patients may be due to an inclination among the latter group to be casual about weight reduction. To forestall this possibility, every effort was made to make the treatment appear "official" but no validation of the success of this effort was undertaken. Furthermore, it is perhaps noteworthy that the results were obtained with no evidence of psycho-

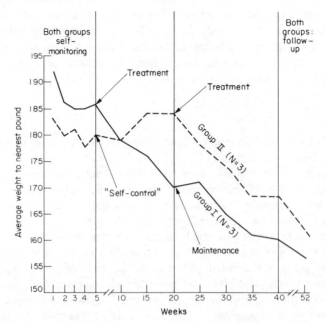

FIG. 1. Weight changes in two groups of women undergoing
behavior therapy for overeating.

logical stress in a patient population which was regarded as "well-adjusted" at
the start and termination of treatment.

To validate these procedures in any definitive manner, extensive replication is
needed using careful experimental control procedures applied to a far more
diverse population than was used in this pilot study. Research such as that
recently completed by Penick *et al.* (1970) has made important strides in this
direction. It is only through experimentation that the vast amount of "faddism
and quackery (Gordon, 1969, p. 148)" which characterizes the broad field of
obesity control can be replaced by a scientifically validated set of procedures.

References

AGRICULTURAL RESEARCH SERVICE, U.S. DEPARTMENT OF AGRICULTURE
(1969) *Food Intake and Nutritive Value of Diets of Men, Women and Children in the
United States, Spring* 1965: *A Preliminary Report.* (ARS 61–18), Washington, D.C.:
United States Government Printing Office.
AMERICAN ACADEMY OF PEDIATRICS, COMMITTEE ON NUTRITION (1967) Obesity
in childhood. *Pediatrics* **40**, 455–465.
BANDURA, A. and KUPERS, C. J. (1964) Transmission of patterns of self-reinforcement
through modeling. *J. abnorm. soc. Psychol.* **69**, 1–9.
BERNARD, J. L. (1968) Rapid treatment of gross obesity by operant techniques. *Psychol.
Rep.* **23**, 663–666.
BIJOU, S. W. and BAER, D. M. (1961) *Child Development I: A Systematic and Empirical
Theory.* Appleton-Century-Crofts, New York.

BLOOM, W. L. and EIDEX, M. F. (1967) The comparison of energy expenditure in the obese and lean. *Metabolism* 16, 685–692.

BORTZ, W. (1969) A 500 pound weight loss. *Am. J. Med.* 47, 325–331.

BRAY, G. A. (1969) Effect of caloric restriction on energy expenditure in obese patients. *Lancet* 2, 397–398.

BRUCH, H. (1964) The psychosomatic aspects of obesity. *Am. Practnr. Dig. Treat.* 5, 48–49.

CAPPON, D. (1958) Obesity. *Can. Med. Assoc. Jl* 79, 568–573.

CATTELL, R. B. and EBER, H. W. (1957) *Handbook for the Sixteen Personality Factor Questionnaire.* The Institute for Personality and Ability Testing, Champaign, Ill.

CAUFFMAN, W. J. and PAULEY, W. G. (1961) Obesity and emotional status. *Penn. Med. Jl.* 64, 505–507.

CAUTELA J. R. (1967) Covert sensitization. *Psychol. Rep.* 20, 459–468.

CAUTELA, J. R. (1969) Behavior therapy and self-control: Techniques and implications. In *Behavior Therapy: Appraisal and Status* (Ed. C. M. FRANKS). McGraw-Hill, New York.

CONRAD, S. W. (1954) The problem of weight reduction in the obese woman. *Am. Practnr. Dig. Treat.* 5, 38–47.

COOPER, K. H. (1968) *Aerobics.* Bantam Books, New York.

CORNELL CONFERENCES ON THERAPY (1958) The management of obesity. *N. Y. S. J. Med.* 58, 79–87.

DEBRY, G., ROHR, R., AZOUAOU, G., VASSILITCH, I. and MOTTAZ, G. (1968) Study of the effect of dividing the daily caloric intake into seven meals on weight loss in obese subjects. *Nutritio Dieta* 10, 288–296.

DURNIN, J. V. G. A. and PASSMORE, R. (undated) The relation between the intake and expenditure of energy and body weight. *Problemes Actuels D'Endocrinologie et de Nutrition* (Serie No. 9), 136–149.

FERSTER, C. B. (1965) Classification of behavior pathology. In *Research in Behavior Modification* (Eds. L. KRASNER and L. P. ULLMANN). Holt, Rinehart & Winston, New York.

FRANKLIN, R. E. and RYNEARSON, E. H. (1960) An evaluation of the effectiveness of diet instruction for the obese. *Staff Meet. Mayo Clin.* 35, 123–124.

GLUCKSMAN, M. L., HIRSCH, J., McCULLY, R. S., BARRON, B. A. and KNITTLE, J. L. (1968) The response of obese patients to weight reduction: A quantitative evaluation of behavior. *Psychosom. Med.* 30, 359–373.

GORDON, E. S. (1969) The present concept of obesity: Etiological factors and treatment. *Med. Times* 97, 142–155.

HAMBURGER, W. W. (1951) Emotional aspects of obesity. *Med. Clin. N. Am.* 35, 483–499.

HANLEY, F. W. (1967) The treatment of obesity by individual and group hypnosis. *Can. Psychiat. Ass. J.* 12, 549–551.

HARRIS, M. B. (1969) Self-directed program for weight control—A pilot study, *J. abnorm. Psychol.* 74, 263–270.

HASHIM, S. A. and VAN ITALLIE, T. B. (1965) Studies in normal and obese subjects with a monitored food dispensary device. *Ann. N. Y. Acad. Sci.* 131, 654–661.

HOLLAND, J. G. and SKINNER, B. F. (1961) *The Analysis of Behavior.* McGraw-Hill, New York.

HOMME, L. E. (1965) Perspectives in psychology: XXIV. Control of coverants, the operants of the mind. *Psychol. Rec.* 15, 501–511.

KANFER, F. H. (1971) Self-monitoring: Methodological limitations and clinical applications. *J. consult. clin. Psychol.* in press.

KANFER, F. H. and MARSTON, A. R. (1963) Conditioning of self-reinforcement responses: An analogue to self-confidence training. *Psychol. Rep.* 13, 63–70.

KAPLAN, H. I. and KAPLAN, H. S. (1957) The psychosomatic concept of obesity. *J. nerv. ment. Dis.* 125, 181–201.

KONISHI, F. (1965) Food energy equivalents of various activities. *J. Am. Diet. Ass.* 46, 186–188.

KORNHABER, A. (1968) Group treatment of obesity. *G.P.* 5, 116–120.

KROGER, W. S. (1970) Comprehensive management of obesity. *Am. J. clin. Hypnosis* 12, 165–176.

MACCUISH, A. C., MUNRO, J. F. and DUNCAN, L. J. P. (1968) Follow-up study of refractory obesity treated by fasting. *Br. Med.* 1, 91–92.

MAYER, J. (1967) Inactivity, an etiological factor in obesity and heart disease. In *Symposia of the Swedish Nutrition Foundation, V: Symposium on Nutrition and Physical Activity* (Ed. G. BLIX). Almqvist & Wiksells, Uppsala, Sweden.

MAYER, J. (1968) *Overweight: Causes, Cost and Control.* Prentice-Hall, Englewood Cliffs, N.J.

MEES, H. L. and KEUTZER, C. S. (1967) Short term group psychotherapy with obese women. *NW Med.* 66, 548–550.

METROPOLITAN INSURANCE COMPANY (1969) New weight standards for men and women. *Statistical Bulletin* 40, 1–8.

MEYER, V. and CRISP, A. H. (1964) Aversion therapy in two cases of obesity. *Behav. Res. & Therapy* 2, 143–147.

MODELL, W. (1960) Status and prospect of drugs for overeating. *J. Am. Med. Ass.* 173, 1131–1136.

NEWBURGH, L. H. and JOHNSTON, M. W. (1930) The nature of obesity. *J. clin. Invest.* 8, 197–213.

NISBETT, R. E. (1968) Taste, deprivation, and weight determinants of eating behavior. *J. person. soc. Psychol.* 10, 107–116.

NISBETT, R. E. and KANOUSE, D. E. (1969) Obesity, food deprivation, and supermarket shopping behavior. *J. person. soc. Psychol.* 12, 289–294.

PENICK, S. B., FILION, R., FOX, S. and STUNKARD, A. (1970) Behavior modification in the treatment of obesity. Paper presented at the annual meeting of the Psychosomatic Society, Washington, D.C.

POWELL, J. and AZRIN, N. (1968) The effects of shock as a punisher for cigarette smoking. *J. Appl. Behav. Anal.* 1, 63–71.

RAMSAY, R. W. (1968) Vermageringsexperiment, Psychologisch Labratorium van de Universiteit van Amsterdam, *Researchpracticum* 101, voorjaar 1968.

SCHACHTER, S. (1968) Obesity and eating. *Science* 161, 751–756.

SCHACHTER, S., GOLDMAN, R. and GORDON, A. (1968) Effects of fear, food deprivation, and obesity on eating. *J. person. soc. Psychol.* 10, 91–97.

SCHACHTER, S. and GROSS, L. P. (1968) Manipulated time and eating behavior. *J. person. soc. Psychol.* 10, 98–106.

SELTZER, C. C. and MAYER, J. (1965) A simple criterion of obesity. *Postgrad. Med.* 38, A101–A106.

SHIPMAN, W. G. and PLESSET, M. R. (1963) Anxiety and depression in obese dieters. *Archs gen. Psychiat.* 8, 26–31.

SILVERSTONE, J. T. and SOLOMON, T. (1965) The long-term management of obesity in general practice. *Br. J. clin. Pract.* 19, 395–398.

SIMON, R. I. (1963) Obesity as a depressive equivalent. *J. Am. Med. Ass.* 183, 208–210.

STANLEY, E. J., GLASER, H. H., LEVIN, D. G., ADAMS, P. A. and COOLEY, I. C. (1970) Overcoming obesity in adolescents: A description of a promising endeavour to improve management. *Clin. Pediat.* 9, 29–36.

STOKES, S. A. (1969) Fasting for obesity. *Am. J. Nurs.* 69, 796–799.

STUART, R. B. (1967) Behavioral control of overeating. *Behav. Res. & Therapy* 5, 357–365.

STUART, R. B. (1971) Situational versus self control. In *Advances in Behavior Therapy* (Ed. R. D. RUBIN). Academic Press, New York, in press.

STUART, R. B. and DAVIS, B. (1971) *Behavioral Techniques for the Management of Obesity.* Research Press, Champaign, Ill., in press.

STUNKARD, A. (1959a) Eating patterns and obesity. *Psychiat. Q.* 33, 284–295.

STUNKARD, A. (1959b) Obesity and the denial of hunger. *Psychosom. Med.* 21, 281–289.

STUNKARD, A. (1968) Environment and obesity: Recent advances in our understanding of regulation of food intake in man. *Fed. Proc.* 6 1367–1373.

STUNKARD, A., LEVINE, H. and FOX, S. (1970) The management of obesity. *Archs intern. Med.* **125**, 1067–1072.

STUNKARD, A. and McLAREN-HUME, M. (1959) The results of treatment for obesity. *Archs intern. Med.* **103** 79–85.

SUCZEK, R. F. (1957) The personality of obese women. *Am. J. Clin. Nutr.* **5**, 197–202.

UNITED STATES PUBLIC HEALTH SERVICE (undated) *Obesity and Health*. (Publication No. 1495), United States Department of Health, Education and Welfare, Washington, D.C.

UNITED STATES SENATE, SELECT COMMITTEE ON NUTRITION AND HUMAN NEEDS (1970) *Nutrition and Human Needs*–1970. Parts I, II & III. U.S. Government Printing Office, Washington, D.C.

WAGONFIELD, S. and WOLOWITZ, H. M. (1968) Obesity and self-help group: A look at TOPS. *Am. J. Psychiat.* **125**, 253–255.

WANG, R. I. H. and SANDOVAL, R. (1969) Current status of drug therapy in management of obesity. *Wis. Med. J.* **68**, 219–220.

YUDKIN, J. (Spring, 1969) Sucrose and heart disease. *Nutrition Today* **4**, 16–20.

CHAPTER 36

Effectiveness of Group Therapy Based upon Learning Principles in the Treatment of Overweight Women[1]

JANET P. WOLLERSHEIM[2]

University of Illinois

Summary— Following an 18-wk. base-line period, 79 motivated overweight female students were randomly assigned from stratified blocks, on percentage overweight, to one of four experimental conditions: (a) positive expectation—social pressure; (b) nonspecific therapy; (c) focal therapy based upon major learning principles; or (d) no-treatment—wait-control. Four therapists (two males and two females) each treated one group of 5 Ss in each of the three treatment conditions for 10 sessions extending over a 12-wk. period. At both posttreatment and the 8-wk. follow-up, the focal group was superior in weight reduction and reduction of reported frequencies of various eating behaviors. Evidence for "symptom substitution" was lacking. While significant differential weight reduction occurred for the various treatments, it did not occur for the different therapists or for the various therapist-treatment combinations.

One of the major difficulties encountered in conducting psychotherapy outcome research is the selection of a dependent variable which not only can be objectively measured, but which also represents a relevant criterion of change. The treatment of obesity involving designation of actual body weight as the dependent variable represents a measure which is not only completely objective, but which also thoroughly defines the criterion, as reduction in body weight represents the primary and specific goal of treatment. Additionally, since obesity is a condition which affects from 23% to 68% of women in the United States (United States Department of Health, Education, and Welfare, 1967), it constitutes a significant health problem which in its own right should merit serious attention.

Reprinted with permission from the *Journal of Abnormal Psychology*, 1970, 76, 462–474.

[1] This article is based upon a dissertation submitted in partial fulfillment of requirements for the Ph.D. at the University of Illinois. Gratitutde is expressed to Gordon L. Paul, dissertation chairman, and to the other committee members, John S. Werry, Leonard P. Ullmann, Donald R. Peterson, Merle B. Karnes, and Wesley C. Becker for their support and valuable suggestions.

[2] Requests for reprints should be sent to the author, who is now at the University of Missouri, Department of Psychology, University of Missouri, Columbia, Missouri 65201.

While psychology and psychiatry have contributed a plethora of theories concerning the cause of obesity, the majority of these theories (Alexander & Flagg, 1965; Bruch, 1963; Fenichel, 1945) view obesity and overeating as a symptom of some underlying "psychic abnormality" and imply or directly contend that treatment must focus upon the underlying cause. Emphasis has been placed upon the presumed deviant personality characteristics which distinguish overweight from normal weight individuals. These deviant personality characteristics together with the symptom of overeating are then construed as a basic syndrome which must be treated by dealing with the presumed underlying causes.

Yet, on the basis of a recent review of the relevant literature, as well as from the evidence of an assessment study which they conducted, Wollersheim, Paul, and Werry[3] concluded that while from a physiological point of view, obesity may result from multiple etiologies, overeating has been the only behavioral or personality characteristic consistently distinguishing the obese from the nonobese. In the great majority of cases, successful weight reduction would depend upon reducing the positive energy balance which results from overweight individuals simply *eating too much* for their activity level.

Of the hundreds of papers published on the treatment of obesity, few give even slight attention to specifically helping the client learn to modify his eating practices, although some professionals have stressed the importance of directly focusing upon a change in eating practices (Ferster, Nurnberger, & Levitt, 1962; Goldiamond, 1965). Even more discouraging is the fact that the overwhelming majority of studies fail to meet even minimal standards of experimental control and scientific reporting, making it impossible to replicate the study or to make definitive statements concerning treatment. In the most comprehensive review of the treatment of obesity, covering the medical literature for the previous 30 yr., Stunkard and McLaren-Hume (1959) found that, in general, only 25% of patients lost a significant amount of weight. A review of group attempts at weight reduction yielded nearly identical results (see Suczek, 1955). More precise estimates of the results of treatment are precluded because of the unfortunate state of affairs characterizing this literature. Investigators have been further discouraged by high attrition rates showing that from 20% to 80% of patients beginning weight reduction programs abandoned them before completion (see Stunkard, 1957).

The theoretical orientation of this study derives from learning principles and views eating behavior and *overeating* as essentially similar to any other learned behavior patterns in terms of development, maintenance, and change (see Ullmann & Krasner, 1965). While behavior modification techniques derived from learning principles are becoming more popular among psychologists, even within

3 J. P. Wollersheim, G. L. Paul, & J. S. Wherry. Correlates of obesity: Clarification and suggestions for treatment. Manuscript in preparation.

the learning principles framework, experimental studies designed to establish cause-effect relationships between treatment procedures and weight loss have been lacking.

The primary purpose of this investigation was to develop a group therapy program for obesity based upon learning principles and to evaluate the effectiveness of this program in an experimental design including adequate control groups which would control for the effects of time, season, and intercurrent life experiences (i.e., no treatment); nonspecific effects of undergoing treatment, such as attention, "faith," rational conceptualizations, "ritual," and expectation of relief (i.e., non-specific treatment); and a control for positive expectation and social pressure, minimizing other nonspecific effects. This latter type of control group is viewed as desirable in an obesity study as the elements of positive expectation and social pressure appear to be the major ingredients in the nationwide Take Off Pounds Sensibly (TOPS) weight-reducing clubs (see Toch, 1965), which, to the best of the investigator's knowledge, have not been evaluated by controlled investigations.

Method

DESIGN AND PROCEDURE

The general experimental design and procedure are presented in Fig. 1. Seventy-nine motivated, overweight female Ss completed an assessment battery, including body weight, at the beginning and end of an 18-wk. base-line period. Following the second assessment, Ss were randomly assigned from stratified blocks, on percentage overweight, to one of four experimental conditions: (a) positive expectation-social pressure (SP); (b) nonspecific therapy (NS); (c) focal therapy (FT); (d) no-treatment–wait-control (C). Since percentage overweight, rather than actual weight, is indicative of degree of obesity, this procedure insured equating the degree of obesity across experimental conditions. Four

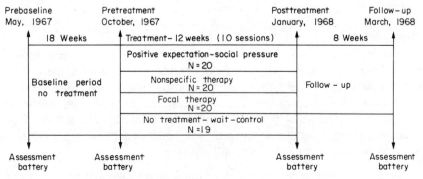

FIG. 1. General experimental design and procedure

therapists (two males and two females) each treated one group of 5 Ss in each of the three treatment conditions for a total of 10 sessions spanning a period of 12 wk. (mid-October to mid-January). Treatment sessions within all conditions were designed such that any S could miss one session without missing new material. The relative efficacy of the treatments in producing weight loss and changes in eating patterns was then evaluated on the basis of posttreatment and an 8-wk. follow-up administration of the assessment battery.

ASSESSMENT INSTRUMENTS

The assessment battery administered at the four assessment periods included: height (to the nearest inch without shoes) and weight (to the nearest pound in indoor clothing without shoes) obtained on standard physician's balance scales; an Eating Patterns Questionnaire (EPQ; see footnote 3), providing historical data on obesity and yielding six factor scores concerning specific eating practices (Factor 1 — emotional and uncontrolled overeating; Factor 2 — eating response to interpersonal situations; Factor 3 — eating in isolation; Factor 4 — eating as reward; Factor 5 — eating response to evaluative situations; Factor 6 — between-meal eating); Wollersheim *et al.*'s (see footnote 3) modification of Schifferes' (1966) Physical Activity Scale, yielding a 5-point classification of activity level (1, sedentary, to 5, exceptionally active) based upon reported frequency of six specific types of activities during a 24-hr. period; the Pittsburg Social Extra-version-Introversion Scale (Bendig, 1962); the IPAT Anxiety Scale Questionnaire (Cattell, 1957); and 10 situation-specific anxiety scales ("Speech Before a Large Group", "Job Interview", "Final Course Examination", "Night Before Big Dance", "Entering Lecture Hall for Large Class", "Discussing College Experience with Parents", "Talking to Attractive Boy at Party", "Chatting with Girl Friends", "Home Watching TV on Saturday Night", "Doing Homework in Study Area"), following the format of the S-R Inventory of Anxiousness (Endler, Hunt, & Rosenstein, 1962). In addition, at the termination of treatment, Ss rated therapist competence and likeability.

Therapists

Four therapists (two males and two females), including the investigator, participated in the study.[4] All were Ph.D. candidates in clinical psychology who had completed all clinical training and preliminary examination requirements at the time of the investigation. Each therapist had at least 2 yr. supervised experience in conducting psychotherapy (both individuals and group). Their orientations were cognitive-behavioral, with formulations of psychotherapy based upon learning principles being influential.

[4]Gratitude is expressed to Judy Martin, Robert Marx, and Ralph Trimble who served as therapists for this research.

Treatment

Each *S* assigned to positive expectation — social pressure, nonspecific, or focal treatment — was treated in a closed group of 5. All therapists understood that the criterion of improvement was to be weight reduction. Each of the four therapists treated one group of 5 *S*s within each treatment, for a total of 15 *S*s each, therefore holding constant potentially important effects of therapist characteristics such as sex, personality, and physical attributes.

Prior to treatment contact, each therapist studied four treatment manuals[5] written for this project by the investigator and met for a total of 7 hr. of intensive training in the specific treatment conditions. The "Therapist General Orientation Manual for Weight Reduction Study" described the purpose of the investigation, presented an overview of each treatment condition, and detailed procedures common to all forms of group therapy which were to be used in all three treatments.

Besides the General Orientation Manual, therapists were provided with a manual for each of the three treatment conditions which explicitly delineated all procedures to be followed, including the time to be spent in various activities and the rationale to be given *S*s. All therapy sessions within each treatment were recorded and monitored weekly by the investigator to insure consistent and appropriate application of procedures.

The *S*s in all treatment conditions were presented the same factual information pertaining to obesity, health, nutrition, and weight reduction, and all were told that successful weight reduction depended upon either increased activity or decreased caloric intake. Additionally, *S*s in all three treatment conditions were urged to decrease their caloric intake to between 1000 and 1500 calories daily, in a manner appropriate to their general living circumstances. They were encouraged to lose 2 lb. a week by reducing their caloric intake and were provided with identical booklets listing the caloric value of over 2600 foods. Students in each treatment were told that they were assigned to the treatment in which they should be most successful, on the basis of personality characteristics. Sessions for the positive expectation — social pressure treatment were limited to 15–20 min., while nonspecific and focal sessions were 90 min. each.

POSITIVE EXPECTATION–SOCIAL PRESSURE (GROUP SP)

The main purpose of SP treatment was to foster in *S*s a high positive expectation for losing weight and to *foster* and *use* social pressure in helping

[5] The four treatment manuals have been deposited with the National Auxiliary Publications Service. Order Document No. 01251 from the National Auxiliary Publications Service of the American Society for Information Science, c/o CCM Information Sciences, Inc., 909 3rd Avenue, New York, New York 10022. Remit in advance $5.00 for photocopies or $2.00 for microfiche and make checks payable to Research and Microfilm Publications, Inc.

each *S* reduce. The rationale presented to *S*s assigned to this treatment was that the outstanding variable to which success could be attributed is the motivational one, that is, the fact that *S* makes a commitment to lose weight and has a group of fellow students and the therapist checking upon the outcome of this commitment in terms of weekly "weigh-ins" before the group. Each session consisted of weighing each *S* before the group, announcing her weight, and noting her loss or gain from the previous week. The therapist and group administered mild negative reinforcers (e.g., "What a shame!") and encouragement (e.g. "But you'll show us next week, won't you?") for weight gains and positive reinforcers (e.g., "This gal is really going places!") for weight losses. Those who gained weight from the previous week were required to wear a red tag drawn in the form of a pig throughout the session. Those whose weight remained constant wore a green sign reading "TURTLE", while yellow stars were worn by those who lost weight. The member who lost the most weight that week wore a star and a crown.

After the "weigh-ins", commendations and "playful ribbing" were continued, or group discussions centered upon factual questions relating to obesity, health, nutrition, or weight loss. If *S*s began to inquire about specific ways to decrease overeating, the therapist emphasized that the important thing was to reduce daily caloric intake and that each person should do this in a manner appropriate to her particular living circumstances. In the event the group discussion continued on the topic of specific ways to reduce overeating, the therapist diverted attention away from this topic by posing questions or commenting upon factual information concerning obesity, nutrition, or weight reduction.

NONSPECIFIC THERAPY (GROUP NS)

The main purpose of this treatment was, at the minimum, to control for effects of undergoing group treatment resulting from such nonspecific factors as increased attention, "faith", expectation of relief, and presentation of a treatment rationale and meaningful "ritual". The rationale presented to *S*s assigned to this treatment was that it would be important for them to develop insight into the "real and not readily recognizable underlying reasons" for their behavior and to discover the "unconscious motives" underlying their "personality make-up." It was explained that as each individual obtained insight and better understanding of the "real motives and forces" operating within her personality, she would find it easier to accomplish her goals and to lose weight.

The first 15–20 min. of these sessions employed the procedures used in the SP treatment. The next 20–30 min. were devoted to a control use of relaxation training following the training procedures reported by Paul and Shannon (1966), with the rationale being to help *S*s feel at ease so they could "better develop insight". The remaining 40–55 min. of NS therapy sessions were devoted to discussion focused upon hypothetical *underlying causes* for their behavior, not only in the area of eating, but broadly extending into other areas as well. Historical elaboration was encouraged rather than emphasizing current events. In order to structure this treatment condition to provide an internally consistent conceptual framework which would be maximally specific and acceptable to Ss, therapy procedures utilized a psychoanalytically oriented game model superficially similar to that of Eric Berne's (1964).[6] "Games" were introduced as a way of more clearly conceptualizing the underlying causes of behavior. In the NS treatment, discussion frequently strayed from a game model, obesity, and any current behavior to such topics as movies seen or an experience one had with a grade school teacher. If group discussion turned to specific ways to modify eating patterns, the therapist used his clinical skill in diverting the group's attention away from overt behavior and to underlying causes and historical material. The treatment manual provided 22 suggested games as well as specific interpretive principles to be applied.

FOCAL THERAPY (GROUP F)

The major purpose of this treatment was to identify and shape current eating behavior by applying techniques derived from learning principles. The Ss receiving this treatment were told that their eating practices were learned patterns of behavior. Just as they had learned inappropriate eating patterns, they could, by application of appropriate principles, learn appropriate eating practices which would promote weight loss and make effective maintenance of the loss possible. Extensive use was made of instrumental learning techniques.

Procedures used in the SP treatment were employed during the first 15–20 min. of each session, followed by a discussion period lasting from 40 to 55 min. The remaining 20–30 min. were devoted to training and instruction in the use of deep relaxation after Paul and Shannon (1966). Unlike the control use of relaxation in Group NS, Ss were told that learning to become deeply relaxed was a skill, and that as they learned this skill they would be instructed in how to use relaxation to counter tension in many situations which in the past might have typically resulted in eating behavior.

During the discussion phase of the first session, Ss were instructed in methods of recording their eating behavior in a small notebook provided for this purpose. In the following sessions, references were made to the eating records to provide a basis for individual functional analyses of stimuli controlling eating behavior. The first half of the discussion phase in Session 2–6 was devoted to a review of techniques already presented and discussed in previous sessions, with the second half used to introduce new techniques. The therapist's most important task was to help each S specifically identify discriminative, reinforcing, and eliciting stimuli related to overeating and to implement self-control techniques in the

---

[6]Grateful acknowledgment is made to the late D. C. Ober for suggesting the use of a game model in NS treatment.

circumstances arising in her individual mode of living. The following is a synopsis of the techniques introduced in each session: Session 1 — building positive associations concerning eating control; Session 2 — developing appropriate stimulus control of eating behavior and manipulation of deprivation and satiation by shaping and fading; Session 3 — rewarding oneself for developing self-control in eating, and developing and using personally meaningful ultimate aversive consequences of overeating; Session 4 — obtaining reinforcers from areas of life other than eating and establishing alternative behaviors incompatible with eating; Session 5 — utilization of chaining; Session 6 — supplementary techniques involving aversive imagery. All techniques were introduced and discussed by the end of the sixth session, with the remaining four sessions devoted to continued discussion of each Ss utilization of the techniques and the correction of misunderstandings and misapplications.

NO-TREATMENT–WAIT–CONTROL (GROUP C)

The major purpose of this condition was to provide control for such factors as intercurrent life experiences, time of year, effects of testing and other potentially influential variables not related to treatment *per se*. The Ss in this condition followed the same procedures, under the same conditions, as Ss in the treatment groups, with the exception of treatment itself. A few days before their first scheduled group session, Ss were contacted by telephone and told that because of unexpected increase in clinical and research responsibilities, Dr. _____ , their therapist, was unable to serve in the program. They were assured, however, that treatment would be definitely provided for them the following semester as soon as therapist time became available. At the time of posttreatment assessment, the investigator contacted these Ss by telephone and told them that treatment would be available, but it would first be necessary to again take the assessment battery. After these posttreatment measures were taken, these Ss were given treatment and hence were not available for the 8-wk. follow-up assessment.

SUBJECTS

A total of 79 female students at the University of Illinois ranging in age from 18 to 36 yr. (*Mdn* = 19) participated in the study. These Ss were selected on motivation for treatment and percentage overweight from a population requesting treatment for obesity, following announcement of program availability in the university newspaper and bulletin boards. The weight criteria were based upon the 1959 Metropolitan Life Insurance Company norms for desirable weight for women (United States Department of Health, Education, and Welfare, 1967). Desirable weight was determined by taking the lowest weight given for a person of medium frame and 2 in. taller than the S in the Metropolitan norms.[7] A woman was considered overweight only if her actual weight was *at least* 10% above her desirable weight at the time of initial contact (i.e., pre-base line).

Students were further screened for motivation by attendance at pretreatment assessment and a consequent brief interview (10—15 min.) with the investigator. The purpose of the interview was to establish common expectations for all *S*s and to exclude those who felt they did not overeat, were not sufficiently concerned to attend weekly sessions, or those who were currently receiving any type of psychotherapy or treatment for weight reduction.

The average percentage overweight of the resulting sample of 70 *S*s at pre-base line was 28.63%, ranging from 10% to 70%. These *S*s reported continuous obesity for 1—24 yr. (*Mdn* = 5 yr.). All *S*s reported unsuccessful attempts to lose weight, with 76% of the sample reporting nearly continuous attempts at weight reduction which resulted in considerable discouragement. In general, these *S*s were characteristic of the "hard core" group of obese persons discussed in the literature (see Mendelson, 1966; National Dairy Council, 1965; Young, Berresford, & Moore, 1957) in that most had been obese since childhood or adolescence and the degree of obesity was considerable with many previous unsuccessful attempts at weight reduction which resulted in significant discouragement. The fact that *S*s were all female was also an unfavorable prognostic indicator (see Stunkard & McLaren-Hume, 1959).

Results

ATTRITION

Of the 70 *S*s participating in the study at pretreatment (20 *S*s in each of the treatment groups and 19 *S*s in the control group), 76 remained at posttreatment (Group F lost 2 and Group C 1). The attrition rate was less than 4% for the total sample. The amount of attrition was not significant, as evaluated by Fisher's test of exact probability for all possible combinations of the four experimental groups (all *p*s > .21). At follow-up, only 3 treated *S*s (2 from Group SP and 1 from Group NS) were lost as they had left school. The *S*s not available for postassessment were dropped from all subsequent analyses, with the consequent *N* for the total sample being 76. The *N* for each group was as follows: SP = 20; NS = 20; F = 18; C = 18. Analyses involving follow-up data involved a total *N* of 55 (SP = 18; NS = 19, F = 18).

---

[7]The lower end of the weight range was appropriate for determining desirable weight since the Metropolitan norms are for women over age 25 who are expected to weigh more than the younger women in the present sample where only three were age 25 or over. Two inches were added to height as the Metropolitan norms are based upon height measurements taken with shoes on and *S*s height was measured with shoes off in the present study. This procedure tended to make the estimate of the degree of obesity conservative.

COMPARATIVE TREATMENT EFFECTS: WEIGHT

Detailed analyses of actual weight and percentage overweight demonstrated that the four experimental groups were equated on these variables at pre-base line and pretreatment and that there were no significant changes in these measures over the base-line period (Wollersheim, 1968, p. 211).

Major analyses on· actual weight and the other assessment measures were performed on the basis of residual change scores for each S, consisting of the difference between the obtained score at posttreatment and that predicted on the basis of multiple linear regression from pre-base line and pretreatment, thus providing a base-free measure of change (see DuBois, 1957). Since the sample of Ss changed from posttreatment to follow-up because of the loss of control Ss and three treated Ss, separate residual change scores were computed for post-treatment and follow-up data, using pre-base line and pretreatment to predict posttreatment scores with a sample of 76 and using pre-base line and pretreatment to predict follow-up scores with a sample of 55.

The means and standard deviations of the four groups on actual weight at pre-base line, pretreatment, posttreatment, and follow-up are presented in Table 1. Results from the one-way analysis of variance on treatments on post-

TABLE 1. Means and standard deviations of experimental groups for actual weight across all time periods

	Group											
Time	Social pressure			Nonspecific			Focal			Control		
	M	SD	N	M	SD	N	M	SD	N	M	SD	N
Pre-base line	157.80	21.15	20	161.35	25.29	20	154.11	18.70	18	157.72	22.58	18
Pretreatment	160.15	23.91	20	159.20	25.13	20	153.61	19.06	18	156.39	22.54	18
Posttreatment	154.75a	22.44	20	152.30b	21.03	20	143.28ab	16.69	18	158.78ab	28.40	18
Follow-up	156.61a	23.24	18	152.68b	18.72	19	145.00ab	16.11	18	–	–	–

Note:– Subscript symbols refer to means which differ significantly in residual change score analyses. If any two means within a row share the same symbol, it means that significantly different changes from pretreatment were revealed ($p < 0.5$, Duncan's multi-range test).

residual change scores are presented in Table 2. The treatment effect for actual weight was highly significant ($p < .001$), indicating differential changes between groups. For the measures of actual weight, ratings involving rate reduction, and the factor scores on eating practices, differences between treatment means were tested with a more refined analysis utilizing Duncan's multiple-range tests, corrected for unequal Ns (Kramer, 1956) with α equal to .05, using one-tailed comparisons for differences in the hypothesized direction. (The hypothesized order of treatment effects for weight was that most weight reduction would be shown by Group F, then Group NS, then Group SP, and then Group C. For factor scores on eating practices, the hypothesized order of treatment effects was that most reduction· in reported frequency of eating behaviors would be shown by Group F, followed by Group NS or SP and then Group C.)

TABLE 2. One-way analyses of variance on postresidual change scores for actual weight, eating patterns questionnaire factor scores, and physical activity scale (PAS)

Measure	Source	df	MS	F
			Analyses	
Weight	Treatment	3	524.64	11.58***
	error	72	46.49	
Factor 1 (Emotional and uncontrolled overeating)	Treatment	3	527.09	6.01**
	error	72	87.65	
Factor 2 (Eating response to interpersonal situations)	Treatment	3	23.18	1.46
	error	72	15.92	
Factor 3 (Eating in isolation)	Treatment	3	107.99	9.87***
	error	72	10.95	
Factor (Eating as reward)	Treatment	3	25.10	3.49*
	error	72	7.20	
Factor 5 (Eating response to evaluative situations)	Treatment	3	2.19	.29
	error	72	7.46	
Factor 6 (Eating between meals)	Treatment	3	33.53	4.38**
	error	72	7.65	
PAS	Treatment	3	.89	2.08
	error	72	.43	

Note.—N = 76.
*$p < .05$.
**$p < .01$.
***$p < .001$.

Duncan's tests on postresidual change score treatment means showed that all three treatment groups evidenced significant weight reduction in contrast to Group C. Additionally, Group F differed significantly from Group NS and Group SP, while the latter two did not differ significantly from each other (Wollersheim, 1968, pp. 44–50). An additional analysis of variance demonstrated that therapist and therapist-by-treatment effects were nonsignificant (Wollersheim, 1968, p. 223).

Further analyses showed a slight increase in weight for all groups from posttreatment to follow-up (Wollersheim, 1968, p. 227). However, from posttreatment to follow-up, there were no significant differential weight changes by treatments or therapist-treatment groups.

Residual change scores of treated Ss at follow-up were subjected to a two-way analysis of variance, summarized in Table 3. With the control group absent, and treatment effects of the SP and NS groups similar to each other, the analyses of variance revealed no significant effects. However, Duncan's multiple-range tests performed on the means of the treatment groups revealed that while Groups NS and SP did not differ significantly, Group F was significantly different from *both* of these treatments indicating that at the time of the follow-up, Ss in the focal treatment condition still showed a significantly greater weight loss from pretreatment than either of the other two treatment groups. The results of the Duncan's multiple-range tests for the analyses on residual change scores are indicated in Table 1 with reference to raw score means, since raw score means and mean changes in raw scores are more meaningful from an interpretive point of view than residual change scores.

TABLE 3. Two-way analyses of variance on follow-up residual change scores for actual weight, eating patterns questionnaire factor scores and physical activity scale (PAS)

Source	df	Actual weight		Factor 1		Factor 2		Factor 3		Factor 4		Factor 5		Factor 6		PAS	
		MS	F	MS	F	MS	F	MS	F	MS	F	MS	F	MS	F	MS	F
Treatment	2	137.49	2.89	236.94	1.78	8.28	.39	75.41	6.08*	19.22	2.16	.82	.12	15.44	1.73	.53	1.17
Therapist	3	97.08	2.04	208.48	1.57	12.56	.59	18.50	1.49	6.86	.77	4.14	.61	2.43	.27	.93	2.07
Treatment X Therapist	6	27.87	.59	98.96	.74	6.43	.30	8.70	.70	14.11	1.59	7.60	1.12	6.19	.69	.17	.39
Error	43	47.63		133.11		21.22		12.40		8.89		6.77		8.94		.45	

Note.—$N = 55$.
*$p < .01$

Mean change in actual weight from pretreatment to posttreatment and follow-up for each experimental group is graphically presented in Fig. 2. From pretreatment to posttreatment, Group C gained 2.39 lb., Group SP lost 5.40 lb., Group NS lost 6.90 lb., while Group F showed a 10.33-lb. reduction. From pretreatment to follow-up, weight losses were less than those at posttreatment for all groups, but Group F still maintained a significantly greater weight loss from pretreatment than the other groups, with weight loss for Group F being 8.61 lb., for Group SP, 3.44 lb., and for Group NS, 6.52 lb.

INDIVIDUAL SUBJECT IMPROVEMENT

Because clinical workers are frequently more concerned with percentage improvements in individual cases than with mean group differences and because negative treatment effects would be more easily identified from data on individuals, all data concerning weight reduction were further evaluated on the

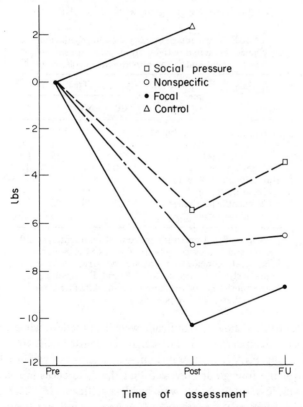

FIG. 2. Mean change in actual weight from pretreatment to posttreatment and follow-up.

basis of individually significant change scores. In evaluating significant change in weight from pretreatment to posttreatment, an individual case was classified as showing a "significant loss" if the pretreatment-posttreatment reduction in weight was 9 lb. or more. Likewise, an individual case was classified as showing a "significant gain" if the pretreatment-posttreatment increase in weight was 9 lb. or more. These criteria were derived empirically in the following manner: a cumulative frequency distribution was made of "absolute change in weight for each S from pre-base line to pretreatment ($N = 76$); absolute change in weight at the ninety-fifth percentile was 12 lb. (absolute change in weight at the fiftieth percentile was 3 lb.) over the 18-wk. base-line period, meaning that the change in weight of 95% of the Ss was less than $\frac{2}{3}$ lb./wk.; treatment (pretreatment–posttreatment) extended over 12 wk., so 95% of the Ss could be expected to show less than an 8-lb. weight change; hence, 9 lb. was used as indicating a significant change in weight.

Improvement rates from pretreatment to posttreatment are presented in Table 4. Particularly striking is the finding that not a single case in any treatment group evidenced a significant weight gain, while 11% of the control Ss did. Only

TABLE 4. Percentage of cases showing significant change in actual weight from pretreatment to posttreatment and from pretreatment to follow-up

Time	Treatments[1]			
	SP	NS	F	C
Pretreatment–Posttreatment				
Significant loss	25	40	61	6
No significant change	75	60	39	83
Significant gain	0	0	0	11
Pretreatment–follow-up				
Significant loss	33	21	50	–
No significant change	61	79	50	–
Significant gain	6	0	0	–

Note.– From pretreatment to posttreatment, Ns = 20, 20, 18, and 18, respectively, for Groups SP, NS, F, and C. From pretreatment to follow-up, Ns = 18, 19, and 18, respectively, for Groups SP, NS and F. Classifications were empirically derived from base-line data (see text).
[1] Numbers given are percentages.

6% of the control Ss showed significant weight reduction, while 25% of Ss in Group SP lost a significant amount of weight, contrasted with 40% in Group NS and 61% in Group F. A Kruskal-Wallis one-way analysis of variance by ranks on these data over the four groups revealed that the differences in cases showing a significant gain, loss, or no change were highly significant ($H = 23.71, p < .001$).

Table 4 also presents the percentage of cases who still met the 9-lb. criterion of significant loss or gain in weight from pretreatment to follow-up. At follow-up, the highest improvement rate was still obtained by Group F(50%), while only 21% of the Ss in Group NS and 33% in Group SP had lost 9 lb. or more from pretreatment to follow-up. A Kruskal-Wallis one-way analysis of variance by ranks on these data over the three groups showed that the differences in percentages were highly significant ($H = 9.79, p < .01$).

COMPARATIVE TREATMENT EFFECTS: EATING BEHAVIOR AND PHYSICAL ACTIVITY

Results from the one-way analyses of variance on treatments on the postresidual change scores for the factor measures and the physical activity scale are presented in Table 2. The following four factors showed significant treatment effects: Factor 1, emotional and uncontrolled overeating ($p < .01$); Factor 3, eating in isolation ($p < .001$); Factor 4, eating as reward ($p < .05$); and Factor 6, between-meal eating ($p < .01$). Analyses by means of Duncan's tests revealed that on Factors 1, 3, and 4, Group F showed a significantly greater reduction in the defined eating behaviors than did any of the other three groups whose changes did not differ significantly from each other. On Factor 6, the reduction for Group F was again significantly greater than that of the other three groups and Group SP showed a significantly greater reduction than Group C, although the reductions shown by Group SP and Group NS did not differ significantly from each other. No differential changes occurred in reported level of physical activity. Thus, while all treated groups showed significant pretreatment—posttreatment weight reduction in contrast to the control group, only Group F showed systematic reduction in the reported frequency of various eating behaviors as defined by the factor scores.

Next, follow-up residual change scores on the factor measures and activity scale were subjected to two-way analysis of variance summarized in Table 3. Only the treatment effect on Factor 3, eating in isolation, reached statistical significance ($p < .01$), with Duncan's tests showing that Group F showed significantly greater reduction than the other two groups whose changes did not differ significantly from each other. Duncan's tests were also performed on Factors 1, 4, and 6 since these measures showed significantly different changes among treatment groups at posttreatment. These analyses at follow-up revealed no differential changes on Factors 1 and 6, but on Factor 4, eating as reward, Group F showed a significantly greater reduction than either of the other two groups whose changes did not differ significantly from each other.

Supplementary analyses (Wollersheim, 1968, pp. 64–73) for therapists and therapist-treatment combinations indicated that the differential changes in reported frequency of eating behaviors which did occur were the results of the different treatments rather than different therapists or therapist-treatment combinations, with focal treatment resulting in significantly greater reductions in the reported frequencies of various eating behaviors than the other groups from both pretreatment to posttreatment and from pretreatment to follow-up.

GENERALIZATION EFFECTS OF TREATMENT AND "SYMPTOM SUBSTITUTION"

Although none of the other personality or anxiety scales in the assessment battery were concerned with the specific target behaviors of treatment, they were included to aid in identifying the sample and to check on the generalization effects of treatment or, conversely, "symptom substitution". From the learning framework underlying focal treatment, no change or mild positive changes would be expected on the measures of these secondary variables. The *disease-analogy* model, however, would interpret the reduction in weight achieved by Groups F and SP as merely symptomatic and the result of suggestion or positive transference (see Paul, 1967). This model would also expect Groups F and SP to manifest harmful results as a result of "symptomatic weight reduction". In addition, the disease-analogy model might possibly predict "symptom substitution", not only for these two groups but for Group NS as well, since in this project Group NS was not designed to be truly representative of traditional psychodynamic treatment but instead served as a control condition, adding to social pressure elements nonspecific factors such as presentation of a treatment rationale and a "ritual" meaningful for Ss. In this investigation, the measures of extraversion, general anxiety, and situation-specific anxiety (SR scales) served to check on the "symptom substitution" hypothesis.

Analyses of variance of the residual change scores of these secondary measures at posttreatment and follow-up revealed no evidence for "symptom substitution" (Wollersheim, 1968, pp. 72–83). Additionally, detailed correlational analyses indicated that reduction in weight and in reported frequencies of eating behavior were related to reductions on anxiety measures (Wollersheim, 1968, pp. 98–101). Thus, rather than providing evidence for "symptom substitution", the data supported the learning framework model which would expect specificity of treatment effects with perhaps some degree of generalization of positive effects.

SUBJECT RATINGS

An analysis of variance (Treatment X Therapists) of Ss' ratings of therapists on the scale of likeability (unlikeable, likeable, or very likeable) revealed no significant differential effects (Wollersheim, 1968, pp. 85–86). All therapists were rated as "likeable" or "very likeable" by everyone of their clients. Ratings of therapists on the competency scale (incompetent, competent, very competent) revealed a significant treatment effect ($p < .05$), while treatment and Therapist X Treatment effects were nonsignificant. While every S rated her therapist as competent or very competent, Ss in Group SP rated their therapist competent more often than very competent, while Ss in the other two groups rated their therapist as very competent more often than competent (Wollersheim, 1968, pp. 85–87).

PREDICTION OF IMPROVEMENT

The ability to predict which persons respond to treatment was not of major interest in this investigation. However, as such information would be of considerable value in both clinical practice and future research, possible relationships between the pretreatment assessment measures and weight reduction were investigated (Wollersheim, 1968, p. 107). Each pretreatment measure was correlated with posttreatment and follow-up residual change scores for weight. The results of these correlational analyses were totally nonsignificant. Of the 38 coefficients computed, not even one attained significance at the 5% level. Thus, for the sample included in the present study, measures of extraversion–introversion, general anxiety, situation-specific anxiety, physical activity, and reported frequencies of various eating behaviors were all unable to predict specific responsiveness to treatment.

Discussion

The results of the present study demonstrate the superiority of focal treatment based on learning principles over nonspecific and social pressure treatment. Focal therapy produced greater weight loss and greater reduction in reported frequencies of various eating behaviors, not only at the termination of treatment but at an 8-wk. follow-up as well. Evidence for symptom substitution was totally lacking. While significant differential weight reduction occurred for the various treatments, it did not occur for the different therapists or for the various therapist-treatment combinations. It is quite possible that when treatment techniques are explicitly specified and that when skilled therapists are trained in the therapeutic procedures and consistently apply them, treatment outcome becomes more a function of the treatment techniques utilized rather than the therapists using them. In addition to developing a feasible group therapy for obesity and demonstrating its effectiveness, the present study, in contrast to the weight-reduction studies reported in the literature, was characterized by an extremely low attrition rate. Making acceptance into treatment contingent upon a firm commitment to attend sessions regularly and emphasis throughout the sessions of the importance of attendance to their own success and the success of their fellow group members were seemingly the factors most responsible for preventing "drop-outs"

The specificity of effects with focal treatment is considerably enhanced by comparison with the effects of nonspecific treatment which contained both

N

social pressure and "placebo" elements. Not only did focal treatment produce significantly greater weight reduction, but it also produced significantly greater reductions in reported frequencies of various eating behaviors over the control group. The findings suggest that while Ss in Group F were systematically reducing the frequencies of their eating behavior, Ss in the NS and SP groups were generally not changing their eating behavior in any systematic way. The weight loss of these latter two groups may well have resulted from erratic, temporary, and fluctuating caloric intake. Yet, the weight losses of both of these groups were as good as and even better than many of the losses reported for therapy groups in the literature. It should be further noted that Group C did not constitute a "pure control" in the sense that a no-treatment, no-contact group would have. Group C received extra attention in the form of four telephone calls, a short interview, and participation in three testing and weighing sessions. If no-treatment control groups are actually therapy groups as stated by some investigators (Bergin, 1963), then the control group in the present study represents a conservative control measure. The finding that all three treatments produced significant weight loss in contrast to the control group is encouraging in an area so characterized by pessimism (see Stunkard & McLaren-Hume, 1959) and in view of the fact that the sample of Ss in the present investigation were characteristic of the "hard core" group of obese persons described in the literature.

To the investigator's knowledge, the present study represents the first group psychotherapy study concerning weight reduction designed with the controls necessary to establish cause-effect relationships between therapeutic techniques and treatment outcome. Two studies published after the completion of the present investigation (Harmatz & Lapuc, 1968; Harris, 1969) and a report of eight case studies (Stuart, 1967) all strongly point to the potential effectiveness in the ultilization of learning principles in the treatment of obesity. These studies together with the present investigation reported rates of weight loss which would be considered highly favorable by members of the health professions (see United States Department of Health, Education, and Welfare, 1967). The results for Group F in the present study are among the most care-fully validated and successful results reported to date in the psychological treatment of obesity. These results take on even greater significance when it is realized that both psychologists and physicians (see Meyer & Crisp, 1964; Rynearson & Gastineau, 1949) have pointed out that the psychological treatment of obesity, although discouraging, is impressive when compared to other methods of treatment such as dieting alone or endocrine therapy.

Groups NS and SP deserve further comment. Since Group NS did not lose significantly more weight than Group SP, seemingly it would be of questionable value to treat obesity in relatively lengthy nonspecific therapy sessions when using 15–20-min. sessions of positive expectation—social pressure seems to be just as effective. The social pressure treatment of the present study is highly similar to the nationwide TOPS weight reducing groups. Usually, however, TOPS groups employ a more complex reinforcement system for weight loss than does the social pressure group (e.g., monetary fines for weight gain, slogans and songs, local and national conventions). TOPS groups, however, average about 30 persons per group (Toch, 1965). Although to the investigator's knowledge, the effectiveness of TOPS has not yet been scientifically investigated, it is suspected that it would be about as effective as Group SP in the present study in promoting weight loss of members who do not drop out. At any rate, from a clinician's viewpoint, weight loss may be just as great for a client who is referred to TOPS as for one who is involved in nonspecific forms of psychotherapy.

The most notable limitation of the present investigation is that the treatment period was relatively short in relation to the degree of the Ss' obesity. Weight loss requires time and should be gradual if it is to be sound from the viewpoint of physical health. Since Ss in this study were considerably obese, even the majority of those who lost a significant amount of weight during the treatment period still were considerably overweight. When treatment terminated, group reinforcement for weight loss also terminated, and perhaps most Ss had not lost enough of their excess weight to warrant sufficient reinforcement from their own appearance, family, and friends to motivate them to endure the hardships of continued caloric restriction. It is suspected that all groups would have evidenced better maintenance if they had continued to meet at regular intervals after the tenth session merely for 15–20 min. for use of the positive expectation–social pressure techniques alone. Ten sessions appeared to be adequate in instructing Ss in focal treatment in the implementation of learning principles, but subsequent additional sessions involving only social pressure techniques and social reinforcement would most likely have promoted further weight loss.

Two further limitations of this study deserve comment. The first revolves around the fact that the focal treatment herein developed and evaluated represents a treatment *package* including many techniques derived from learning principles. Only subsequent research can specifically delineate the more potent elements of this package. For example, research is not in progress to test the hypothesis that the use of deep relaxation could be subtracted from the focal treatment package without decreasing its effectiveness. Second, the extrinsic validity (see Campbell & Stanley, 1966) of the present investigation would be extended by employing nonlearning theory-oriented therapists in the implementation of the techniques of focal therapy.

In conclusion, in that the present investigation obtained carefully validated and highly positive results in an area so characterized by failure, replication certainly seems warranted. Beyond its specific contribution to the treatment of obesity, this study represents an attempt to contribute to more sophisticated therapy outcome research by focusing upon the establishment of cause-effect relations between therapeutic techniques and treatment outcome.

References

ALEXANDER, F. & FLAGG, G. W. The psychosomatic approach. In B. J. Wolman (Ed.), *Handbook of clinical psychology*. New York: McGraw-Hill, 1965.

BENDIG, A. W. Pittsburg scale of social extraversion-introversion and emotionality. *Journal of Psychology*, 1962, 53, 199–210.

BERGIN, A. E. The effects of psychotherapy: Negative results revisited. *Journal of Counseling Psychology*, 1963, 10, 244–250.

BERNE, E. *Games people play: The psychology of human relationships*. New York: Grove Press, 1964.

BRUCH, H. Disturbed communication in eating disorders. *American Journal of Orthopsychiatry*, 1963, 33, 99–104.

CAMPBELL, D. T. & STANLEY, J. C.: *Experimental and quasiexperimental designs for research*. Chicago: Rand McNally, 1966.

CATTELL, R. B. *The IPAT Anxiety Scale*. Champaign, Ill.: Institute for Personality and Ability Testing, 1957.

DUBOIS, P. H. *Multivariant correlational analysis*. New York: Harper, 1957.

ENDLER, N. S., HUNT, J. McV., & ROSENSTEIN, A. J. An S-R inventory of anxiousness. *Psychological Monographs*, 1962, 76, (17, Whole No. 536).

FENICHEL, O. *The psychoanalytic theory of neuroses*. New York: Norton, 1945.

FERSTER, C. B., NURNBERGER, J. I., & LEVITT, E. E.. The control of eating. *Journal of Mathetics*, 1962, 1, 87–109.

GOLDIAMOND, I. Self-control procedures in personal behavior problems. *Psychological Reports*, 1965, 17, 851–868.

HARMATZ, M. G. & LAPUC, P. Behavior modification of overeating in a psychiatric population. *Journal of Consulting and Clinical Psychology*, 1968, 32, 583–587.

HARRIS, M. B. Self-directed program for weight control: A pilot study. *Journal of Abnormal Psychology*, 1969, 74, 263–270.

KRAMER, C. Y. Extension of multiple range tests to group means with unequal numbers of replications. *Biometrics*, 1956, 12, 307–310.

MENDELSON, M. Psychological aspects of obesity. *International Journal of Psychiatry*, 1966, 2, 599–611.

MEYER, V., & CRISP, A. H. Aversion therapy in two cases of obesity. *Behaviour Research and Therapy*, 1964, 2, 143–147.

NATIONAL DAIRY COUNCIL. Obesity and its management. *Dairy Council Digest*, 1965, 36, 13–18.

PAUL, G. L. Insight versus desensitization in psychotherapy two years after termination. *Journal of Consulting Psychology*, 1967, 31, 333–348.

PAUL, G. L. & SHANNON, D. T. Treatment of anxiety through systematic desensitization in therapy groups. *Journal of Abnormal Psychology*, 1966, 71, 124–135.

RYNEARSON, E. H. & GASTINEAU, C. F. *Obesity*. Springfield Ill: Charles C. Thomas, 1949.

SCHIFFERES, J. J. *What's your caloric number?* New York: Macmillan, 1966.

STUART, R. B. Behavioral control of overeating. *Behavior Research and Therapy*, 1967, 5, 357–365.

STUNKARD, A. J. The dieting depression. *The American Journal of Medicine*, 1957, 23, 77–86.

STUNKARD, A. J. & McLAREN-HUME, M.: The results of treatment for obesity: A review of the literature and report of a series. *Archives of Internal Medicine*, 1959, 103, 79–85.

SUCZEK, R. F. Psychological aspects of weight reduction. In E. S. Eppright, P. Swanson, & C. A. Iverson (Eds.), *Weight control: A collection of papers presented at the Weight Control Colloquium*. Ames: Iowa State College Press, 1955.

TOCH, H. *The social psychology of social movements*. New York: Bonns-Merrill, 1965.

ULLMANN, L. P. & KRASNER, L. (Eds.) *Case studies in behavior modification*. New York: Holt, 1965.

UNITED STATES DEPARTMENT OF HEALTH, EDUCATION, AND WELFARE. *Obesity* and health: A source-book of current information for professional health personnel, Arlington, Va.: United States Public Health Service, 1967.

WOLLERSHEIM, J. P. The effectiveness of learning theory-based group therapy in the treatment of overweight women. Unpublished doctoral dissertation, University of Illinois, 1968.

YOUNG, C. M., BERRESFORD, K., & MOORE, N. S. Psychologic factors in weight control. *American Journal of Clinical Nutrition*, 1957, **5**, 186–191.

Group Therapy versus Bibliotherapy in Weight Reduction[1]

RICHARD L. HAGEN[2]

University of Illinois, Urbana, Illinois

Summary— Eighty-nine coeds were treated for obesity under three conditions: (a) group therapy, (b) use of a written manual (bibliotherapy), (c) group therapy and bibliotherapy combined. All treatment conditions produced significantly more weight loss than that observed in the control group ($p < .01$), but the treatment groups did not differ significantly from each other. Subjects who attended group meetings reported their treatments to have been significantly more helpful ($p < .05$) than did subjects who received the manual only. No differences were observed in therapist effectiveness, and a 4-week follow-up revealed no significant changes in weight. While change in physical activity did not differ across groups, changes in eating habits were significantly different across groups ($p < .05$).

The recent emphasis upon therapeutic intervention without the involvement of trained professionals (e.g., Lang, 1966, 1968; Melamed & Lang, 1967; Kahn & Baker, 1968; Bandura & Menlove, 1968; Cassell, 1965; Hogan & Kirchner, 1968; Gilbert & Ewing, 1965) represents a movement not only of theoretical interest but also of great practical significance. The movement, however, has provided little evaluative data bearing on (a) the question of the importance traditionally assigned the "personal relationship" between client and therapist and (b) the efficacy of written materials in producing change.

The personal relationship between therapist and client has been described as the heart of the therapeutic process (Brammer & Shostrom, 1960) and has long been considered the critical factor in psychotherapy (Gilbert & Ewing, 1965). However, studies designed to provide data relevant to the validity of this assumption have failed to affirm a major role of the personal relationship in the treatment of phobias (Kahn & Baker, 1968; Melamed & Lang, 1967; Hogan & Kirchner, 1968) or in the counseling of university freshmen (Gilbert & Ewing,

Reprinted with permission from *Behavior Therapy*, 1974, 5, 222–234. Copyright © 1974 by Academic Press, Inc.

[1] This article is based upon a dissertation submitted in partial fulfillment of requirements for the Ph.D. at the University of Illinois. Gratitude is expressed to Gordon L. Paul, dissertation chairman, for his support and valuable suggestions.

[2] Requests for reprints should be sent to Richard L. Hagen, Department of Psychology, Florida State University, Tallahassee, Florida 32306.

1965). If the face-to-face client-therapist encounter is not absolutely essential, therapy via written materials (bibliotherapy) suggests an inexpensive and widely available treatment method. Bibliotherapy has been seen by some as useless in bringing about behavior change (Brammer & Shostrom, 1960) and even as potentially harmful and dangerous (Brower, 1952), but at the present time, there exists little data from which to evaluate such statements. What data are available provide encouragement for further research using bibliotherapy (Gilbert & Ewing, 1965).

In the present investigation, obesity was selected as a clinical problem on which to evaluate the importance of the face-to-face contact between client and therapist and the general effectiveness of a treatment program involving biblio-therapy. The prevalence of obesity provides for a large population of subjects, body weight represents a reliable, nonreactive dependent variable, and recent studies involving learning principles in the treatment of obesity (Stuart, 1967; Ferster, Nurnberger & Levitt, 1962; Homme, 1965; Goldiamond, 1965; Wollersheim, 1970) suggest a treatment program of sufficient detail for the personal contact variable to be systematically included or excluded.

The treatment program outlined by Wollersheim (1970) is particularly well suited for the development of a written weight reduction manual. Her study showed that a treatment based on learning principles produced significantly more weight loss over a 10-week treatment period than did social-pressure or insight-oriented therapy. However, the learning theory group also received a great deal of personal attention from the therapist. The question which now becomes important is whether the content or information will produce the desired results when the relationship factor is considerably reduced.

Data relevant to the latter question were obtained in the study reported below, which focused specifically on the following questions: (a) can a written presentation of principles previously found effective in the treatment of obesity produce significant weight reduction without a face-to-face encounter between client and therapist or therapy group? (b) Does attendance in a therapy group, which includes personal contact, make a contribution to treatment over and above principles provided through written communication?

Method

SUBJECTS

A total of 90 female subjects requesting treatment for obesity after an announcement of program availability in the university newspaper were selected on motivation and percent overweight. All were students at the University of Illinois, varying in age from 17 to 22. Using the same procedure as Wollersheim (1970), the weight criteria were based upon the 1959 Metropolitan Life

Insurance Company norms for desirable weight for women (U.S. Dept. of Health, Education, and Welfare, 1967). A subject was included in the program only if her actual weight was at least 10% above her desirable weight at the time of initial contact.

ASSESSMENT INSTRUMENTS

The assessment battery administered at pretreatment included height (to the nearest inch without shoes) and weight (to the nearest pound in indoor clothing without shoes) obtained on a standard physician's balance scales; the Pittsburgh Social Extroversion-Introversion and Emotionality Scale (Bendig, 1962); and Eating Patterns Questionnaire (Wollersheim, 1970); and a modification of Schifferes' (1966) Physical-Activity Scale. Assessment instruments at post-treatment and follow-up included all of the above measures except height and the Pittsburgh scales.

THERAPISTS

Three male therapists, including the investigator, participated in the study.[3] All were Ph.D. candidates in clinical psychology and had completed clinical training and preliminary examination requirements at the time of the investigation.

TREATMENTS

The principles involved in all treatment programs are the principles found in Wollersheim's (1970) most effective treatment, that which involved the use of learning principles. Furthermore, order of introduction and time spent on these principles in theory groups were equated with her treatment; thus, the differences systematically studied in the present experiment involved differences in manner of presentation of the material and the presence or absence of a therapy group and therapist as represented in the following groups: Manual Only (principles and feedback presented via written communication); Manual Plus Contact (written communication of the principles plus face-to-face contact within a group setting); Contact Only (replication of Wollersheim's Focal Therapy involving both presentation of principles and feedback with a group setting); and No-treatment—Wait Control. In order to insure consistency among the three therapists in carrying out the prescribed treatment procedures, all sessions were taped and monitored by the investigator who provided corrective feedback when necessary.

[3] Gratitude is expressed to Edward Craighead and Robert Marx who served as therapists for the research.

MANUAL ONLY

The manual was based largely on Wollersheim's (1970) therapist training manual but was modified for consumption by laymen.[4] Each week for 10 weeks, lessons were mailed out to the subjects. Subjects returned homework which was corrected and returned with the following lesson.

MANUAL PLUS CONTACT

This group received the 10 lessons on a weekly basis, but the exchange of lessons and assignments took place at a weekly therapy session rather than via the mail. The therapy session was 1 hr long, following as closely as possible the format presented by Wollersheim (1970) for the first 60 min of her Focal Therapy Group, which included weighing in, use of charts and social pressure, and discussion of principles and techniques in weight reduction with individual application.

CONTACT ONLY

The Contact Only group was conducted in an effort to provide as close a replication as possible of Wollersheim's (1970) Focal Therapy Group including all of the above plus relaxation training. These subjects did not receive the manual; rather, all communication of principles and techniques involved in weight reduction took place in the 90-min weekly therapy group meeting.

NO-TREATMENT–WAIT CONTROL

Subjects in this condition followed the same procedures, under the same conditions, as subjects in the treatment groups, with the exception of treatment itself. Shortly before treatment was scheduled to begin for the other three groups, control subjects were informed by letter that on the basis of their personality scores they had been assigned to a group which would receive bibliotherapy beginning 10 weeks later. They were also told that two more assessments would be necessary, one in 10 weeks and one in 14 weeks. After the follow-up assessment, these subjects were given the treatment manual *in toto*.

GENERAL PROCEDURE

Students responding to program announcements were asked to attend a pretreatment assessment session where they were measured and weighed and given the assessment instruments. They were told that the purpose of the study was to investigate the relationship between height and weight and psychological

---

[4] The weight reduction manual may be found in the complete dissertation copy which is on file at the University Microfilms, Dissertation Copies, P.O. Box 1764, Ann Arbor, Michigan 48106. Order No.: 70–20, 973, $4.00 micro., $10.60 Xerox, 231 pages.

characteristics and to determine "which people benefit most" from different types of psychological procedures utilized in treating weight problems. Students were also told that assignment to groups would be made on the basis of scores on personality tests.

As a further screening device, 2 weeks before treatment began, students were sent a questionnaire asking for their schedules. Those who had met the selection criteria at the prescreening assessment and who returned their schedules were stratified on the basis of percent overweight and randomly assigned from blocks of four to one of the four experimental conditions.

Within each of the two treatments involving therapy groups (Manual Plus Contact and Contact Only), subjects were again stratified on the basis of percent overweight and were assigned from blocks of three to one of the three therapists. Each of the three therapists treated one group of six subjects in both of these conditions.

Treatment via therapy groups and/or correspondence was conducted during the ensuing 11-week period, allowing for 10 treatment sessions and/or correspondence lessons and 1-week vacation period.

Posttreatment assessment was made after the last week of treatment. All subjects were informed of the time and place for the 4-week follow-up at the posttreatment assessment and were also contacted by telephone several days before they were scheduled for the follow-up assessment.

Results

ATTRITION

Out of ninety subjects originally in the study, only one, a member of the control group, dropped out and thus could not be included in the data analysis.

EQUATION OF GROUPS

One-way analyses of variance were performed to ascertain whether or not the groups differed before treatment began on the following 15 variables: age; number of friends in the study; number of friends in the same treatment condition; extroversion, emotionality and lie scales on the Pittsburgh Social Extroversion—Introversion and Emotionality Scale; Physical Activity Scale; six factors from the Eating Patterns Questionnaire; percent overweight, and actual weight. These analyses revealed that the groups were well equated (all $p > .20$).[5] Similar analyses revealed that the therapist groups ($n = 6$) within each of the Contact Only and Manual Plus Contact treatment groups were also well equated (all $p > .20$).

[5] Complete tables of *MS* and *F* values on all analyses contained in the results section of this paper are contained in the complete dissertation (see footnote 4).

TABLE 1. Means and standard deviations for treatment groups on actual weight across all time periods[1]

Time	Contact only (N = 18)		Manual plus contact (N = 18)		Manual only (N = 18)		Control (N = 35)	
	M	SD	M	SD	M	SD	M	SD
Pretreatment	153.94	21.20	153.06	21.42	152.83	17.97	153.20	20.38
Posttreatment	142.00^x	21.48	138.06^y	19.13	140.83^z	17.82	151.40^{xyz}	20.15
Follow-up	141.67^x	21.42	139.72^y	18.72	142.33^z	18.36	153.09^{xys}	21.66

[1] Superscript symbols refer to means which differ significantly in residual change score analyses. Means which differ significantly within each row ($p < .05$, Duncan's Multiple Range Test) share the same symbol.

COMPARATIVE TREATMENT EFFECTS: WEIGHT

The single most important dependent variable was actual body weight, since a change in body weight represented the primary and specific goal of treatment. The means and standard deviations of the four experimental groups at pretreatment, posttreatment, and follow-up are presented in Table 1. Mean change in actual weight from pretreatment to posttreatment and follow-up for each experimental group is presented in Fig. 1.

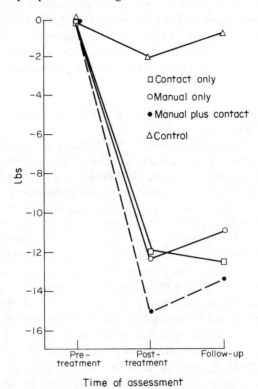

FIG. 1. Mean change in actual weight from pretreatment to posttreatment and follow-up.

Major analyses on actual weight and other assessment measures were performed on residual change scores, consisting of the difference between obtained scores and the scores predicted by linear regression from pretreatment to posttreatment and from pretreatment to follow-up. The treatment effect for actual weight was significant ($p = .00000$). Differences between treatment means were tested utilizing Duncan's Multiple Range Test (Kramer, 1956). While all experimental group means differed significantly from the control group ($p < .01$), the three experimental groups did not differ significantly from each other.

To test for differences in therapist effectiveness, a supplementary analysis for therapist effects was performed using Contact Only and Manual Plus Contact subjects and subjecting posttreatment and follow-up residual change scores to two-way analyses of variance (Treatments X Therapists). Therapist and Treatments X Therapists effects were non-significant on both sets of scores ($p > .25$).

Insignificant Trial and Treatment X Trial effects on posttreatment and follow-up raw weight scores indicated that there was no significant weight change during the 4 weeks after the termination of treatment.

Using raw weight scores of Contact Only and Manual Plus Contact subjects, a three-way analysis of variance (Treatments X Therapists X Trials), was also performed to test for a Therapist X Trials interaction or a three-way interaction involving Treatments, Therapists and Trials. Neither interaction was significant.

COMPARATIVE TREATMENT EFFECTS: EATING BEHAVIOR AND PHYSICAL ACTIVITY

The Eating Patterns Questionnaire (Wollersheim, 1970) yields six factor scores concerning specific eating practices: (1) emotional and uncontrolled overeating; (2) eating response to interpersonal situations; (3) eating in isolation; (4) eating as reward; (5) eating in response to evaluative situation; (6) between meal eating. Analyses on pretreatment to posttreatment residual change scores for these factors showed significant treatment effects on factors 1 ($p = .003$); 3 ($p = .001$); 4 ($p = .04$); and 6 ($p = .04$). Duncan's tests revealed that on factors 1 and 3 all treatment groups differed significantly from the control group ($p < .01$) but the three treatment groups did not differ significantly from each other. On Factor 4 the Manual Plus Contact and Manual Only groups differed significantly from the control group ($p < .05$) but not from the Contact Only group. Contact Only and Control groups did not differ significantly. A similar pattern was found for Factor 6 but with Manual Only and Contact Only exchanging places in the rank order of means. Manual Plus Contact and Contact Only groups differed significantly from the Control group ($p < .05$) but not from the Manual Only group. Manual Only and Control groups did not differ significantly from each other.

A one-way analysis of variance across groups on physical activity residual change scores revealed no significant differences in physical activity. Furthermore, analyses for therapist effects on the eating patterns factor scores and activity measure (Treatments X Therapists) revealed no significant therapist effects or treatments by therapists interaction on any of the measures.

INTERRELATIONSHIPS AMONG VARIABLES

In order to investigate relationships among changes which occurred on various instruments, residual change scores on the Physical Activity Scale, on the six factor scores of the Eating Patterns Questionnaire and on weight were intercorrelated.

Inspection of Table 2 reveals that in all cases, changes on the eating patterns factor scores correlated positively with changes in weight (10 of the 12 correlations were significant at $p < .01$) attesting to the validity of the Eating Patterns Questionnaire and providing confirmation for the efficacy of the treatment program in bringing about changes in patterns of eating. These correlations are positive, indicating that a decrease in weight was related to a decrease in frequency of eating. Correlations of the Physical Activity Scale with other measures were not significant, indicating that changes in physical activity were related neither to changes in eating patterns nor to changes in weight.

EVALUATION OF TREATMENT BY SUBJECTS

At the time of posttreatment assessment, each treated subject was asked to rate, on a scale of 1 to 5 (a) how much she liked the program and (b) how helpful the program was. In each case, the higher scores indicated the more positive rating.

A one-way analysis of variance on scores for Question 1 (how much the subject liked the program) revealed no significant differences among the treatment groups ($p = .22$). However, the analysis for Question 2 (how helpful the program was) did reveal significant differences among the groups ($p = .04$). Duncan's Multiple Range Test showed that subjects in the Contact Only and Manual Plus Contact groups rated their treatments as not significantly different in helpfulness but as significantly more helpful than did subjects in the Manual Only group ($p < .05$).

Regardless of treatment, one would expect subjects who lost weight to rate the programs more positively on both scales than would subjects who did not lose weight. Thus, negative correlations would be predicted between scores on each scale and weight residual change scores. In all cases, significant negative correlations were found.

Discussion

When viewed by itself, without reference to Wollersheim's (1970) study, the present investigation might be criticized as not containing a placebo control group. Were this true, effectiveness of treatment packages apart from placebo effects could not be established since the treatments did not produce significant differences in weight even though all treatments were effective as compared with the control group. Such a criticism, however, is not a valid one. In the present investigation, Wollersheim's Focal Therapy package, a treatment of demonstrated effectiveness over a placebo control, was replicated for comparison with

TABLE 2. Intercorrelations of residual change scores on each measure ($N = 89$)

	(1)	(2)	(3)	(4)	(5)	(6)	(7)	(8)	(9)
(1) Eating Patterns, Factor 1 pretreatment to posttreatment	—								
(2) Eating Patterns, Factor 2 pretreatment to posttreatment	.36**	—							
(3) Eating Patterns, Factor 3 pretreatment to posttreatment	.44**	.51**	—						
(4) Eating Patterns, Factor 4 pretreatment to posttreatment	.48**	.56**	.55**	—					
(5) Eating Patterns, Factor 5 pretreatment to posttreatment	.37**	.28**	.18	.40**	—				
(6) Eating Patterns, Factor 6 pretreatment to posttreatment	.47**	.32**	.50**	.39**	.26*	—			
(7) Weight pretreatment to posttreatment	.49**	.34**	.49**	.38**	.21*	.44**	—		
(8) Weight pretreatment to follow-up	.39**	.27**	.40**	.34**	.14	.40**	.79**	—	
(9) Physical Activity Scale pretreatment to posttreatment	.05	-.08	-.20	-.08	.07	-.12	-.12	.09	—

*$p < .05$ (two-tailed).
**$p < .01$ (two-tailed).

other treatment packages, thus eliminating the necessity for a placebo control group. Such an orientation is necessary for a proper interpretation of the results of this study.

An affirmative answer has been provided to the question concerning the possibility of treating obesity via written communication with the minimal personal contact. The treatment group which received only the written manual lost significantly more weight ($p < .01$) than the control group, which received no formal treatment.

The second major question to be considered in this investigation is that of the extent to which face-to-face "personal contact" with a therapist or therapy group would make a contribution to treatment over and above principles provided through written communications. In an effort to provide some data bearing on this question, the Manual Plus Contact group was included. These subjects received the same written program the Manual Only subjects received, including weekly written comments by the investigator, but, in addition, they met for 1 hr each week with a trained therapist during which time the traditional group therapy devices of reflection, clarification, praise, etc., were used. The difference in weight loss between the Manual Only and the Manual Plus Contact groups was not statistically significant; therefore, evidence was not provided to affirm a contribution to treatment by the group experience over and above that of the principles provided via by the written manual.

Other studies in the literature have produced data consonant with those of the present investigation. Melamed and Lang (1967) reported no significant difference between desensitization conducted by a live therapist and automated desensitization presented by Lang's Device for Automated Desensitization; however, personal contact as a significant variable of change in their automated group cannot be entirely ruled out. Gilbert and Ewing (1965) found, with incoming university freshmen, that Programmed Counseling (personal relationship absent) and Simulated Programmed Counseling (personal relationship present), while more effective than no counseling at all, produced no significant differences on their dependent measures.

The analysis for change in weight over the 4 weeks between posttreatment and follow-up produced no significant gain or loss; however, there was a mean weight gain across all groups of 1.24 lb. Wollersheim (1970) reported a mean weight gain for all groups of 1.36 during an 8-week follow-up period. Stollak (1967) found that 8 weeks after treatment not one experimental treatment group showed a significant weight reduction from pretreatment even though one group had significantly lost weight during treatment. Thus, previous follow-up reports are discouraging, and long-term follow-ups of these studies are highly desirable.

Wollersheim postulated that the gain in weight could be accounted for by the termination of group reinforcement when treatment terminated. With that in mind, one might predict that subjects who had been in therapy groups would show a weight gain when this support was removed while subjects who had learned to lose weight apart from a group (Manual Only subjects) would continue to show a weight loss or would hold their own after treatment. This prediction was not borne out.

On the secondary measures, interesting comparisons can be made with the results of Wollersheim, who found significant treatment effects on four of the six factor scores from the Eating Patterns Questionnaire: Factor 1, Emotional and Uncontrolled Overeating; Factor 3, Eating in Isolation; Factor 4, Eating as Reward; and Factor 6, Between Meal Eating. On these same four factors, and only on these four, significant treatment effects were also found in the present investigation, a replication which lends a measure of validity to the Eating Patterns Questionnaire. Furthermore, as in Wollersheim's study, the present investigation revealed no significant change in physical activity across treatment groups. Thus, analyses on these two measures, Physical Activity Scale and Eating Patterns Questionnaire, indicate that the treatment programs were instrumental in bringing about changes in patterns of eating, the major thrust of all treatments, while changes in physical activity were not significantly influenced by treatment.

One other study has appeared in which subjects were asked to rate in terms of helpfulness, bibliotherapy against traditional counseling. Students who received face-to-face counseling rated their program as more helpful than did students who were assigned to read a self-counseling manual at home (Gilbert & Ewing, 1965). In the present investigation, the same results were obtained. The Manual Only treatment condition was rated as being significantly less helpful than either of the other treatment conditions, both of which involved face-to-face contact. However, in the Gilbert and Ewing study and in the present study, dependent measures revealed no significant differences in treatment outcomes among the various treatments. Thus, in both investigations, subjects thought they were receiving more help when treatment involved a face-to-face encounter but such differential help was not reflected in dependent measures.

While in the Gilbert and Ewing study subjects may truly have received differential help which was not assessed in the dependent measures, such an interpretation would, indeed, be difficult to apply to the present study since subjects expressly entered the program to lose weight and weight loss was the basic dependent measure. It seems more likely that subjects have learned to expect more help from face-to-face counseling than from written materials and that these expectations were reflected in the ratings for both investigations.

In conclusion, the present investigation has provided evidence that: (a) a written manual has been derived which is effective in the treatment for obesity; (b) the importance traditionally assigned the face-to-face personal-contact aspect of treatment, at least for obesity, may have been overrated. The findings of the present investigation point to the possibility of a treatment for obesity available at nominal cost to all who can read.

References

BANDURA, A. & MENLOVE, F. L. Factors determining vicarious extinction of avoidance behavior through symbolic modeling. *Journal of Personality and Social Psychology*, 1968, 8, 99–108.

BENDIG, A. W. Pittsburgh scale of social extroversion-introversion and emotionality. *Journal of Psychology*, 1962, 53, 199–210.

BRAMMER, L. M. & SHOSTROM, E. L. *Therapeutic psychology*, Englewood Cliffs, New Jersey: Prentice-Hall, 1960.

BROWER, D. *Progress in clinical psychology*, Vol. VI. New York: Grune & Stratton, 1952.

CASSELL, S. Effect of brief puppet therapy upon the emotional responses of children undergoing cardiac cathaterization. *Journal of Consulting Psychology*, 1965, 29, 1–8.

COLBY, K. M., WATT, J., & GILBERT, J. P. A computer method of psychotherapy. *Journal of Nervous and Mental Disease*, 1966, 142, 148–152.

FERSTER, C. B., NURNBERGER, J. I., & LEVITT, E. E. The control of eating. *Journal of Mathetics*, 1962, 1, 87–109.

GILBERT, W. M. & EWING, T. N. An investigation of the importance of the personal relationship and associated factors in teaching machine procedures. Student Counseling Service, University of Illinois, Champaign, Illinois, 1965.

GOLDIAMOND, I. Self-control procedures in personal behavior problems. *Psychological Reports*, 1965, 17, 851–868.

HAGEN, R. L. Group therapy versus bibliotherapy in weight reduction. Unpublished doctoral dissertation, University of Illinois, 1969.

HOGAN, R. A. & KIRCHNER, J. H. Implosive, eclectic verbal and bibliotherapy in the treatment of fears of snakes. *Behaviour Research and Therapy*, 1968, 6, 167–171.

HOMME, L. E. Perspectives in psychology: XXIV. Control of coverants, the operants of the mind. *Psychological Record*, 1965, 15, 501–511.

KAHN, M. & BAKER, B. Desensitization with minimal therapist contact. *Journal of Abnormal Psychology*, 1968, 73, 198–200.

KRAMER, C. Y. Extension of multiple range tests to group means with unequal numbers of replications. *Biometrics*, 1956, 12, 307–310.

LANG, P. J. The transfer of treatment. *Journal of Consulting Psychology*, 1966, 30, 375–378.

LANG, P. J. Fear reduction and fear behavior. *Research in Psychotherapy*, 1968, 3, 90–102.

MELAMED, B. & LANG, P. Study of the automated desensitization of fear. Paper presented at the Midwestern Psychological Association Convention, Chicago, Illinois, May, 1967.

PAUL, G. L. *Insight versus desensitization in psychotherapy*. Stanford: Stanford University Press, 1966a.

PAUL, G. L. The specific control of anxiety: "Hypnosis" and "conditioning." Symposium paper read at annual meeting of the American Psychological Association, New York, September, 1966b.

PAUL, G. L. & SHANNON, D. T. Treatment of anxiety through systematic desensitization in therapy groups. *Journal of Abnormal Psychology*, 1966, 71, 124–135.

SCHIFFERES, J. J. *What's your caloric number?"* New York: Macmillan, 1966.

STOLLAK, G. E. Weight loss obtained under different experimental procedures. *Psychotherapy: Theory, Research and Practice*, 1967, 4, 61–64.

STUART, R. B. Behavioral control of overeating. *Behaviour Research and Therapy*, 1967, 5, 357–365.

U.S. Department of Health, Education and Welfare. *Obesity and health: a sourcebook of current information for professional health personnel.* Arlington, Va. U.S. Public Health Service, 1967.

WOLLERSHEIM, J. P. Effectiveness of group therapy based upon learning principles in the treatment of overweight women. *Journal of Abnormal Psychology*, 1970, 76, 462–474.

CHAPTER 38

Self-directed Program for Weight Control: a pilot study

MARY B. HARRIS[1]

Stanford University

Summary— A treatment program was designed to enable Ss to lose weight through the use of self-monitored techniques for changing their eating behaviors. All Ss who participated in the program achieved a stable loss in weight, and their mean loss was significantly greater than the change shown by a group of similarly motivated control Ss. No additional effects due to a few sessions of aversive counter-conditioning were demonstrated, and no general mood changes accompanied the weight loss. The Ss did report a decreased temptation to overeat. It was suggested that similar programs of gradual habit change through self-control of stimulus conditions and reinforcement contingencies might be applied to the treatment of other addictive behaviors, which are also very refractory to change.

Attempts to deal with the undesirable behavior of overeating have been spectacularly unsuccessful. Although a great number of causal agents or correlates have been postulated, such as depression (Simon, 1963), anxiety (Cauffman & Pauley, 1961), power orientation (Suczek, 1967), a variety of other personality problems (Bruch, 1957; Kaplan & Kaplan, 1957, who list twenty-eight suggested meanings of obesity; Shipman & Plesset, 1963), insufficient exercise (Mayer, 1955), presence of night-eating syndrome (Stunkard, 1959a), lack of correlation between report of hunger and gastric motility (Stunkard, 1959b), obesity of parents (Cappon, 1958), more dependence on external stimuli such as flavors and time of day to regulate hunger (Schachter, 1967), and no doubt many others, no clear causal relationships have been substantially detailed. An equally large variety of treatments have been tried, ranging from such nonacademic means as low-calorie products, exercise salons, yoga, and reducing clubs to hypnosis (Erickson, 1960), dietary instruction (Young *et al.*, 1955), appetite depressants and other drugs (Silverstone & Solomon, 1965), general medical advice (Stunkard, 1958), psychoanalysis and

Reprinted with permission from the *Journal of Abnormal Psychology*, 1969, **74**, 263–270.

[1]The author wishes to express her appreciation to Albert Bandura for his generous assistance with all phases of the study. Request for reprints should be to the author, Department of Educational Foundations, University of New Mexico, Albuquerque, New Mexico 87106.

other forms of psychotherapy (Bruch, 1957), group discussion of physical and emotional factors (Harmon, Purkonen, & Rasmussen, 1958), aversion-relief therapy (Thorpe *et al.*, 1964), recording all eating (Ferster, Nurnberger, & Levitt, 1962; Stollak, 1966), self-control (Ferster *et al.*, 1962; Goldiamond, 1965), aversive counterconditioning with shock (Stollak, 1966; Wolpe, 1958), operant conditioning with shock (Meyer & Crisp, 1964), and aversive counter-conditioning with nausea (Cautela, 1966).

In general, the reported attempts to treat overweight people fall into two categories: case histories of techniques which proved successful with one or a very few patients (Cautela, 1966; Erikson, 1960; Ferster *et al.*, 1962; Goldiamond, 1965; Meyer & Crisp, 1964; Thorpe *et al.*, 1964; Wolpe, 1958) and survey studies of patients in a medical setting, most of which have reported a general lack of success in effecting any long-range weight reduction (Franklin & Rynearson, 1960; Harmon *et al.*, 1958; Shipman & Plesset, 1963; Silverstone & Solomon, 1965; Young *et al.*, 1955). An experimental study by Stollak, using aversive counterconditioning therapy with electric shock and adequate control groups, reported the same poor results (a mean net loss of less than 5 lb.). The inadequacy of treatment has been nicely summarized by Stunkard (1958) — "most obese persons will not stay in treatment for obesity. Of those who stay in treatment, most will not lose weight and of those who do lose weight, most will regain it [p. 79]." The evidence to disconfirm this description has not yet appeared.

An examination of the contingencies governing addictive behavior in general and overeating in particular shows several reasons why this type of behavior should be so resistant to change. Addictive behaviors such as overeating provide immediate positive reinforcement for the individual, while the reinforcement for refraining from eating is usually extremely delayed. Moreover, the aversive consequences of overeating are typically delayed for weeks or even years. As Eysenck (1960) has pointed out, therapies based on pairing aversive reinforcement with the performance of the undesirable behavior are likely to be ineffective in the long run, because the fear of the negative consequences will tend to be extinguished when the behavior is performed without the negative reinforcement following. In addition, there are two other variables which make overeating behavior particularly resistant to alteration. Both Ferster *et al.* (1962) and Goldiamond (1965) have pointed out that eating behavior occurs in a very wide range of situations and is under the control of many stimuli other than those physiological ones causing hunger. A second factor, one unique to over-eating among the addictions, is that one cannot be delivered from temptation. Drugs, cigarettes, sexual perversions, and alcohol can all be given up completely and the stimuli association with them can be avoided; however, everyone must eat at least two or three times a day, and it is impossible to avoid exposure to situations and performance of behaviors one wishes to avoid. Thus the control of eating shares elements with the control of other undesirable appetitive behaviors but is further complicated by the facts that the stimuli for eating are ubiquitous and that some eating behaviors must be performed several times a day.

The study to be discussed attempted to use some of the specific procedures and methods of analysis which have been found useful in controlling both over-eating and other undesirable behaviors. Many of these techniques, particularly those of Ferster *et al.* (1962) and Goldiamond (1965), place a very strong emphasis on the development of self-control through altering the stimulus conditions under which the behavior occurs and generating self-produced consequences for the behavior. A second major influence was the use of aversive conditioning, both operant (Meyer & Crisp, 1964) and classical (Stollak, 1966; Wolpe, 1958), particularly the nausea conditioning of Cautela (1966). For the present study, nausea has several advantages over electric shock. It is completely under the individual's control, can be used in any situation, and is a response directly antagonistic to eating. In addition, a group setting was used in this research, primarily because of convenience, but also to take advantage of any slight increase in motivation which group discussion and support might generate.

Because long-term control of eating has been so refractory to change, it was felt that there was little to be gained by employing an attention-placebo control group in addition to a no-treatment control group. For the same reason it was decided to study the efficacy of a treatment approach combining several different components rather than comparing different techniques. The study was thus designed as a broad program to produce change by use of all the procedures which might assist an individual in attaining control of his own eating behavior by gradually approximating the eating pattern he eventually wanted to maintain. Drugs, lists of forbidden foods, or rigid rules of only three meals per day were not used, as they were felt to be useless in the maintenance of permanent habits. Although the procedures used were often geared to the individual's specific problems with eating, the type of approach should prove amenable to extension to dealing with other types of addictive behaviors.

Method

SUBJECTS

The *S*s for this study were both men and women who had answered an advertisement in the Stanford University newspaper, who were at least 15 lb. overweight, and who were not being medically treated for overweight or any serious illness. Two individuals who spontaneously began to discuss their psychiatric problems in a 10-min. interview with *E* were not included in the study. From the pool of satisfactory *S*s, two sections of three men and five women each who had the same available time for meetings were selected, along with a random group of three men and five women from the remaining potential *S*s to serve as a control group.

CONTROL GROUP

The members of the control group were truthfully told that the experimental groups would not be meeting during their available hours. They were then asked if they would attempt to lose weight on their own and if they would consent to be reweighed at the conclusion of the experiment. All Ss agreed. They were then weighed without shoes on a commercial bathroom scale, to the nearest half pound, given a calorie chart, and reminded that the only way to lose weight was to change their eating habits permanently.

TREATMENT PROCEDURE

The two experimental sections of eight Ss each met with E twice a week for approximately 2 mo. until the end of the school quarter. At the beginning of every meeting Ss were weighed individually without shoes on a commercial bathroom scale to the nearest half pound. The Ss were all given calorie charts and asked to keep a record of their normal eating habits for 1 wk. and of their daily intake, including place and time, for the next several months. At the first meeting and approximately every 3 wk. thereafter Ss completed a brief questionnaire consisting of eight rating scales. Four of the scales concerned their levels of tension and depression both generally and with specific reference to eating; three scales concerned temptations to eat rich foods, large meals, and snacks; and one concerned time thinking about food. One purpose of this questionnaire was to ascertain whether any mood changes would accompany or result from the process of weight reduction, as is suggested by such theories as "obesity as a depressive equivalent" (Simon, 1963). Another purpose of the rating scale was to see whether changes in the temptation to eat would accompany changes in eating behavior.

Three very general aspects of the program were discussed thoroughly with Ss. It was stressed that the program was designed to enable each individual to develop permanent eating habits he could maintain indefinitely. For this reason no arbitrary restrictions were placed on diet, and the individual was urged to consider what type of permanent eating pattern he would like to maintain. Along with the emphasis on establishing permanent habits there was an emphasis on awareness of what one was eating, especially caloric content and food value, and of the reasons for eating and the situation in which the eating occurred. A third general aspect of the treatment program was its emphasis on making only gradual changes. It was felt that making drastic changes, although perhaps producing greater immediate loss, would make it too difficult to maintain the changes indefinitely. The Ss were urged to make only small changes which they were sure they could maintain and which were in the direction of the permanent eating pattern they desired to establish.

TECHNIQUES

Three general types of techniques for approaching their goal of altered eating habits were recommended to *S* during the first 2 mo. of the program. First, *S*s were told about the concepts of positive and negative reinforcement, and it was explained to them how eating behavior was controlled by immediate positive reinforcement and only very delayed negative reinforcement. All *S*s were asked to consider the positive outcomes maintaining their eating and to hand in a list of the aversive consequences causing their desire to lose weight. In group discussions suggestions were made as to methods useful for making reward for refraining from eating more immediate and for making aversive consequences come immediately after beginning to eat; among the suggestions were the reciting of the list of reasons for losing weight when tempted to overeat, the viewing of an unattractive picture of oneself in a bathing suit when tempted, self-rewards of money, movies, clothes, etc. for every day or week of good eating habits or for every pound lost. It was emphasized that food should not be used as a reward.

The second group of techniques concerned the stimulus control of eating behavior and attempted to limit the situations which were associated with eating. The *S*s were asked to analyze the stimuli governing their eating behavior and were given suggestions about limiting the number of situations in which they eat and of stimuli connected with eating. Among these suggestions were many concerning limitations of place and time of eating — for example, try to eat sitting in only one chair at the same table or in as few places as possible; never eat while standing or in the office, bedroom, living room, etc.; try to eat meals and planned snacks only at certain definite times during the day. Other suggestions concerned the limitation of the availability of other reinforcements for eating and of tempting foods — for example, don't eat while reading, watching television, studying, etc.; try to avoid walking past candy machines, snack bars, etc. The *S*s were also informed of some Schachter's research (Schachter, 1967) demonstrating the control of eating behavior by external rather than internal stimuli in overweight people.

The third general group of suggestions dealt with the actual behaviors involved in eating. It was pointed out that many overweight people, particularly people on diets, eat much more rapidly than people of normal weight, and that it takes at least 15 min. after beginning to eat before one begins to feel the effects of the food. It was thus suggested that *S*s try to break up the chain of eating by not putting any more food on the fork until they had finished chewing and swallowing the last bite, that they chew their food very slowly and with great attention to taste and texture like a gourmet, that they practice taking short breaks of not eating during a meal, and that they begin to try out all of these suggestions only near the end of a meal when they are not so hungry that these behaviors would become aversive. It was also recommended that they attempt to practice leaving a little bit of every food on their plate, rather than automatically eating it all.

Throughout the presentation and discussion of all these techniques for controlling eating habits, it was emphasized that these were all methods for self-control of these behaviors. Although each technique should prove to be useful in some cases, it was recognized that certain techniques would be differentially useful for certain individuals; for this reason, each S was asked to try out all techniques which he felt might be appropriate for regulating his own behaviors and to try to commit himself to one small change at a time in the direction of his permanent eating habits. After the above meetings were completed, so that Ss had learned principles and techniques of reinforcement and self-control of eating behaviors, they were given a paper summarizing these principles and techniques. A list of low calorie foods and beverages suggested for cooking and eating was also given to them.

Two additional aspects of the treatment procedure were the discussion of nutrition and training in relaxation. A nutritionist spoke to Ss about diet in general, answered many questions about the nutritional and caloric values of various foods, and made brief verbal and written comments to Ss about the nutritional adequacy of their individual eating records. The Ss were also given training in relaxation exercises by listening to a tape and reading a manual designed by E to accompany the tape. The relaxation exercises were presented as an alternative to eating in dealing with tension, depression, and boredom.

DIFFERENTIAL TREATMENT OF SUBGROUPS

After a period of approximately 2½ mo. and following a change of schedule for those Ss who were university students, each of the two earlier experimental sections was subdivided into an aversive conditioning subgroup and a continuation subgroup. As two participants had withdrawn from the program, only the remaining 14 Ss were subdivided. The division was made into two subgroups such that each had 4 from one original section and 3 from the other, each had three males and four females, three good friends were put in one subgroup, each had about the same number of those who showed regular attendance in earlier meetings, and each had approximately the same mean weight loss for men and for women up to that time. A random selection was then made as to which of the two subgroups would be designated the continuation subgroup and which the aversive counterconditioning subgroup. Two hours per week were chosen at times when the continuation Ss were free, and these Ss were told that they could attend group meetings at one or both of these times. At these meetings, discussion centered around current problems Ss were having with eating and included suggestions and support from the other group members. The aversive counterconditioning Ss, on the other hand, did not have further group meetings, although a few of these Ss attended one or two of the continuation subgroup meetings. Instead, the aversive counterconditioning was carried out in individual meetings with E, which were held approximately weekly.

AVERSIVE COUNTERCONDITIONING

The procedures used in conditioning were based on a report by Cautela (1966). The Ss who were not able to relax sufficiently after the group instructions in relaxation were given further individual instruction until they were able to experience a moderate degree of relaxation. Each E was then given a thorough explanation of and rationale for aversive counterconditioning including the fact that the response was completely under his control and that the nausea conditioning would only be applied to certain foods in certain situations in which he was sure he did not want to eat. As work with two Ss in a preliminary study had demonstrated that nausea conditioning could also be effectively applied to reduce the positive valence of such behaviors as eating all the food on one's plate or eating more than one cookie, these were also mentioned as possibilities. Each S then chose a specific food in a specific situation where he desired to refrain from eating and was asked to describe the situation to E in great detail. The S was also asked to recall the last time he felt nauseous and vomited and to describe to E the sensations associated with nausea. Surprisingly, these varied a great deal among Ss.

During the actual nausea conditioning session, S sat comfortably in a chair with eyes closed and tried to visualize and imagine as vividly as possible the scene E described to him. The E then described in detail the situation S had chosen and described S's eating the food, feeling more and more nauseous and sick with every bite, and then vomiting. On alternate trials, S was described as about to eat the food, realizing how he didn't really want it, deciding not to eat the food, and then relaxing and feeling very happy. All but one S reported that their imagery and feelings of nausea were extremely vivid. One S (who had lost 20 lb.) reported at the next meeting that he did not want to undergo nausea conditioning again, because he had found it unpleasant. All the other Ss reported that they felt the experience was very effective. Usually two aversive and two relief trials were given in each session. Some Ss chose different situations for each aversive counterconditioning session; some practiced aversive counterconditioning at home; some did neither or both. Due to the approaching end of the academic year and because some Ss required lengthier instruction in relaxation exercises than others and some were unable to meet with E each week, each S had only one to three sessions of aversive counterconditioning.

FINAL WEIGHING

A final meeting was held approximately 4 mo. after the study began in order to get a final weight for all experimental and control Ss. All Ss who could not attend the meeting were contacted and final weights were obtained for all but the two Ss who had previously stopped participating and one control S who repeatedly broke appointments and finally could not be located. At the time of the final weighing, the experimental program was discussed with control Ss, and they were given copies of the paper on suggestions for weight reduction, the list of low calorie foods, and the manual of relaxation exercises.

Results

The weights for individual experimental and control Ss are reported in Table 1. All 14 Ss who remained in the study as well as the 2 who dropped out lost weight, with the difference between pretest and posttest weights being highly significant ($t = 5.19, p < .001$). These losses are represented graphically in Fig. 1.

TABLE 1. Weight losses for individual experimental and control subjects

	Original weight	Loss at 2½ mo.	Final weight	Total change	Percentage of change
Aversive counterconditioning subgroup					
Male	196.5	−15.5	176.0	−20.5	−10
Male	197.0	−20.5	171.0	−26.0	−13
Male	198.0	−3.5	194.5	−3.5	−2
Female	135.0	−3.5	124.5	−10.5	−8
Female	143.0	−2.5	137.5	−5.5	−4
Female	159.0	−6.0	152.0	−7.0	−4
Female	135.0	−5.0	130.0	−5.0	−4
Mean for males	197.2	−13.2	180.5	−16.7	−8
Mean for females	143.0	−4.3	136.0	−7.0	−5
Mean for subgroup	166.2	−8.1	155.1	−11.1	−7
Continuation subgroup					
Male	190.0	−8.0	175.0	−14.5	−8
Male	218.5	−11.5	208.0	−10.5	−5
Male	214.0	−14.0	193.0	−21.0	−10
Female	155.5	−7.5	146.5	−9.0	−6
Female	143.0	+0.5	137.0	−6.0	−5
Female	152.0	−7.0	145.5	−6.5	−4
Female	129.5	−2.5	127.5	−2.0	−2
Mean for males	207.5	−11.2	192.2	−15.3	−7
Mean for females	145.0	−4.1	139.1	−5.9	−4
Mean for subgroup	171.7	−6.9	161.9	−9.9	−6
Mean for treatment males	202.4	−12.2	186.4	−16.0	−8
Mean for treatment females	144.0	−4.3	137.6	−6.5	−5
Mean for treatment group	169.0	−7.5	158.5	−10.5	−6
Control Ss					
Male	181.0		179.5	−1.5	−1
Male	178.5		166.5	−12.0	−7
Male	238.0		254.5	16.5	7
Female	149.0		144.0	−5.0	−3
Female	147.0		159.0	12.0	8
Female	143.0		155.0	12.0	8
Female	146.5		150.0	3.5	2
Mean for control males	199.2		200.2	1.0	0.5
Mean for control females	146.4		152.0	5.6	4
Mean for control group	169.0		172.6	3.6	2

Tables 2 and 3 show the results of analyses of variance for pounds lost and percentage weight loss, respectively, for all experimental Ss versus the controls. The effect of the experimental treatment is highly significant using both measures ($p < .001$), and the effect of sex is significant at the $p < .05$ level for pounds lost and at the $.05 < p < .10$ level for percentage weight loss. Clearly, the sample is too small to allow definite conclusions to be reached about

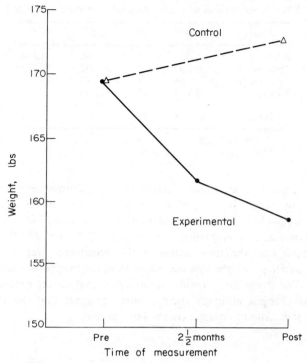

FIG. 1. Mean weights for experimental and control Ss.

whether men are likely to lose more weight than women independent of original weight. A t test on the difference between the additional weight losses of the aversive conditioning and continuation Ss during the last month and a half, when aversive conditioning Ss were receiving the extra treatment, revealed no significant differences ($t = .201$) between the two experimental subgroups.

The questionnaire data generally did not show large changes in the mood indexes over time. Only the data from those 12 Ss who had taken the questionnaire both in late January and in mid April were analyzed, as fewer Ss completed questionnaires in May and June. General level of tension or depression as well as

TABLE 2. Summary of analysis of variance for pounds lost

Source	SS	df	MS	F
Sex	322.32	1	322.32	5.51*
Treatment	938.15	1	938.15	16.04**
Interaction	27.86	1	27.86	<1
Within	994.41	17	58.49	
Total	2282.74	20		

*p $<$ .05
**p $<$ .001

TABLE 3. Summary of analysis of variance for percentage weight loss

Source	SS	df	MS	F
Sex	67.06	1	67.06	4.03*
Treatment	304.02	1	304.02	18.25**
Interaction	.58	1	.58	<1
Within	283.29	17	16.66	
Total	654.95	20		

* $.10 > p > .05$.
** $p < .001$.

tension or depression specifically related to eating showed only nonsignificant decreases from beginning to end of the experiment and no relationship to amount of weight loss. Both the temptation to eat large meals ($t = 2.34, p < .05$) and a general index of temptation to overeat ($t = 2.22, p < .05$) showed significant decreases over the time course of the experiment, but the correlation between percentage weight loss and decrease in temptation was not significant ($r = .186$). The study thus provides no evidence that dieting necessarily causes large mood changes, although there is some evidence that this program can reduce the temptation to overeat over a 3-mo. period.

Discussion

The minimal requirement for a weight reduction routine is that it enable people to lose weight and keep it off for a moderate amount of time without causing serious disruption of the individual's daily life or health. More desirable attributes would be the production of permanent weight loss with minimal expense of time or money and with the new eating pattern becoming both habitual and satisfying, so that the individual is not constantly troubled by desires to eat. It is clear that the program described in this study does satisfy the minimal requirements. All Ss showed a decrease in weight, a loss which was significantly greater than zero and than the slight gain shown by control Ss. Expense in money was nil and time spent attending meetings varied from about 10 to 20 hr.

Several of the less essential but desirable features are also found in this program. All Ss expressed satisfaction with the program and stated that they had found it extremely helpful. The low dropout rate of 12.5% compares very favorably with those reported in the literature, such as 39% not returning after one visit (Stunkard, 1959c), 33% not answering questionnaires after 6 mo. (Franklin & Rynearson, 1960), 66% dropping out within 1 yr. (Silverstone & Solomon, 1965), 27% after one meeting (Shipman & Plesset, 1963). Of the Ss who received aversive conditioning only one was not enthusiastic about the technique. This was the only instance of any S objecting to any aspect of the procedure; part of the success of the program may have been that *S*s were free to choose the techniques and eating patterns which suited them best rather than being forced to conform to rigid rules.

The questionnaire data show no significant mood changes as a result of the program, although the changes are in the direction of greater happiness and relaxation. The only changes which were significant were those indicating a lesser desire to overeat at meals and a decrease in general temptation to overeat at meals, eat sweets, and eat between meals. It seems likely that 3 mo. is not a sufficient time for large changes in affective values of eating to occur. It is also possible that questions dealing with eating behaviors rather than attitudes would reveal more significant changes.

The data appear to indicate that the program may be more effective for males than females, a difference also reported in a study by Stunkard (1959c). Although the possibility of physiological differences is not ruled out, the variables of awareness and motivation probably contribute to the sex differences found. In general, the men participating in this study were less aware of the caloric and nutritional values of various foods and of what their own eating habits were than were the women; moreover it is possible that the commitment to a group weight-reduction program represents a greater degree of motivation for men than for women, who often have a long history of going on diets with "the girls." A larger study will be necessary to discover the extent and causes of these sex differences, which were not quite significant when percentage weight lost rather than pounds lost was used as the measure.

The most crucial test of a weight reduction program or indeed of any therapy program is the permanence of its changes. Although long-term data are very difficult to obtain on members of a fluctuating university population, some data are available on *S*s who participated in a preliminary study of many of the techniques used in this final program. Twelve female *S*s originally began the pilot study; two dropped out very early, one for medical reasons and pregnancy. Eight of the *S*s met with *E* in two groups; two of the *S*s met individually with *E* and received aversive conditioning. All *S*s learned about stimulus control procedures. Each *S* kept daily eating records before and during the period of the experiment. Most of the *S*s met regularly with *E* for only 2 to 3 mo., although follow-up data were gathered on all available *S*s about 6–7 mo. after the start of the study. All but one *S* lost weight after 2–3 mo. with the mean short-term and also long-term loss for all pilot *S*s being 6 lb. Thus it does appear, for this preliminary study, that some of the effects of this program do last for at least 6 or 7 mo. Other long-term data are provided by *E*, who lost about 27 lb., regained about 12 lb. and has lost about 7 of those, 12 mo. after the beginning of the original study. However, in view of the extremely poor long-term results of other weight-reduction programs, it is clear that no conclusion can be drawn about the permanence of these changes.

It is possible that several variables may have contributed to the success of this particular study besides the planned experimental procedures. The modeling effect of E, who went from fat to moderate with the pretest Ss and from moderate to thin with Ss in the final study, was commented upon by many of the Ss. Many of the Ss stated that participating in a research project where data they provided were important increased their motivation. The majority of these Ss, moreover, were college educated, which may have made it easier for them to assimilate such concepts as reinforcement, stimulus control, and caloric values.

It is also possible that certain of the variables in this program, such as the group interaction, might make no additional contribution beyond that of the other procedures. It is possible that certain procedures, such as eating only when sitting down at the table, might be effective for all Ss whereas others, such as rewarding oneself monetarily for every day of good eating habits, might be of no use to any S. A much more controlled study in which various techniques and combinations of procedures are isolated would be necessary to discover their differential effects. In this study no additional effect of a very few sessions of aversive conditioning was found, although most Ss reported that it had reduced or eliminated their desires for those foods and the two pretest Ss given aversive conditioning continued to lose weight at least over a period of 6 mo. It is conceivable that aversive conditioning, both classical and operant, will turn out to be a useful tool for Ss who do have cravings for certain foods or for eating everything set before them, although it may well be useless for Ss whose problem is lack of awareness of their eating habits and caloric values. One might expect the effects of aversive counterconditioning used as an adjunct to such a program as the one described in this study to be much more enduring than the effects of aversive counterconditioning sessions alone. In short, the study was designed to see if any program for long-term weight reduction through change of eating habits could be achieved; future studies will be necessary to discover the contributions of specific variables, and the permanence of the weight losses achieved.

References

BRUCH, H. *The importance of overweight*. New York: Norton, 1957.

CAPPON, D. Obesity. *Canadian Medical Association Journal*, 1958, 79, 568–573.

CAUFFMAN, W. J. & PAULEY, W. G. Obesity and emotional status. *Pennsylvania Medical Journal*, 1961, 64, 505–507.

CAUTELA, J. R. Treatment of compulsive behavior by covert sensitization. *Psychological Record*, 1966, 16, 33–41.

ERICKSON, M. A. The utilization of patient behavior in the hypnotherapy of obesity: Three case reports. *American Journal of Clinical Hypnosis*, 1960, 3, 112–116.

EYSENCK, H. J. *Handbook of abnormal psychology*. New York: Basic Books, 1960.

FERSTER, C. B., NURNBERGER, J. I. & LEVITT, E. E. The control of eating. *Journal of Mathetics*, 1962, 1, 87–109.

FRANKLIN, R. E. & RYNEARSON, E. H. An evaluation of the effectiveness of dietary instruction for the obese. *Staff Meetings of the Mayo Clinic*, 1960, 35, 123–131.

GOLDIAMOND, I. Self-control procedures in personal behavior problems. *Psychological Reports*, 1965, 17, 851–868.

HARMON, A. R., PURKONEN, R. A. & RASMUSSEN, L. P. Obesity: A physical and emotional problem. *Nursing Outlook*, 1958, 6, 452–456.

KAPLAN, H. I. & KAPLAN, H. S. The psychosomatic concept of obesity. *Journal of Nervous and Mental Disorders*, 1957, 125, 181–201.

MAYER, J. Exercise does keep the weight down. *Atlantic Monthly*, 1955, 196, 63–66.

MEYER, V. & CRISP, A. H. Aversion therapy in two cases of obesity. *Behavior Research and Therapy*, 1964, 2, 143–147.

SCHACHTER, S. Obesity as a cognitive error. Speech presented at Stanford Medical School, February 14, 1967.

SHIPMAN, W. G. & PLESSET, M. R. Anxiety and depression in obese dieters. *Archives of General Psychiatry*, 1963, 8, 530–535.

SILVERSTONE, J. T. & SOLOMON, T. The long-term management of obesity in general practice. *British Journal of Clinical Practice*, 1965, 19, 395–398.

SIMON, R. I. Obesity as a depressive equivalent. *American Medical Association Journal*, 1963, 183, 208–210.

STOLLAK, G. E. Weight loss obtained under various experimental procedures. Paper presented at the meeting of the Midwestern Psychological Association, Chicago, May 1966.

STUNKARD, A. J. The management of obesity. *New York State Journal of Medicine*, 1958, 58, 79–87.

STUNKARD, A. J. Eating patterns and obesity. *Psychiatric Quarterly*, 1959, 33, 284–295. (a)

STUNKARD, A. J. Obesity and the denial of hunger. *Psychosomatic Medicine*, 1959, 21, 281–289. (b)

STUNKARD, A. J. The results of treatment for obesity. *Archives of Internal Medicine*, 1959, 103, 79–85. (c)

SUCZEK, R. F. The personality of obese women. *American Journal of Clinical Nutrition*, 1957, 5, 197–202.

THORPE, J. G., SCHMIDT, E., BROWN, P. T. & CASTELL, D. Aversion relief therapy: A new method for general application. *Behavior Research and Therapy*, 1964, 2, 71–82.

WOLPE, J. *Psychotherapy by reciprocal inhibition*. Stanford: Stanford University Press, 1958.

YOUNG, C. M., MOORE, N. S., BERRESFORD, K., EINSET, B. McK. & WALDNER, B. G. The problem of the obese patient. *Journal of the American Dietetic Association*, 1955, 31, 1111–1115.

CHAPTER 39

Self-directed Weight Control through Eating and Exercise

MARY B. HARRIS and ERIN S. HALLBAUER

The University of New Mexico, Albuquerque, New Mexico, 87131, U.S.A.

Summary— A weight control program using a written contract and other self-control behavior modification techniques for changing eating habits was compared with a similar program concentrating on both eating and exercise behavior and with an attention-placebo control condition. Participants in all three programs lost weight during the 12 week program, with no significant differences between groups. A seven-month follow-up revealed that Ss in the two behavior modification groups lost more than those in the control group and that those in the eating plus exercise group lost more than those in the group dealing only with eating behavior.

The treatment of obesity has, until very recently, been a severely discouraging endeavour. Medical treatments have included various diets, drugs, fasting and psychotherapy, generally leading to the same sad conclusion that more dieters fail than succeed (Feinstein, 1960). Considering the ineffectiveness of the above approaches and that it is almost universally accepted that caloric intake must be reduced in order for weight loss to occur, psychologists and physicians have recently become interested in using behavior modification techniques to control overeating (Stuart and Davis, 1972; Stunkard, 1972; Levitz, 1973). Most procedures rely on aversive counter-conditioning using electric shock (Meyer and Crisp, 1964) or nauseous odors (Foreyt and Kennedy, 1971), or on covert sensitization to particular foods (Cautela, 1966; Lick and Bootzin, 1971). These approaches seem to have enjoyed some success, but have not been tested on a large number of subjects, and, except for Cautela's treatment, are limited to a laboratory setting.

Two additional behavioral techniques have been tried with some degree of success: (1) contingency management, involving self-control procedures (Ferster et al., 1962; Goldiamond, 1965; Stuart, 1967; Harris, 1969; Penick et al., 1971; Wollersheim, 1970; Harris and Bruner, 1971; Hall, 1972; Stuart and Davis, 1972) and (2) a contract system (Harris and Bruner, 1971; Mann, 1971; Hall, 1972; Jeffrey et al., 1972). Both of these techniques have been shown to produce substantial weight losses, with the contract system producing a slightly greater weight loss in the Harris and Bruner study as well as in Hall's work.

Since both the contract and self-control procedures have been shown to be

Reprinted by permission from *Behaviour Research and Therapy*, 1973, **11**, 523–529.

effective in producing weight loss, it was decided to determine what effect a combination of the two would have. As noted by Harris and Bruner, the contract seems to weed out those who are not serious about losing weight and provide an incentive for weight loss during the contract period. It was hypothesized that combining the contract with self-control techniques would serve to effect significant weight loss for those who are willing to sign the contract and make a "meaningful" monetary deposit.

In most of the treatment procedures for obesity, exercise is momentarily considered and then discounted completely, usually on the basis that it takes entirely too much activity to produce a significant weight loss by exercise alone (Feinstein, 1960). Complicating the problem are the common misconceptions that exercising expends relatively little energy and that at all caloric levels, increasing physical activity will automatically cause an increase in appetite, thereby inadvertently causing weight gain (Mayer and Stare, 1953; Mayer, 1955; Mayer, 1968). Actually, it has been shown that subjects at a truly sedentary level of activity eat more than those who participate in regular moderate activity (Mayer, 1968). Stuart (1967) notes that in studying obese persons only two common characteristics can be found: overeating and underexercising. In addition, studies of adolescent girls indicate that their relative inactivity is significant in perpetuating their obesity (Bullen et al., 1964); Mayer (1968) reports similar findings for both boys and girls. Similarly, Stimbert and Coffey (1972) imply in their review that lack of exercise may contribute significantly to obesity in children and adolescents.

These facts would seem to indicate that a program incorporating both restriction of caloric intake and moderate exercise should be effective in reducing weight. This has been suggested by many (e.g. Douthwaite, 1936; Johnson et al., 1959; Konishi, 1965; Stuart and Davis, 1972); but actual programs seem to be few in number. One study has been done using treadmill walking in conjunction with diet restriction in a hospital setting; results indicated the combination was effective in producing substantial weight loss (Buskirk et al., 1963).

This study was designed to show the effect of including exercise in a self-control/contract program for weight reduction. It was hypothesized that a self-control/contract/exercise group would lose more weight than a self-control/contract group, and that both would lose substantially more than an attention-placebo control group.

Method

GENERAL PROCEDURE

Subjects were solicited by means of advertisements placed in the local and campus newspapers. Thirty-five females and eleven males ranging in age from 14 to 50 years and in weight from 119 to 295 lb were recruited; all reported the need to lose at least 15 lb. Of these 56 potential subjects, 50 actually attended at least one meeting. These 50 consisted of 21 full-time students, eight students who worked part-time, 12 housewives, 14 professional or semi-professional workers, and one unemployed semi-professional worker. *S*s were randomly assigned to the experimental and control groups, with pairs of friends or relatives being assigned to the same group; consideration was given to *S*s' available times for meeting. Twenty were assigned to the self-control/contract for eating group (E-1); 22 to the self-control/contract/exercise group (E-2); and 14 to the control group. All subjects were reported to be in good health and were taking no weight-reducing drugs or participating in other programs concurrently.

Subjects met in groups for a 12-week period from mid-March to early June with a female graduate student serving as *E*. At the initial meeting all *S*s were advised of the experimental nature of the program and were informed that the specific procedures to be followed had been successful in the past. They were also reminded that overeating, rather than any physical factors, is usually the cause of obesity, and even those few with metabolic problems still have to eat less in order to lose weight. *S*s were informed that their weight would be recorded weekly during the 12-week experimental period on a commercial bath-room scale and follow-up weight checks would be made. *S*s were given sheets on which to record all food consumed daily, compute caloric values, and note the circumstances involved in their eating behavior. At the second meeting, after recording and discussing current eating behavior, *S*s were asked to follow a sensible, nutritional diet with the intention of losing about 2 lb per week. At one meeting a nutritionist from the New Mexico Dairy Council spoke to each group on proper nutrition and its effect on dieting. In addition, all *S*s were given hand-outs of low-calorie recipes and calorie counts of native New Mexican foods.

Eating behavior only group (*E*-1). The treatment for this group consisted of a two-pronged approach: use of self-control behavior modification techniques to control eating in conjunction with a contract. Both approaches are almost identical to those used by Harris and Bruner (1971).

The actual behavior modification techniques used for self-control were given to *S*s at eight group meetings during which the basic principles of behavior therapy were explained and discussed; particular attention was paid to operant and respondent conditioning techniques and their application to weight control. Lessons were designed to teach *S*s to use these techniques to alter their eating behavior. For example, *S*s were asked to make a list of all personal aversive consequences of eating and to use this list to help counteract positive reinforcement from eating. They were also instructed to use positive reinforcements (other than food) for attaining long and short-range goals, such as not snacking while watching television for 1 week. Schachter's hypothesis of external stimulus control (1971) and related research were discussed, and suggestions were made for techniques to limit and control the stimuli which provoke eating. One lesson dealt with the principle of chaining, and suggestions were given to help break down and lengthen the chain of actions involved in getting food from plate to mouth to stomach. Group discussion was encouraged by E, especially in attempts to find solutions to individual problems.

At the first meeting Ss were given a copy of the contract; the contract procedures were explained and the reinforcing power of money, both positive and negative, was discussed. Ss were asked to decide on a reasonable amount of weight to lose in 12 weeks (N), to determine how much each pound was worth (X), and to make a deposit of XN dollars. It was emphasized that X should be a reasonable and meaningful amount for each S; $1.00 per pound was suggested, but any amount really meaningful to S was considered acceptable. The deposit was to be returned by E at the rate of X dollars per pound, during the week following the weight loss, provided the weight loss had been maintained. According to the contract stipulations, the remaining deposit was automatically forfeited if S dropped from the program or failed to lose the complete N pounds. Ss were told that all forfeited monies would be divided equally among the remaining participants at the end of the 12-week period, and this was done. Ss were given 1 week to consider the terms of the contract before making a definite commitment.

Eighteen Ss attended the first meeting ($\overline{X}$ of the 17 who stayed to be weighed = 168.5 lb; range = 125—202 lb). Eleven Ss, all female, attended the second meeting ($\overline{X}$ = 173.3 lb; range was 125—202 lb); all signed contracts to lose an average of 19.5 lb (range 11—25 lb) and made deposits ranging from 10¢ to $1.00 per lb ($\overline{X}$ = $0.77 per lb). The initial weight for the Ss who attended only the first meeting was 159.8 lb, with a range of 129—188 lb.

Eating and exercise group (E-2). The treatment for this group was identical to that of group E-1 with the exception that exercise was included in the treatment. During the second meeting, the importance of physical activity in determining total caloric needs was discussed (Stuart and Davis, 1972), as was Mayer's repudiation of the common belief that an increase in activity always results in increased appetite (Mayer, 1953; 1955; 1968). It was stressed that at the sedentary level food intake may actually increase, suggesting that for every person "a critical point might be reached at which food consumption would be at its low point relative to energy expenditure" (Stuart and Davis, 1972, p. 169). Ss were asked to commit themselves to some sort of daily exercise program; it was emphasized that the exercise undertaken should be enjoyable and should represent an increase over normal energy output (but not be so strenuous as to lead to exhaustion and/or discouragement). Suggestions of possible starting programs were given: parking two blocks farther from the office, using the stairs rather than the elevator; a daily walk or bicycle ride, ten sit-ups per night, etc. Ss were asked to slightly increase their individual programs each week until an optimal level appears to have been reached. In addition to a regular exercise program, *S*s were asked to critically examine their life styles and determine where they could increase caloric expenditure as a part of daily living. It was also suggested that additional exercise could be used to overcome effects of excessive calories consumed during weak moments. *S*s were given information on estimated caloric expenditures of various daily and recreational activities. The same suggestions for changing eating behavior given to *S*s in group E-1 were also given to these *S*s.

Nineteen *S*s attended the first meeting ($\overline{X}$ = 184.7 lb; range was 119–295 lb). Twelve attended the second meeting and all but two signed contracts to lose an average of 20.0 lb (range was 14–30 lb) and made deposits ranging from 5¢ to $2.00 per lb ($\overline{X}$ = $0.73 per lb). The two *S*s who requested another week to consider the contract did not return the following week. For the three males and seven females signing contracts, $\overline{X}$ initial weight was 171.0 lb with a range of 119–218 lb; for those not attending at least three meetings, $\overline{X}$ weight was 199.9 lb with a range of 149–295 lb.

Control group. Thirteen *S*s, twelve of whom stayed to be weighed, with an average weight of 154.5 lb (range 123.5–200.5 lb) attended the first meeting. They were informed that their specific treatment would consist of a combination of group discussion of dieting problems and individual counseling with *E*. Nine *S*s were present at the second meeting, and of these, 6 *S*s ($\overline{X}$ = 146.5; range was 123.5–198 lb; one male, five females) continued to report on a regular basis for weekly weight checks and pseudo-counseling. Other than weight recording and encouraging *S*s to keep accurate diet records, no specific techniques or recommendations were given. The $\overline{X}$ initial weight of the 6 non-participants was 161.4 lb with a range of 125–200.5 lb.

Measures. At the end of the 12-week period all *S*s who could be contacted were weighed; these weights constituted the post-test measure. Approximately 7 months after the beginning of the study *S*s were again contacted and weighed, with these weights serving as the follow-up measure. For purposes of comparisons, *S*s within each of the treatment groups were divided into participants (those who attended at least three meetings) and non-participants.

Results

Table 1 represents the mean number of pounds lost at the 12-week post-test and the 7-month follow-up for *S*s assigned to the three treatment groups who did and did not participate in the study. None of the differences in pounds lost at the post-test between treatment groups participants and non-participants, or any combination of the above were significant, although the participants did lose a significantly greater percentage of body weight (4.3%) than the non-participants (1.5%) at this point (t = 2.25, df = 40, $p < 0.05$).

Data from the 7-month follow-up indicated that all participants in the program lost more weight than non-participants (t = 3.38, df = 31, $p < 0.01$),

TABLE 1. Mean pounds lost and Ns for Ss in the treatment groups

	Post test	(n)	Follow-up	(n)
Participants				
Eating (E-1)	−6.9	(11)	−8.8	(9)
Exercise (E-2)	−9.1	(10)	−13.1	(7)
Control	−6.8	(6)	+0.2	(5)
Non-participants				
Eating	−3.3	(5)	−0.6	(4)
Exercise	−1.9	(4)	+1.7	(3)
Control	−2.0	(6)	+3.4	(5)
Combined				
Eating	−5.8	(16)	−6.3	(13)
Exercise	−7.0	(14)	−8.7	(10)
Control	−4.4	(12)	+1.8	(10)
Combined				
Experimental				
Group participants	−7.9	(21)	−10.7	(16)
All participants	−7.7	(27)	−8.1	(21)
Non-participants	−2.4	(15)	+1.6	(12)

that participants in both experimental groups combined lost more weight than participants in the control group ($t = 2.22$, df = 19, $p < 0.05$), and that all Ss in the experimental group combined lost more weight than all Ss in the control group ($t = 3.46$, df = 31, $p < 0.01$). In addition, participants in group E-2 tended to lose more weight than those in group E-1 ($t = 2.06$, df = 14, $0.10\ p < 0.05$), and the mean loss of all Ss assigned to treatment E-2 was greater than that shown by all Ss in group E-1 ($t = 2.28$, df = 21, $p < 0.05$).

Discussion

The results indicate that although all three programs led to short-term weight loss with no significant differences between them and only a weak tendency for participants to lose more than non-participants, the behavior modification programs were superior to the attention-placebo control in leading to long-term maintenance of the weight loss. In addition, the program which stressed control of exercise behavior as well as eating appeared more successful than that dealing with eating habits alone. Since most behavior modification programs for weight control have either ignored long-term results or reported relatively unsuccessful ones (Harris and Bruner, 1971; Jeffrey et al., 1972), the long-term success of this program is particularly encouraging. In fact, informal conversations with the participants at the time of the follow-up indicated that those who had maintained their weight loss or continued to lose indicated that they had continued to utilize the self-control techniques suggested, particularly the use of eating records.

A question that often arises in studies dealing with the effects of psychotherapy, as well as weight-control programs specifically, is that of evaluating the data of non-participants or drop-outs. Although it seems that people who drop out of a program without exposure to the entire treatment do not provide an adequate test of the treatment, it also seems biased to look at scores of only those motivated *S*s who finish a program, particularly in an area where a substantial number of *S*s do not complete the treatment. For that reason, the present study compared scores of participants and drop-outs and analyzed the data both including all *S*s originally assigned to each condition and excluding those who did not attend at least three meetings. Although the non-participants appeared to lose less weight than the participants, the differences between treatment groups on the follow-up test are the same regardless of whether or not scores of drop-outs are concluded. It is possible, of course, that the *S*s who could not be located for the post-test and follow-up were different from those who were weighed, since of the 48 who were weighed originally, only 42 were available for the post-test and 33 for the follow-up. However, the percentages of *S*s who were weighed seem reasonably large, particularly in view of the fact that several *S*s had mentioned that they would be leaving town between the post-test and follow-up.

Even though the combined self-control and contract program, particularly when dealing with exercise as well as eating behavior, did enable *S*s to lose weight, it was certainly not an unqualified success. The amounts of weight lost by the time of the follow-up although statistically significant, do not seem to be large in absolute terms, indicating that the program is not achieving the goal of producing extensive weight loss. Since participants in the experimental group lost far more during the 3 months of the study than during the 4 months following (and non-participants and control group members showed a mean weight gain during this latter period), it would appear that providing subjects with information about techniques is not adequate to ensure their continued use of these techniques when encouragement and reinforcement for doing so are no longer available from the *E* or other participants. Either one or more extensions of the contract, periodic check-ups, or continued group meetings might serve to motivate *S*s to attempt to lose weight consistently after the formal treatment program has ended. Only a program which leads to permanent maintenance of the participants at their desired weight, which this one did not, can be considered truly successful.

References

BRUCH, H. (1957) *The Importance of Overweight.* W. W. Norton, New York.

BULLEN, B. A., REED, R. B. and MAYER, J. (1964) Physical activity of obese and nonobese adolescent girls appraised by motion picture sampling. *Am. J. clin. Nutr.* **14**, 211–223.

BUSKIRK, E. R., THOMPSON, R. H., LUTWAK, L. and WHEDON, G. D. (1963) Energy balance of obese patients during weight reduction: Influence of diet restriction and exercise. *N. Y. Acad. Sci. Ann.* **110**, 918–939.

CAUTELA, J. R. (1966) Treatment of compulsive behavior by covert sensitization. *Psychol. Rec.* **16**, 33–41.

DOUTHWAITE, A. H. (1936) The treatment of obesity. *Br. Med. J.* **2**, 344–346.

FEINSTEIN, A. R. (1960) The treatment of obesity: An analysis of methods, results and factors which influence success. *J. chronic Disease* **11**, 349–393.

FERSTER, C. B., NURNBERGER, J. and LEVITT, E. E. (1962) The control of eating. *J. Mathetics* **1**, 87–109.

FOREYT, J. P. and KENNEDY, W. A. (1971) Treatment of overweight by aversion therapy. *Behav. Res. & Therapy* **9**, 29–34.

GOLDIAMOND, I. (1965) Self-control procedures in personal behavior problems. *Psychol. Rep.* **17**, 851–868.

HALL, S. M. (1972) Self-control and therapist control in the behavioral treatment of overweight women. *Behav. Res. & Therapy* **10**, 59–68.

HARRIS, M. B. (1969) Self-directed program for weight control: A pilot study. *J. abnorm. Psychol.* **74**, 263–270.

HARRIS, M. B. and BRUNER, C. G. (1971) A comparison of a self-control and a contract procedure for weight control. *Behav. Res. & Therapy* **9**, 347–354.

JEFFREY, D. B., CHRISTENSEN, E. R. and PAPPAS, J. P. (1972) A case study report of a behavioral modification weight reduction group: Treatment and follow-up. Paper presented at the Rocky Mountain Psychological Association Meeting.

JOHNSON, M. L., BURKE, B. S. and MAYER, J. (1959) Relative importance of inactivity and overeating in the energy balance of obese high school girls. *Am. J. clin. Nutr.* **4**, 37–44.

KONISHI, F. (1965) Food energy equivalents of various activities. *J. Am. diet. Ass.* **46**, 186–188.

LEVITZ, L. S. (1973) Behavior therapy in treating obesity. *J. Am. diet. Ass.* **62**, 22–26.

LICK, J. and BOOTZIN, R. (1971) Covert sensitization for the treatment of obesity. Paper presented at the Midwestern Psychological Association Convention.

MANN, R. A. (1971) The use of contingency contracting to control obesity in adult subjects. Paper presented at the Western Psychological Association Convention.

MAYER, J. and STARE, F. J. (1953) Exercise and weight control: Frequent misconceptions. *J. Am. diet. Ass.* **29**, 340–343.

MAYER, J. (1955) Exercise does keep the weight down. *Atlantic Monthly* **196**, 63–66.

MAYER, J. (1968) *Overweight: Causes, Cost and Control.* Prentice-Hall, Englewood Cliffs, New Jersey.

MEYER, V. and CRISP, A. H. (1964) Aversion therapy in two cases of obesity. *Behav. Res. & Therapy* **2**, 143–147.

PÉNICK, S., FILION, R., FOX, S. and STUNKARD, A. (1971) Behavior modification in the treatment of obesity. *Psychom. Med.* **33**, 49–55.

SCHACHTER, S. (1971) Some extraordinary facts about obese humans and rats. *Am. Psychol.* **26**, 129–144.

STIMBERT, V. E. and COFFEY, K. R. (1972) Obese children and adolescents: A review. *Res. Relating to Child (ERIC)*, **30**, 1–30.

STUART, R. B. (1967) Behavioral control of overeating. *Behav. Res. & Therapy* **5**, 357–365.

STUART, R. B. and DAVIS, B. (1972) *Slim Chance in a Fat World: Behavioral Control of Obesity.* Research Press Company, Champaign, Illinois.

STUNKARD, A. (1958) The management of obesity. *N.Y. St. J. Med.* **58**, 79–87.

STUNKARD, A. (1972) New therapies for the eating disorders. *Archs. gen. Psychiat.* **26**, 391–398.

WOLLERSHEIM, J. P. (1970) Effectiveness of group therapy based upon learning principles in the treatment of overweight women. *J. abnorm. Psychol.* **76**, 462–474.

CHAPTER 40

Behavior Modification in the Treatment
of Obesity

SYDNOR B. PENICK, ROSS FILION, SONJA FOX and ALBERT J. STUNKARD
Department of Psychiatry, University of Pennsylvania, Philadelphia, Pa.

   Summary— Current interest in behavior modification has extended to the
treatment of obesity and the results of two recent applications of this technology
have been encouraging. The present study compared behavior modification in groups
with traditional group psychotherapy in a sample of 32 obese patients. Each of two
groups treated with behavior modification lost more weight than a matched control
group treated with traditional group therapy. Furthermore, 13% of the patients
treated by behavior modification lost more than 40 pounds and 53% lost more than
20 pounds, results which rank with the best in the medical literature. We conclude
that behavior modification may represent a significant advance in the treatment of
obesity.

"Most obese persons will not stay in treatment for obesity. Of those who stay
in treatment most will not lose weight and of those who do lose weight, most
will regain it."[1] Until recently, this summary of the results of outpatient
treatment for obesity has been unchallenged. Reports in the medical literature
agree that no more than 25% of obese persons entering treatment will lose as
much as 20 pounds and only 5% will lose as much as 40 pounds.

The current interest in behavior modification and the evidence of its
effectiveness in the control of several conditions rendered inevitable its application to the problems of overeating and obesity. Yet the results of the first such
application, by Ferster,[2] were disappointing. The modal weight loss of the 10
patients in his program was only 10 pounds, with a range from 5 to 20.[3] A
second study reported significantly greater weight losses among a group treated
behaviorally than among a no-treatment control group; few of these patients
were really obese, however, and only 21% of those remaining in treatment lost as
much as 20 pounds.[4]

Reprinted with permission from *Psychosomatic Medicine*, 1971, 33, 49−55.

Supported in part by NIMH grant MH-15383-04.
Presented in part at the Annual Meeting of the American Psychosomatic Society,
Washington, DC, March 22, 1970.
Address for reprint requests: Albert J. Stunkard, MD, Department of Psychiatry,
University of Pennsylvania, Philadelphia, Pa 19104.

Against this background, Stuart's recent report on *Behavioral Control of Overeating* stands out.[5] Eighty per cent of patients who began treatment (and all who continued) lost more than 20 pounds and 30% lost more than 40 pounds — the best results of outpatient treatment for obesity yet reported. These results persuaded us to assess the effectiveness of behavior modification in the treatment of obesity.

Methods and Materials

The assessment of behavior modification was carried out in a day-care program for the treatment of obesity which is described more fully elsewhere.[6] Duration of treatment was 3 months, carried out once a week from 10:30 am to approximately 3 pm. Activities consisted of an exercise period, preparation and eating of a low calorie lunch, and group therapy.

Thirty-two patients, all at least 20% overweight,[7] comprised the study group. Median per cent overweight of patients treated by behavior therapy was 78%; that of the control patients was 80%. Median age of the behavior therapy patients was 39 (range 22–61); that of the control group was 44 (range 15–61). Most of the subjects were middle-class private patients referred for weight reduction, while 6 were lower-class persons referred by a state rehabilitation agency. Twenty-four were women and 8 were men.

Two cohorts were studied, the first composed entirely of private patients, the second containing also the rehabilitation patients. Patients from each source were randomly assigned to either a behavior therapy or a control group. Private patients paid in advance for the entire program and the fees were not refundable; welfare patients' fees were paid by the state.

Therapy of both groups lasted about 2 hours and was carried out by a man-and-woman team. The control group received supportive psychotherapy, instruction about dieting and nutrition and, upon demand, which was infrequent, appetite suppressants. The male therapist (SP) was an internist with long experience in the treatment of obesity. He is currently undertaking residency training in psychiatry, which has given him considerable additional training in group therapy. The female therapist was a research nurse with long association with her co-therapist, but no previous experience in group therapy.

The behavior modification therapists had had experience with group therapy only once before, in a 2-month pilot study of a group of obese women. The male therapist (RF), an experimental psychologist, had a strong background in learning theory but little clinical experience. The female therapist (SF), a research technician, had had extensive experience in clinical research, particularly in obesity. No appetite suppressants were used with these groups. The behavioral program is described below.

Results

THE BEHAVIORAL PROGRAM

The behavioral program was similar to that described by earlier writers and involved four general principles.

1. *Description of the behavior to be controlled.* The patients were asked to keep daily records of the amount, time and circumstances of their eating. The immediate results of this time-consuming and inconvenient procedure were grumbling and complaints. Eventually, however, each patient reluctantly acknowledged that keeping these records had proved very helpful, particularly in increasing his awareness of how much he ate, the speed with which he ate, and the large variety of environmental and psychologic situations associated with eating. For example, after 2 weeks of record-keeping, a 30-year-old housewife reported that for the first time in her life, she recognized that anger stimulated her eating. Accordingly, whenever she began to get angry, she left the kitchen and wrote down how she felt, thereby decreasing her anger and aborting her eating.

2. *Modification and control of the discriminatory stimuli governing eating.* Most of the patients reported that their eating occurred in a wide variety of places and at many different times during the day. They were accordingly encouraged to confine their eating, including snacking, to one place. In order not to disrupt domestic routines, this place was usually the dining room. Further efforts to control the discriminatory stimuli included the use of a distinctive table setting, including an unusually colored place mat and napkin. Patients were encouraged to make eating a pure experience, unaccompanied by any other activity, particularly reading, watching television or arguing with their families.

3. *Development of technics which control the act of eating.* Specific technics were utilized to help patients decrease the speed of their eating, to become aware of the various components of the eating process, and to gain control over these components. Exercises included counting each mouthful of food eaten during a meal, and placing utensils on the plate after every third mouthful until that mouthful was chewed and swallowed.

4. *Prompt reinforcement of behaviors which delay or control eating.* A reinforcement schedule, utilizing a point system, was devised for control of eating behavior. Exercise of the suggested control procedures during a meal earned a certain number of points; devising an alternative to eating in the face of strong temptation earned double this number of points. Points were converted into money which was brought to the next meeting and donated to the group. At the beginning of the program, the group decided how the money should be used, and, to our surprise, highly altruistic courses were chosen. Each week, the first group donated its savings to the Salvation Army; the second, to a needy friend of one of the members, a widow with 14 children.

In addition to positive reinforcement, negative reinforcement was utilized. For example, control over snacking was facilitated by "doctoring" favorite snack foods with castor oil or other aversive taste. Furthermore, failure to exercise control resulted in the loss of points.

Our program differed from previous behavioral methods in at least two ways: (a) infrequent weighings and (b) separate reinforcement schedules for exercise of self-control and for weight loss.

(a) Previous workers, ourselves included, had weighed patients more frequently, and had attached contingencies to weighings as frequently as four times a day. Such short-term weight fluctuations, however, may result from physiologic factors such as fluid shifts, and are therefore probably imperfectly related to the exercise of behavioral control of eating. Their reinforcement could thus be counter-productive at times.

(b) The primary objective of this program was the development of self-control of eating, and weight loss was considered a consequence of the adaptive behaviors resulting from self-control. Separate reinforcement systems were therefore established for self-control and for weight loss. Reinforcements for self-control have been described. Various reinforcements for weight loss were devised by individual patients and therapists. An example of a popular and effective method utilized by all group members was purchase of a pound of suet which was cut into 16 pieces and placed in a plastic bag in a prominent place in the refrigerator. The patient attempted to visualize this fat on his body. For each pound lost, he removed 1 ounce of fat from the bag and tried to imagine its disappearance from his body. If he gained weight, he took home an ounce of fat for each pound gained and added it to his fat bag. When a patient had lost the entire fat bag, a prize such as a book or cosmetics was presented to him by the group, along with lavish praise.

WEIGHT LOSS

The results of treatment of the two cohorts are summarized in Table 1. The weight losses in the control group are comparable to those reported for a variety of treatments in the medical literature; none lost 40 pounds and 24% lost more than 20 pounds. By contrast, 13% of the behavioral modification group lost more than 40 pounds and 53% lost more than 20 pounds. Although neither of the differences between behavior modification and control groups for weight losses of over 20 and 40 pounds is statistically significant, that for weight losses of over 30 pounds is ($p = 0.015$ by Fisher exact probability test).

The weight losses for each subject are plotted in Figs. 1 and 2. Two findings should be noted. First, in each cohort the median weight loss for the behavior modification group was greater than that of the control group — 24 versus 18 pounds for the first cohort and 13 versus 11 pounds for the second. The second

TABLE 1. Results of treatment: percent of groups losing
specified amounts of weight

Weight	Behavior modification groups (%) (N =15)	Control therapy groups (%) (N = 17)	Average medical literature (%)
More than 40 pounds	13	0	5
More than 30 pounds	33	0	–
More than 20 pounds	53	24	25

finding is the far greater variability of the results of the behavior modification groups ($f = 4.38$, $p < 0.005$). The 5 best performers belonged to these groups as did the single least effective one, the only patient who actually gained weight during treatment. Because of this great variability, the overall differences in weight loss between the behavior modification and the control groups did not reach statistical significance.

Follow-up of the two cohorts at 6 and 3 months, respectively, provided evidence of the continuing influence of treatment, in contrast to the usual experience of rapid regaining of weight after treatment. Table 2 reveals that the number of persons in the behavior modification group who lost more than 40 pounds doubled after termination of treatment (from 2 to 4), and 3 have actually lost more than 50 pounds. The control group similarly showed an increase in the number of persons losing large amounts of weight, a finding which attests to the effectiveness of this treatment. The median weight losses of the groups again showed differences favoring behavior modification: 18.5 versus 13.5 pounds for the first cohort and 22 versus 15 pounds for the second cohort.

TABLE 2. Follow-up at 3–6 months: percent of groups
losing specified amounts of weight

Weight	Behavior modification groups (%) (N = 15)	Control therapy groups (%) (N = 17)
More than 40 pounds	27	12
More than 30 pounds	40	18
More than 20 pounds	53	29

Discussion

This study showed that behavior modification, devised by a team with little experience in this modality, was more effective in the treatment of obesity than was the best alternate program that could be devised by an internist with long

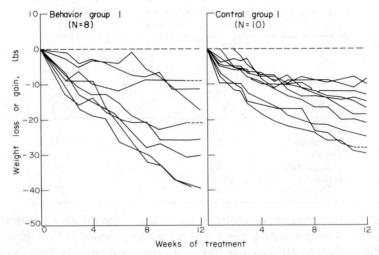

FIG. 1. Weight changes of patients in first cohort. Dotted lines represent interpolated data based upon weights obtained during follow-up. Note greater weight loss of behavior modification group and greater variability of this weight loss as compared with that of control group.

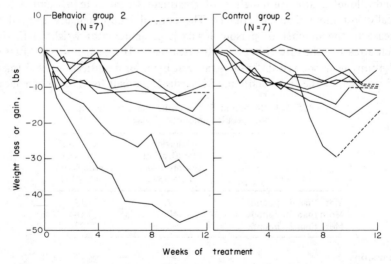

FIG. 2. Weight changes of patients in second cohort. Dotted lines again represent interpolated data. Variability of weight loss of behavior modification group is even larger than that of first cohort, while variability of weight loss in control group is even smaller.

experience in the treatment of this disorder. These results and those of Stuart[5] and of Harris[4] cited earlier, strongly suggest that behavior modification represents a significant advance in the treatment of obesity.

Two factors increase our confidence in the significance of these results. First, the weight losses in the control group are representative of the majority of reports in the medical literature. The difference between behavior modification and control groups is thus not due to decreased effectiveness of treatment in the control group. Second, although the weight losses of the behavior modification group are not as great as those reported by Stuart in his precedent-making report cited earlier, they are a result of only 3 months of treatment, compared with the year's duration of treatment in Stuart's series. Indeed, they are greater than the weight losses after 3 months among Stuart's patients, none of whom had lost as much as 20 pounds at that time. This significant difference ($p = 0.013$ by Fisher exact probability test) suggests that a group setting may increase the effectiveness of behavior modification when compared with individual treatment as utilized by Stuart.

The major limitation of this study must be considered — the use of different therapists *as well as* different therapies. Ideally, each therapist should utilize each modality of therapy in an unbiased manner. Since this ideal cannot be realized, the next best procedure is to control the bias by utilizing frankly biased therapists, some whose bias is for behavior modification and some whose bias is against it. We are now beginning such a study, which is both laborious and time-consuming. Short of such an investment, the design utilized in the present study is the most efficient. Until almost the end of the study, each therapist team believed that the treatment it used was the better, and it was biased in favor of it. Furthermore, SP's experience in the treatment of obesity and as a group therapist was far greater than that of the leaders of the behavior modification groups.

A possible limitation of the study is that the day hospital setting may have had differential effects upon the behavior modification and supportive psychotherapy groups. If the former group responded more favorably to this setting, such an interaction, rather than behavior modification alone, could account for the apparently greater effectiveness of behavior modification.

The great variability in the performance of the patients in the behavior modification groups raises intriguing questions for further research, as both the best and the worst results were obtained in these groups. It appears that behavior modification can be remarkably effective for certain patients and quite ineffective for others. None of the criteria we utilized, primarily our clinical impressions and MMPI data, predicted which patients would respond. A major goal of our further research will be to develop such predictors, as even limited success in this endeavor, coupled with the replication of the current findings, would mean a significant advance in the treatment of obesity. For selected persons, an effective treatment for their obesity would be at hand.

Summary

The effectiveness of behavior modification in the treatment of obesity was assessed in a group of 32 patients divided into two cohorts. Half of each cohort was treated as a group with a behavior modification program, and half received more conventional group psychotherapy. Treatment modalities were compared with each other and with the results of treatment for obesity as reported in the medical literature.

All four treatment groups performed well by accepted standards. In each cohort, however, the weight loss of the behavioral modification group exceeded that of the traditional therapy group, and even in this small sample, this difference reached statistical significance by one criterion. Furthermore, 13% of this group lost more than 40 pounds and 53% lost more than 20 pounds, results which rank with the best reports in the medical literature.

The results of the behavior modification groups were far more variable than those of traditional group therapy programs, with individual patients performing both more and less effectively than those of the traditional therapy groups. Available data were insufficient to distinguish responders to behavior modification from nonresponders. The development of predictors of response to behavior modification, in combination with replication of the current findings, could mean a significant advance in the treatment of obesity.

References

1. Stunkard, A. J. The results of treatment for obesity. *New York State J. Med.* **58,** 79, 1958.
2. Ferster, C. B., Nurnberger, J. I., and Levitt, E. E. The control of eating. *J. Mathetics* **1,** 87, 1962.
3. Ferster, C. B. Personal communication.
4. Harris, M. B. A self-directed program for weight control: a pilot study. *J. Abnorm. Psychol.* **74,** 263, 1969.
5. Stuart, R. B. Behavioral control of overeating. *Behav. Res. Ther.* **5,** 357, 1967.
6. Penick, S. B., Filion, R. D. L., Fox, S. *et al.* A day hospital approach to human obesity. Unpublished data.
7. Metropolitan Life Insurance Company, N.Y. New weight standards for men and women. *Statistical Bulletin*, Vol. 40, Nov.–Dec. 1969, p. 3.

CHAPTER 41

Self-control and Therapist Control in the Behavioral Treatment of Overweight Women

SHARON MARTINELLI HALL[1]

Washington State University, Pullman, Washington, U.S.A.

Summary– Weight changes during two behavioral treatment programs were compared with baseline weights of 10 obese women, median age, 41.5 years, in a single-subject design. Weekly weights were obtained from the TOPS Club of which the *S*s were members for 3 months prior to the beginning of the study. The *S*s monitored their weights for 2 weeks, then monitored both weight and food intake for an additional 2 weeks. The *S*s were then randomly assigned to one of two conditions: In Condition 1, the *S*s were taught self-control principles (SC) for 5 weeks, and then underwent an experimenter controlled reinforcement program (EC) for 5 weeks. The order of treatments were reversed for *S*s in Condition 2. The *S*s weekly weights then were obtained from the TOPS Club for an additional 4 weeks. The results indicated that both SC and EC produced weight losses in overweight women, but only the losses effect by EC were large enough to be of practical value. Weight losses were maintained during follow-up. The results also indicated considerable agreement between self-report of weight and weights obtained by *E*. The implications for the present study for behavior therapy and research were discussed.

Overeating is difficult to modify by traditional methods (Stunkard and McClaren-Hume, 1958) and it requires methods of modification which will be effective when the therapist is not present. As such, it is prototypical for the majority of behavior change attempts. In most therapy, what the patient does in his life situation, when he is not in the presence of the therapist, is the focus of change.

Attempts to eliminate maladaptive eating responses can be roughly divided into two classes: Those techniques where the primary degree of control over the reinforcers employed is with the therapist or *E*, and those techniques where the primary degree of control of the reinforcers employed is with the client or *S*. These two classes are not dichotomous; rather, the difference between them is a matter of degree, rather than kind. In any therapeutic situation both client and therapist have some control over the reinforcers which would change the client's

Reprinted with permission from *Behaviour Research and Therapy*, 1972, **10**, 59–68.

[1] This paper is based upon a doctoral dissertation submitted to Washington State University. The author wishes to thank Warren Garlington, Robert Chapman, James Whipple and Norris Vestre for their assistance, and wishes also to thank Robert G. Hall for reading the manuscript. The author is presently at the Veteran's Administration Hospital, Palo Alto, California.

behavior. However, the distinction made here is between the *primary* locus of control of the techniques. In a behavioral program of the first sort, the contingencies are directly controlled by E and S is virtually dependent upon E for the manipulation of the contingencies which are to effect the therapeutic change. In programs of the second sort, the behavioral program instituted is so designed that the arrangement of the majority of contingencies is left to the client. The client is no longer as dependent upon the therapist for the production of the behavioral contingencies which effect change and is also able to engineer his own contingencies for new programs if he so desires.

Behavioral control of eating responses effected primarily through therapist control of contingencies has been attempted by Wolpe (1958), Meyer and Crisp (1964), Thorpe *et al.* (1964), Stollak (1966), Harmatz and Lapuc (1968), and Kennedy and Foreyt (1968), and Foreyt and Kennedy (1971). With the exception of Harmatz and Lapuc, the experimenter controlled techniques have involved E presenting an aversive stimulus either contingent upon approach behavior to food or as an unconditioned stimulus preceded by food in a classical conditioning paradigm. The Harmatz and Lapuc procedure involved the removal of a positively reinforcing stimulus rather than the presentation of an aversive stimulus. These investigators fined hospitalized schizophrenic men for failure to lose weight. On the whole, experimenter-controlled techniques have produced equivocal results. Wolpe, Foreyt and Kennedy (1971), and Harmatz and Lapuc all reported positive results, while Thorpe *et al.*, Kennedy and Foreyt (1968), Meyer and Crisp, and Stollak reported either equivocal results, positive results that did not last during follow-up, or failure to effect weight loss. These equivocal results may be due to the complexities of designing an effective aversive stimulation paradigm, or they may be the result of the increased emotionality which is produced by aversive stimulation. That is, as Ferster *et al.* (1962) have noted, heightened emotionality results in increased eating among obese women. Because of the occurrence of this phenomenon, the effects of the conditioned aversion to food may be weakened by the increased disposition to eat evoked by the emotionality.

At the opposite end of the continuum from experimenter controlled techniques are the techniques which rely primarily upon the client's arranging his own responses and the stimuli in his environment to alter the probability of problem responses such as overeating. Such techniques rely upon the client's application of concepts such as reinforcement and punishment, stimulus control, weakening of chains of behavior, and development of alternative repertoires to his environment. Such programs have been designed by Ferster *et al.* (1962), Goldiamond (1965), Stuart (1967), Harris (1969), and Wollersheim (1970). Ferster *et al.* and Goldiamond did not report quantitative data; such data were reported in studies by Stuart, Harris and Wollersheim. These studies all indicated that the techniques were successful in producing weight loss. Both Harris and Wollersheim reported significant differences between groups of college students who were taught self-control techniques and those who served as no-contact control subjects, or who received other treatments.

The purpose of the present study was to examine the effects of two different behavioral programs for weight loss. The first program gave control of the reinforcing contingencies primarily to the therapist (EC program). Unlike most of the studies reviewed above, the present study used positive reinforcement for weight loss rather than relying upon noxious stimuli associated with certain foods or approach responses to such foods. The second behavioral program (SC program) was a modification of Stuart's (1967) and Ferster *et al.*'s (1962) self-control programs. The present study used an individual subject design which compared each *S*s performance with her own baseline performance, rather than the traditional group design. The individual subject design was chosen for two reasons: First, the design allowed the assessment of the effects of treatments upon the individual *S*, rather than evaluation of treatment effects by group means. Second, the design used in the present study allowed assessment of the clinical utility of the treatment effects even when such effects were slight. For example, for some women, a slight weight loss might indicate an effective treatment for that *S* for she may be unable to achieve such a weight loss without treatment. The same loss may be inconsequential for other *S*'s whose baseline data indicate they can effect such losses without the aid of intervention.

Method

SUBJECTS

The *S*s were 14 female volunteers who were members of TOPS, a national weight-reducing club. These *S*s were chosen from a subject pool of 30 interested TOPS members on the basis of three criteria: (a) willingness to sign a commitment statement which indicated that *S* would not drop from the study before its completion, (b) membership in TOPS for 3 months prior to the beginning of the study, (c) a statement that *S* had not planned a vacation longer than 1 week for the duration of the study.

The *S*s ranged from 26 to 57 years of age with a median age of 41.5 years. The *S*s weights ranged from 130 to 226 lb with a median weight of 173 lb. None of the *S*s were taking appetite depressants or were participating in any sort of weight-reduction program other than TOPS.

APPARATUS AND MATERIALS

The *E* weighed each *S* on a hospital scale each session. Club weights were obtained by the *S*s at their club meetings on a similar scale. Home weights were obtained daily by each S on her own bathroom scale. The Ss received written material on each self-control technique (Hall, 1971) and data sheets for recording weight and food data.

PROCEDURE

Prior to the beginning of the study, each S's weekly weight from the previous 3 months was recorded from the TOPS club weight records. This 3-month period, which will be referred to as B_0, took place during weeks 1–12. These data provided a pretreatment baseline against which to assess treatment effects. The recording of weight data was explained to the Ss after their regular club meeting at the beginning of week 13. The Ss were instructed to weigh themselves daily before breakfast, in their undergarments only, and to record the date and their weight on the weight data sheet provided by E. During the following 2 weeks, weeks 13–14, Ss weighed themselves daily as instructed. Weeks 13–14 will be referred to as B_1. Two weeks after the first day of B_1, that is, on the first day of week 15, Ss were instructed to begin recording food data in addition to weight data. Again, the proper recording techniques were explained to the Ss at their regular club meeting. The Ss were told to record the date and time of each food intake, what was eaten, the quantity of food eaten, the method of preparation, and the circumstances under which the food was eaten. The Ss were instructed to record both food and weight data for the following 2 weeks of the experiment, weeks 15–16. This 2-week period wherein both food and weight data were collected will be referred to as B_2. These data continued to be collected by the Ss throughout the EC and SC treatment programs. The purpose of B_1 and B_2 was to assess the effects of food and weight monitoring independent of the SC and EC programs, for as Euler (1970) has indicated, self-monitoring alone may alter behavior under some circumstances.

At the end of B_2, Ss were randomly assigned to either Condition 1 or Condition 2. The seven Ss who were assigned to Condition 1 received the SC program for 5 weeks (weeks 17–21) and the EC program for the following 5 weeks (weeks 22–26). The order of the two treatment programs was reversed for Condition 2 Ss. During the 10-week period when Ss were exposed to the EC and SC programs each Ss met with E individually twice per week. At the first meeting during this period, regardless of the condition to which S was assigned, S set a weight loss goal for the 10-week period. This figure was divided in half to determine the weight loss goal for each of the two treatment programs. During each meeting regardless of treatment each S was weighed in street clothes without shoes at the beginning of the interview, and E reinforced any weight loss with approval.

Self-control program. The techniques taught during the self-control treatment included manipulations of emotional responses, manipulation of stimuli to narrow stimulus control over eating, weakening of chains leading to eating, and the development of a prepotent repertory.

Manipulation of emotional responses was accomplished by teaching the Emotional Response Routine (ERR) developed by Chapman and Smith (1970). In using the ERR, the aversive consequences of engaging in the problem behavior are covertly verbalized when the disposition to perform that behavior is present. The S then repeats the pleasant, reinforcing consequences of not performing the problem behavior. The ERR thus constitutes a chain of behavior where the repetition of aversive consequences in the presence of certain stimuli is reinforced by the repetition of pleasant consequences. In order to obtain the aversive consequences most punishing to S, each S was questioned by E as to those features of obesity which S found to be most disturbing. The E urged S to give responses which were as anxiety-provoking as possible. The S was also asked to enumerate at least three positive features accruing to weight reduction. The E emphasized that S should choose statements which produced a great deal of positive affect when S thought about them. These benefits of losing weight were used as the reinforcer for the verbalization of the aversive consequences of obesity. The S was repeatedly drilled on the ERR during the treatment interviews. Each S was instructed initially to repeat the sequence aloud when she felt the urge to eat between meals when alone and to repeat it covertly when with others. As the ERR become "over-learned", S was instructed to use the ERR covertly at all times.

Ferster *et al.* (1962) suggested that, in obese people, eating is under the control of a very large number of stimuli. In the present study, an attempt was made to narrow those stimuli by the introduction of the "pure stimulus act", whereby S is to terminate all other activities while eating. In the present study, this restriction was relaxed when the S was eating outside her own home.

Ferster *et al.* (1962) also suggested that the chain leading to the eating response might be weakened through extending the length of the chain by adding more members to the chain or by lengthening the time required to complete individual members of the chain. In the present study, several techniques were used to extend the chain leading to the eating response. First, the Ss were instructed to remove all food from every place but the kitchen. The purpose of this activity was to lengthen the chain leading to between-meal eating for those Ss who were accustomed to keeping food handy in a purse or drawer. The Ss were also instructed to prepare only one portion of food at a time. The purpose of single portion preparation was to lengthen the chain leading to second portions by requiring a second period or preparation for such portions.

The Ss were instructed to use a plate, cup, glass, or bowl one size smaller than that normally used. The rationale for this technique was that in order to eat a large amount, S must take two platefuls, rather than just one, thus again extending the chain leading to eating larger amounts. Also, the Ss were instructed to take very small bites and to chew them carefully, to replace eating utensils on the table after each bite and to pick them up only after the food had been eaten. Both of these techniques lengthened the chain leading to eating by extending the time needed to complete intermediate members of the chain.

A final method of self-control taught the Ss in the present study was "doing something else" instead of the behavior to be controlled. Danger periods of between meal eating were determined for each S individually from the food data sheets. The S was then instructed to choose some reinforcing activity incompatible with eating and to perform this behavior every day at the time when the disposition to eat was usually quite strong.

During each session, E quizzed S on her knowledge of the techniques presented during the previous session. If S did not appear to understand a technique or its use in controlling overeating, the technique was explained to her again, and she was quizzed on it in the immediately succeeding session. Explanation and oral quizzing were continued in this manner until E felt confident that S understood the technique and its use.

EXPERIMENTER CONTROLLED REINFORCEMENT

During the first interview of the EC program, S was told that she should choose for herself a reinforcer which symbolized weight loss to her, and that cost not more than $20.00. The S was given $5.00 and told to put the item on lay-away. She was also told that if she reached her goal at the end of 5 weeks, she would receive the remaining $15.00 from E. Thus, S sampled the reinforcer in the sense that she was exposed to the visual and tactile cues associated with it. During each of the succeeding nine interviews, S was told how much weight she had left to lose, and the amount of time remaining in which to lose it. Also, during each session, E mentioned to S the reinforcer for which she was working, thus providing a cognitive representation to bridge the gap between reinforcer presentation and weight loss.

At the last session during week 26, regardless of the S's treatment condition, E gave S a postcard and asked S to record her club weights on it for the succeeding 4 weeks and then to return the card to E. These 4 weeks, weeks 27–30, comprise the follow-up period (F).

Results

Of the 14 Ss included in the original experimental sample, one S in each condition dropped from the study during the first 3 weeks; thus, the drop-out rate was approximately 14 per cent. Of the twelve Ss remaining, the data from two Condition 2 Ss are not presented. One S was 3 months pregnant at the start of the study, unbeknownst to E. The other S failed to turn in data sheets and terminated her TOPS membership so that no data were available from this source, either. In addition, she had a physical condition which caused her weight to fluctuate markedly due to abnormal water retention.

RELIABILITY OF SELF-REPORT

Weight measures were available from three sources: Home, club and office. In order to determine the reliability of the Ss' self-report of weight, reported home weights were averaged by week and correlated with office weights averaged by week. The resulting correlations ranged from $r = +0.65$ to $r = +0.98$; the mean correlation was $r = +0.91$.

INDIVIDUAL WEIGHT CHANGES

In order to facilitate an examination of the functional relationships between treatment conditions and individual Ss' weights, weekly weights for each S are presented in Fig. 1. Both weekly club weights and average home weights are presented in Fig. 1. Club data were available for the entire span of the experiment. Unfortunately, however, Ss tended to miss many club meetings, especially during weeks 17–26, and for this reason club data is missing at many points. Therefore, the following procedure was adopted. In examining the pre-experimental baseline data and the follow-up periods, the data referred to will be the club data, since these were the only data available during these periods. However, when examining the two experimental baselines and the two active treatment periods, the data referred to are the home data, as these data were available for each week during the EC and SC treatments.

Weight change rates during B_0 ranged from $+0.42$ to -0.58 lb/wk. The mean weight change during this period was -0.01 lb/wk; the median was $+0.02$ lb/wk. Weight change rates during B_1 ranged from $+0.30$ to -1.20 lb/wk. The mean weight change during this period was $+0.04$ lb/wk; the median weight change per week was $+0.05$ lb/wk. Weekly weight changes during B_2 ranged from $+2.00$ to -0.53 lb/wk. The mean weight change per week was $+0.19$ lb/wk; the median change was $+0.05$ lb/wk. Inspection of Fig. 1 indicates little change in weight for the Ss taken as a group during both B_0, B_1 and B_2, but greater intrasubject variability during B_2 than was manifested during either B_0 or B_1.

During SC (weeks 17–21), the six Condition 1 Ss manifested weights changes rates ranging -0.24 to -0.75 lb/wk, with a mean and a median value of -0.48 lb/wk. During EC (weeks 22–26), Condition 1 Ss manifested weight changes ranging from $+0.60$ to -2.40 lb/wk. The mean weight change was $+0.94$ lb/wk; the median weight change was -0.85 lb/wk.

During SC (weeks 22–26), the four Condition 2 Ss manifested weight changes ranging from $+0.40$ to -2.70 lb/wk. The mean weight change was -0.65 lb/wk; the median weight change was -0.14 lb/wk. During EC (weeks 17–21), weight change rates for Condition 2 Ss ranged from -0.52 to -2.00 lb/wk. The mean weight change was -1.1 lb/wk; the median weight change was -0.94 lb/wk.

Follow-up data were not remitted for $S4$, $S6$ or $S10$. Data collected during F indicated that Condition 1 Ss showed weight changes ranging from $+0.50$ to

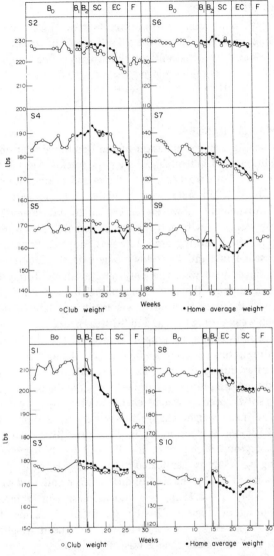

FIG. 1. Weight changes of all subjects during pre-experimental baseline (B_0), weight monitoring only (B_1), weight plus food monitoring (B_2), self-control (SC), experimenter control (EC) and follow-up (F).

−0.65 lb/wk; the mean weight change was −0.09 lb/wk; the median was −0.12 lb/wk. Condition 2 *S*s showed weight change rates ranging from 0 to −0.25 lb/wk. The mean weight change was −0.09 lb/wk; the median change for Condition 2 was zero.

TOTAL WEIGHT CHANGES

To further facilitate an examination of the effects of the experimental programs, the total amount of weight lost during both EC and SC for each S, as determined by E in the interviews, are shown in Table 1, along with weight changes during weeks 8–12 as determined by club weights. The data from weeks 8–12 are presented in order to provide a 5-week period against which to compare the EC and SC treatments.

TABLE 1. Total weight changes during active treatment and comparable baseline periods in pounds

	Subject	Weeks 8–12	Self-control	Experimenter-control
	2	+1.00	− 2.25	−10.50
	4	+3.75	− 6.00	−13.50
Condition 1	5	0.00	− 2.00	+ 0.75
Self-control	6	−0.25	− 1.50	− 4.50
first	7	−2.25	− 3.25	− 6.00
	9	−1.00	− 1.50	+ 4.00
	1	− 1.00	−10.75	−12.25
Condition 2	3	+3.75	− 0.75	− 2.75
Experimenter-	8	+1.50	0.00	− 6.75
control first	10	−0.50	− 3.75	− 7.00

PERCENTAGE CHANGES

To obtain a summary picture of the Ss' performance independent of original weight, median percentage weight changes in club weight from week 1 to the last week of B_0, B_1, B_2 EC, SC and F, respectively, were computed separately for Condition 1 and Condition 2. The results are shown in Fig. 2. Examination of Fig. 2 indicates little change in weight for Ss in either condition from week 1 to the last weeks of B_0 or B_1, but a marked rise in weight by the last week of B_2 for Condition 2 Ss; Condition 1 showed little change. Figure 2 also indicates a modest decrease in weight during SC treatment for both conditions and a markedly steeper decrease during EC for both conditions. Additionally, Fig. 2 indicates a slight decrease in weight for Condition 2 at the last week of follow-up and a slight rise for Condition 1 at the last week of follow-up.

DISCUSSION

The data presented above indicate that both SC and EC produced weight losses in overweight women, and these losses tended to be greater than those occurring during either a pretreatment baseline or periods of weight monitoring and weight plus food monitoring. However, the small median loss achieved during SC suggests that the self-control techniques used in the present study may

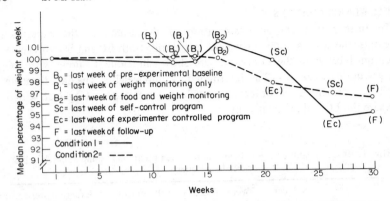

FIG. 2. Median percentage weight change for condition 1 and condition 2 from week 1 to the final weeks of pre-experimental baseline, weight monitoring only, weight plus food monitoring, self-control, experimenter control and follow-up.

be of little practical use for weight losses to be effected over a relatively short period of time. The losses which occurred during EC were large enough to be of clinical use. In fact, the median weight loss of approximately one pound per week achieved during EC would appear to have been one of the largest reported to date in controlled studies of weight reduction with women Ss. The superiority of the EC program occurred regardless of the order in which the treatments were presented.

The SC procedures used in the present study produced a somewhat lower weight loss rate than that achieved by Stuart (1967) or Wollersheim (1970). However, the weight loss rate is approximately equal to that achieved by Harris' (1969) women Ss. The relatively poor showing of the SC procedures in the present study, when compared with the data reported by both Stuart and Wollersheim, may have been due to the relatively greater age of the Ss in the present study, to the short time period during which SC was in effect, or to variation in the techniques included in the self-control programs.

Similarly, the reasons for the differential effectiveness of the two programs in the present study are not entirely clear. It may be that the Ss' natural environments did not provide sufficient reinforcement for weight loss. Therefore, the Ss did not use the self-control techniques, even though they could verbalize them, for weight loss was not sufficiently reinforcing to motivate them to do so. However, EC provided an external reinforcer, and, under these conditions, the Ss developed their own techniques of self-control.

It might be argued that the apparent superiority of the EC program is the result of the experimental design. That is, it could be proposed that the SC program was in effect only after all the SC techniques had been presented to the Ss and, thus, the SC program was only in effect during the last week of the study. This objection cannot be firmly refuted until the techniques are compared over a longer period of time where the initial advantage of EC would be minimized. However, an examination of the data presented in Fig. 1 indicates that the poorer showing of SC was probably not due to this factor. The entire SC program with the exception of the use of the prepotent repertory had been presented to the Ss by the third week of the SC program, and the SC program in its entirety had been presented to the Ss by the fourth week. If knowledge of the entire SC program facilitated weight loss, one might expect the weight loss curves to become increasingly steep during the latter two weeks of the SC treatment. As inspection of Fig. 1 indicates, this was not the case; the curves fail to show increasingly greater weight losses with increasing number of self-control techniques taught the Ss.

The present study has several methodological implications for behavioral therapy. First, the high correlation between the self-report of weight and the office measures indicates that under circumstances such as those which prevailed in the present study; that is, a periodic check on S's veracity, Ss produce self-report data which is generally accurate. A second implication is in the use of club records to obtain a baseline measure. Such baselines are necessarily free from observer effects since the behavior occurred before either E or S had any knowledge that the data would be used in the study. A final implication is in the use of the single-subject design. Such a design, when replicated with a sufficient number of Ss, allows the assessment of the effects of treatments on the individual S and also allows generalizations about the efficacy of the treatment. As mentioned earlier, this design also allows the assessment of the utility of treatments when the treatments produce less than striking effects.

It should be noted that a baseline such as that employed in the present study provides a relatively stringent criteria against which to measure change. Wollersheim (1970) found that a condition which was designed as an analog to TOPS was more effective than no treatment. Had a baseline been obtained from the Ss before club membership, the change might have been more striking. The finding that no-treatment controls generally gain weight during the treatment period (Wollersheim 1970; Harris 1969) indicates that this may indeed have been the case.

References

CHAPMAN, R. F. and SMITH, J. W. (1970) Punishment and self-management training in the elimination of cigarette smoking. Paper presented at the Oregon–Washington State Psychological Association, Richland, Washington.

EULER, H. (1970) Self-monitoring, shaping and competition in the self-management of smoking behavior. Unpublished paper, Washington State University, Pullman, Washington,

FERSTER, C. B., NURNBERGER, J. I. and LEVITT, E. E. (1962) The control of eating. *J. Mathetics* 1, 87–109.

FOREYT, J. P. and KENNEDY, W. A. (1971) Treatment of overweight by aversion therapy. *Behav. Res. & Therapy* 9, 29–34.

GOLDIAMOND, I. (1965) Self-control procedures in personal behavior problems. *Psychol. Rep.* 17, 851–868.

HALL, S. M. (1971) Self-control and therapist control in the treatment of overweight women. Unpublished doctoral dissertation, Washington State University, Pullman, Washington.

HARMATZ, M. G. and LAPUC, P. (1968) Behavior modification of overeating in a psychiatric population. *J. consult. clin. Psychol.* 32, 583–587.

HARRIS, M. B. (1969) Self-directed program for weight control: A pilot study. *J. abnorm. Psychol.* 74, 263–270.

KENNEDY, W. A. and FOREYT, J. P. (1968) Control of eating behavior in an obese patient by avoidance conditioning. *Psychol. Rep.* 22, 571–576.

MEYER, V. and CRISP, A. H. (1964) Aversion therapy in two cases of treatment of obesity. *Behav. Res. & Therapy* 2, 143–147.

STOLLAK, G. E. (1966) Weight loss obtained under various experimental procedures. Papers presented at the meeting of the Midwestern Psychological Association, Chicago. Cited by M. B. HARRIS (1969) Self-directed program for weight control: A pilot study. *J. abnorm. Psychol.* 74, 263–270.

STUART, R. B. (1967) Behavioural control of overeating. *Behav. Res. & Therapy* 5, 357–365.

STUNKARD, A. J. and McCLAREN-HUME, J. (1958) The results of treatment for obesity. *Arch. Int. Med.* 103, 79–85.

WOLLERSHEIM, J. P. (1970) Effectiveness of group therapy based upon learning principles in the treatment of overweight women. *J. abnorm. Psychol.* 76, 462–474.

WOLPE, J. (1958) *Psychotherapy by Reciprocal Inhibition.* Stanford University Press, Stanford, California.

CHAPTER 42

Relative Efficacy of Self-reward, Self-punishment, and Self-monitoring Techniques for Weight Loss[1]

MICHAEL J. MAHONEY,[2] NANCI G. M. MOURA, and TERRY C. WADE

Stanford University

Summary— Obese adults ($N = 53$) were randomly assigned to five groups; (a) self-reward, (b) self-punishment, (c) self-reward and self-punishment, (d) self-monitoring, and (e) information control. All *S*s were given information on effective stimulus control techniques for weight loss. This constituted the sole treatment for control *S*s. Self-monitoring *S*s were asked to weigh in twice per week for 4 weeks and to record their daily weight and eating habits. Self-reward and self-punishment *S*s, in addition to receiving self-monitoring instructions, were asked to award or fine themselves a portion of their own deposit contingent on changes in their weight and eating habits. After 4 weeks of treatment, self-reward *S*s lost significantly more weight than either self-monitoring or control *S*s. At a 4-month follow-up, those *S*s who had received self-reward instructions (Groups a and c) continued to show greater improvement than either the self-punishment or control *S*s. These findings are interpreted as providing a preliminary indication that self-reward strategies are superior to self-punitive and self-recording strategies in the modification of at least some habit patterns.

Despite the fact that self-control strategies have become increasingly popular in clinical and applied settings (Kanfer & Phillips, 1970), there has been an appalling lack of research on the processes and parameters of these techniques (Mahoney, 1972). In particular, there have been neither comparisons among the various techniques nor attempts to isolate their active components. The present study addressed itself to an evaluative comparison of three of the more popular self-control techniques — self-reward, self-punishment, and self-monitoring. Since the latter is also a component of the former, a partial component analysis was also provided.

To provide a stringent test of the efficacy of the above techniques, they were each applied in the modification of a chronic and resistant habit pattern. The pattern chosen was overeating since, in addition to providing observable indices of treatment effectiveness, obesity has been one of the most resistant of

Reprinted with permission from the *Journal of Consulting and Clinical Psychology*, 1973, **40**, 404–407.

[1] The authors would like to thank Albert Bandura for his assistance and suggestions.
[2] Requests for reprints should be sent to Michael J. Mahoney, Department of Psychology, Pennsylvania State University, University Park, Pennsylvania 16802.

maladaptive habit patterns (Stunkard, 1958). Moreover, previous studies have demonstrated that a core of behavioral techniques can − when consistently applied − dramatically improve human weight control (Harris, 1969; Penick *et al.*, 1971; Stuart, 1967, 1971; Wollersheim, 1970). In general, behavior modification approaches to obesity have emphasized the alteration of everyday eating habits by manipulation of eating-related environmental cues (i.e., stimulus control). To date, these techniques have been combined with a variety of auxiliary maintenance strategies such as group support, covert sensitization, and therapist approval. The present study focused on the effectiveness of various self-control strategies in motivating and maintaining individual applications of cue-altering weight-control techniques. Specifically, Ss were instructed to employ self-reward, self-punishment, or self-monitoring techniques in the modification of both their body weight and their eating habits. A control group was provided with identical information on stimulus control techniques, but they did not receive self-regulatory instructions.

Method

SUBJECTS

The Ss were invited by a newspaper ad. to participate in a program for self-managed weight control. Eligibility criteria included (a) a minimum age of 17 years, (b) nonpregnant status, (c) physician's consent, and (d) a minimum of 10% overweight. Applicants who were concurrently enrolled in a reducing club and/or undergoing other treatments for weight loss were ineligible. Also, individuals reporting recent dramatic changes in body weight were excluded. A total of 53 Ss (48 females, 5 males) enrolled and completed the program. Their average age was 39.9 years. Individual body weights varied from 107 to 270 with a mean of 166.3 pounds.

Prior to group assignment, the degree of obesity for each S was computed. This was done by dividing an individual's current weight by his ideal weight (Stillman & Baker, 1967), thereby controlling for height factors. The degree of obesity for all Ss in the study ranged from 13% to 130% with a mean of 48.6%. The Ss were ranked according to degree of obesity and randomly assigned to experimental groups.

PROCEDURE

All Ss were required to place a refundable deposit of $10 with the Es for the duration of treatment (four weeks). A commercially available bathroom scale was employed. At their initial weigh in, all Ss were given a small booklet describing stimulus control approaches to weight loss. Treatment procedures varied as follows:

Self-reward: Group 1 (n = 12). The *S*s in this group were asked to deposit an additional $11 with *E* for purposes of self-reward. They were asked to weigh in biweekly for 7 weigh-ins and to keep a daily graph of their weight at home. The *S*s were provided with a weight chart and a behavioral diary in which they were to record the daily frequency of (a) "fat thoughts" (discouraging self-verbalizations), (b) "thin thoughts" (encouraging self-verbalizations), (c) instances of indulgence (eating a fattening food or excessive quantity), and (d) instances of restraint (refusing a fattening food or reducing food intake). Self-reward was to take place at weigh-ins. Each *S*'s $21 was transformed into 21 shares whose value increased when other *S*s forfeited deposits or self-punished. A type of bank account was set up for each individual. The *S*s began with an empty account and could self-reward by requesting that a deposit be made to their account. Each *S* had access to three shares per weigh in. It was recommended that *S*s self-reward two shares for a weight loss of one pound or more since their last weigh in. The remaining share was to be self-awarded if adaptive behaviors (thin thoughts and restraint) had outnumbered nonadaptive behaviors since the last weigh in. Beyond these recommendations, no external constraints were placed on *S*'s standards or execution of self-reward. When an *S* chose not to self-reward at a weigh-in, his/her shares were placed in a community pool and divided among all other shareholders (thereby increasing the value of a share). The *S* were allowed three absences but were thereafter fined three shares for each absence. At their final weigh-in, they received the amount they had self-rewarded ($1/share) and were later mailed a dividend check covering increases in share value.

Self-punishment: Group 2 (n = 12). Procedures in this group were exactly parallel to those of Group 1 except that *S* began with a full (21-share) account and were instructed to fine themselves shares for lack of weight loss and/or lack of behavior improvement. Self-punished shares were placed in the community pool and divided among all remaining shares. When *S*s did not self-punish at a weigh in, their shares remained in their account and were refunded to them at the final weigh in. The share amounts and goals were identical to those in Group 1.

Self-reward and self-punishment: Group 3 (n = 8). Conditions in this group combined those of Groups 1 and 2. The *S*s began with an empty account and could either deposit to it (self-reward) or fine themselves (self-punish) up to three shares per weigh-in.

Self-monitoring: Group 4 (n = 5). The *S*s in this group were asked to weigh in biweekly and to record their weight and adaptive and nonadaptive eating habits. The standard weight loss and behavior improvement goals used in Groups 1–3 were also suggested for these *S*s. In short, conditions in this group duplicated those in the first three groups with the exception that no additional deposit was required and the self-reward and self-punishment strategies were not discussed.

Information control: Group 5 (n = 16). The *S*s in this group received stimulus control booklets but did not participate in a second weigh in until the four-week

P

treatment period had ended. No self-monitoring materials were provided, and it was recommended that Ss refrain from any weigh ins at home during that time.

Efforts were made to avoid any E approval or disapproval for weight change and to minimize E contact (weigh-ins took 5—10 minutes). After four weeks all Ss were weighed and instructed to continue self-application of their respective techniques. A postquestionnaire inquired about the use of any extraneous methods. Four months after their initial appointment, a follow-up weigh-in was conducted.

Results

Data analyses on the pretreatment degree of obesity for each group revealed no significant differences ($F = .31$, $df = 4/48$). Likewise, the groups did not initially differ on number of pounds overweight ($F = .44$). A posttreatment analysis of number of pounds lost yielded on overall F of 4.49 ($p < .005$). Newman-Keuls comparisons of treatment means showed that the self-reward Ss had lost significantly more pounds than either the self-monitoring ($p < .025$) or the control group ($p < .025$). The self-punishment group did not differ significantly from any other. A difference approaching significance at the .05 level was obtained when Group 3 Ss (self-reward and self-punishment) were compared with those in the self-monitoring group. Average number of pounds lost per individual was 6.4, 3.7, 5.2, .8, and 1.4 for the five groups, respectively.

An analysis of percentage of body weight lost also revealed significant group differences ($F = 3.44$, $p < .025$). Newman-Keuls comparisons indicated that the self-reward group lost significantly more in percentage of body weight than either the self-monitoring ($p < .05$) or the control group ($p < .05$).

An analysis of "follow through" was performed for Groups 1—3 in order to assess any differential tendencies toward self-reward or self-punishment. Since the weigh-ins constituted the most accurately measured and observable behavior of Ss, analyses were done on the consistency with which Ss self-administered rewards or fines for weight change. Using the recommended standard (loss of one pound per weigh-in), Ss were scored on whether they appropriately transacted two shares for success or failure at the above criterion. At first glance the data indicate that follow through was higher for self-reward. There were no instances where an individual made his weight criterion and failed to self-reward, whereas there were numerous instances where individuals failed to make the criterion but failed to self-punish. However, a further analysis revealed quite a few instances where individuals self-rewarded even though they had not met the weight criterion. (It should be recalled that if a self-reward S had not met the criterion and appropriately chosen not to self-reward, he was inadvertently punished by the automatic transfer of his shares to the community pool.) A follow-through analysis using both halves of the dichotomy revealed no significant intergroup differences ($F = .53$, $df = 3/33$). The rate of follow through was 58.1% for self-reward, 57.6% for self-punishment, and 67.1% for the combined group.

In order to control for nonspecific factors associated with weigh-ins, Groups 1–4 Ss who began the study but completed fewer than four (out of seven) weigh-ins were excluded from all data analyses. This restriction affected Group 4 (self-monitoring) more than the others. Only five (out of nine original) Group 4 Ss met the attendance criterion. In the first three groups, attendance was enhanced by levying fines after three absences. An analysis of attendance variations among Ss who did meet the criterion revealed no significant differences ($F = .86$).

Thirty-one Ss appeared for the four-month follow-up weigh-in. Of these, seven had to be excluded because of intervening or attendance factors (e.g., hormone shots, health farms, etc.). Because data were available from only two self-monitoring Ss, this group had to be excluded from follow-up analyses. An analysis of the 4-month data revealed that the self-reward group and the combined group (self-reward plus self-punishment) had both lost greater percentages of their body weight than information control Ss ($p < .05$). Self-punishment Ss did not differ significantly from controls. Because follow-up Ss differed significantly in initial weight, analysis of number of pounds lost had to be converted to a proportion (number of pounds lost divided by number of pounds overweight). After an overall F of 5.03 ($p < .02$), individual Newman-Keuls comparisons showed that both the self-reward and the self-reward plus self-punishment group had lost significantly more weight that either the self-punishment ($p < .05$) or the control group ($p < .05$). No other group comparisons were significant. Over the entire four months, the average number of pounds lost per individual was 11.5 for self-reward, 7.3 for self-punishment, 12.0 for self-reward plus self-punishment, 4.5 for self-monitoring, and 3.2 for controls.

Discussion

The foregoing results provide some preliminary information on the relative effectiveness of several self-control strategies. In general, it would appear that self-reward strategies may provide an effective incentive component in weight loss attempts. Only those groups given self-reward opportunities differed significantly from any others in successful weight loss. Data from information control Ss indicate that the simple provision of relevant information on stimulus control techniques causes only minimal change in body weight. Moreover, variables associated with self-recording, frequent weigh-ins, and E contact failed to produce substantial weight loss. This finding is in contrast with recent evidence on the reactive effects of self-monitoring (e.g., Broden, Hall, & Mitts, 1971; McFall, 1970; McFall & Hammen, 1971). However, subsequent research

(Mahoney, 1973) has suggested that specific self-monitoring applications may vary considerably in their reactivity and in the permanence of their effects.

It should be noted that an empirical comparison of self-reward and self-punishment strategies is complicated by such factors as control for frequency of application (which is, in turn, altered by their relative effectiveness). Moreover, it would be desirable for subsequent studies to motivate *all Ss'* appearance at weigh-ins and follow-up by some form of deposit. Although there were no group differences in drop-out rate, equal deposits are also advisable to insure against pretreatment motivational variations. Finally, care should be taken to avoid *E* punishment of appropriate self-regulation. In the present study, follow-through rates for self-reward *S*s may have been decreased by the fact that these *S*s were adventitiously fined for not self-rewarding (irrespective of goal attainment). A methodologically improved study (Mahoney, 1972) has revealed average self-reward follow-through rates in excess of 90%.

The implications of the present findings are twofold. First, it would appear that self-reward strategies may be superior to self-punishment and/or self-recording techniques in the modification of at least some habit patterns. Second, the parameters and components of successful self-reward strategies need to be investigated. For example, how important are the factors of magnitude, scheduling, and focus in self-reward systems? Can the pattern of the present findings be generalized to behavior problems other than obesity? These and other issues must await clarification by further research in self-control.

References

BRODEN, M., HALL, R. V., & MITTS, B. The effect of self-recording on the classroom behavior of two eighth-grade students. *Journal of Applied Behavior Analysis*, 1971, 4, 191–199.

HARRIS, M. B. Self-directed program for weight control: A pilot study. *Journal of Abnormal Psychology*, 1969, 74, 263–270.

KANFER, F. H. & PHILLIPS, J. S. *Learning foundations of behavior therapy*. New York: Wiley, 1970.

MAHONEY, M. J. Research issues in self-management. *Behaviour Therapy*, 1972, 3, 45–63.

MAHONEY, M. J. Self-reward and self-monitoring techniques for weight loss. *Behaviour Therapy*, 1973 (in press).

McFALL, R. M. The effects of self-monitoring on normal smoking behavior. *Journal of Consulting and Clinical Psychology*, 1970, 35, 135–142.

McFALL, R. M., & HAMMEN, C. L. Motivation, structure, and self-monitoring: The role of non-specific factors in smoking reduction. *Journal of Consulting and Clinical Psychology*, 1971, 37, 80–86.

PENICK, S. B., FILION, R., FOX, S., & STUNKARD, A. J. Behaviour modification in the treatment of obesity. *Psychosomatic Medicine*, 1971, 33, 49–55.

STILLMAN, I. M. & BAKER, S. S. *The doctor's quick weight loss diet*. New York: Dell, 1967.

STUART, R. B. Behavioral control over eating. *Behaviour Research and Therapy*, 1967, 5, 357–365.

STUART, R. B. A three-dimensional program for the treatment of obesity. *Behaviour Research and Therapy*, 1971, 9, 177–186.

STUNKARD, A. J. The management of obesity. *New York State Journal of Medicine*, 1958, 58, 79–87.

WOLLERSHEIM, J. P. The effectiveness of group therapy based upon learning principles in the treatment of overweight women. *Journal of Abnormal Psychology*, 1970, 76, 462–474.

CHAPTER 43

Self-reward and Self-monitoring Techniques for Weight Control[1]

MICHAEL J. MAHONEY[2]

Pennsylvania State University, University Park, Pennsylvania 16802

Summary— Obese adult volunteers ($N = 49$) were randomly assigned to one of four conditions: (1) Self-reward for Weight Loss, (2) Self-reward for Habit Improvement, (3) Self-monitoring, and (4) Delayed Treatment Control. Individuals in the first three groups were given information on basic stimulus control techniques for weight loss and self-monitored their weight and eating habits for a 2-wk baseline. Thereafter, Self-monitoring subjects continued their recording and received standardized weight loss and habit change goals at individual weekly weigh-ins. In addition to the above self-monitoring procedures, Self-reward subjects awarded themselves portions of their own deposit for attainment of either their weight loss (SR-Weight) or their habit improvement (SR-Habit) goals. Control subjects received no treatment during the first 8 wk but thereafter participated in a program which combined the procedures of the previous Self-reward groups. Weight reduction analyses revealed brief and variable losses during the self-monitored baseline. However, even after the addition of goal-setting, these reductions did not prove to be either enduring or significant. When self-reward was added to self-recording, substantial weight loss improvements were observed. These improvements were more pronounced when subjects rewarded themselves for habit change rather than weight loss. A significant relationship was found between successful weight reduction and degree of eating improvement. Clinical implications and contemporary research issues are briefly discussed.

The systematic self-presentation of rewards has become an increasingly popular clinical technique. One of the reasons for this popularity has undoubtedly been its rather consistent success in the treatment of a wide range of behavior problems. To date, self-reward has shown promise as a treatment strategy for the improvement of classroom behaviors, heterosexual relations, study habits, and weight control (Thoresen & Mahoney, 1974). Despite this

Reprinted with permission from *Behavior Therapy*, 1974, 5, 48–57. Copyright © 1974 by Academic Press. Inc.

[1] This article is based on the author's doctoral dissertation at Stanford University. The invaluable assistance and support of Albert Bandura is greatly appreciated. For their efforts above and beyond the call of science, gratitude is also expressed to Nanci Moura, Terry Wade, Lee Appleton, and Fran Mahoney.

[2] Requests for reprints should be sent to Michael J. Mahoney, Department of Psychology, Pennsylvania State University, University Park, PA 16802.

rather surprising unanimity in the effects of self-reinforcement, little research has been addressed to an analysis of its component processes.

Bandura (1969, 1971) and Kanfer (1971) have emphasized three core elements in self-reward operations. First of all, the individual systematically observes his own behavior, hence *self-monitoring* may be contributing to the behavioral outcome. Given this self-recorded information, the individual then compares his performance with the achievement standard adopted for that task. In the course of this comparative process the individual doubtless engages in *self-evaluation*. Performances that match or exceed the goal evoke self-approval. Those which fall short of the goal result in self-dissatisfaction. Finally, if these self-monitoring and self-evaluative operations show performance to match or exceed the chosen standard, the individual may engage in tangible *self-reinforcement*.

The relative contribution of self-monitoring, self-evaluation, and self-reward operations has yet to be investigated. Recent research on clinical self-monitoring suggests that in some instances, this component influence may result in substantial behavior change (McFall, 1970; Johnson & White, 1971; Broden, Hall, & Mitts, 1971). However, the degree and duration of the behavior change can vary considerably (McFall & Hammen, 1971; Mahoney, Moura, & Wade, (1973). Moreover, extant studies on clinical self-regulation have complicated causal interpretations by combining self-monitoring with other treatment strategies (Kazdin, 1974; Mahoney, 1972a). In these investigations it is impossible to determine to what extent any observed behavior change was caused by self-monitoring rather than the supplementary strategies. Finally, the fact that most clinical applications of self-monitoring involve behaviors with explicit evaluative features has precluded attempts to partial out the relative effects of self-monitoring and self-evaluation.

The present research addressed itself to an analysis of the relative effects of self-monitoring, self-evaluation, and self-reward techniques.. Overeating was chosen as the targeted response because it is not only a tenacious behavior problem, but it also provides objective indices of treatment effectiveness. Two basic questions were addressed: (1) whether self-reward operations substantially enhance the effects of self-monitoring and goal-setting in weight control, and (2) whether self-administered rewards are more effective when they are tied to changes in eating habits rather than changes in bodyweight. It was predicted that both of these questions would be answered affirmatively.

Method

SUBJECTS

Subjects were solicited by newspaper advertisement. To be eligible, they had to be at least 18 yr of age, 20% overweight on international standards, and could not be concurrently involved in other obesity treatments (e.g., reducing clubs, drug therapy, etc.). All subjects were ranked according to degree of obesity and randomly assigned from stratified blocks to one of four conditions: (1) Self-reward for Weight Loss (SR-Weight), ($n = 13$), (2) Self-reward for Habit Improvement (SR-Habit) ($n = 11$), (3) Self-monitoring ($n = 14$) and (4) Delayed Treatment Control ($n = 11$). All subjects were female with the exception of one male in the SR-Habit condition and two males in the Control group. Analyses of pre-treatment measures of bodyweight, degree of obesity, pounds overweight, motivation, perceived cause of obesity, and pre-program eating patterns revealed no inter-group differences. Analyses of age and chronicity of weight problems showed that Control subjects were slightly older than subjects in the other three groups and that both Self-monitoring and Control subjects reported their weight problems as being of shorter duration than that of Self-reward subjects. This latter pre-treatment variation, if anything, favored weight reduction by the Self-monitoring and Control groups (Hirsch, in press).

PROCEDURE

Subjects in all four groups were required to leave a refundable deposit of $35 for the duration of the program. This deposit was later used for purposes of self-reward and also to motivate attendance — subjects were fined $5 for absences. In the case of Delayed Treatment Control subjects who received no treatment for the first 8 weeks of the program, the $35 deposit was presented as a means of preserving their place in a second treatment series.

Self-reward and Self-monitoring subjects began their participation by attending group meetings at which they received pamphlets describing basic stimulus control strategies for the alteration of eating habits (e.g., Stuart & Davis, 1972). They were also provided with weight charts and eating habits booklets for daily self-monitoring (Mahoney, 1972b). Eating habits were categorized according to food quality, food quantity, and situational determinants. During 2 baseline weeks, Self-reward and Self-monitoring subjects recorded their daily weight and eating habits and attended individual weekly weigh-ins. To avoid contra-therapeutic expectancies, this self-monitoring was not presented as being preliminary to a more active treatment regimen. Following baseline, differential self-control strategies were recommended. Subjects assigned to the Self-monitoring condition continued their self-recording and, in addition, received standardized weight loss and habit improvement goals at their weekly weigh-ins. Subjects in the two Self-reward conditions likewise received both types of goals and continued their self-monitoring for 6 subsequent treatment weeks. However, in addition, they were instructed to award themselves portions of their own deposit as reinforcement for their weight control progress. In the SR-weight condition, individuals were told to reward attainment of their weekly weight loss goal, while in the SR-Habit condition, attainment of the weekly habit improvement goal was emphasized. After their weigh-in, subjects in the Self-reward conditions had the opportunity to privately reinforce themselves by taking a special envelope from behind a large metal partition. Five envelopes containing cash and gift certificates from local stores were present. Although the experimenter could not monitor subjects' self-rewarding responses, an inventory of remaining envelopes after each subjects' departure served as an objective index of this operation. The privacy partition was present for Self-monitoring subjects but did not conceal self-reward envelopes.

Delayed Treatment Control subjects weighed in at the beginning of the program but were told that they had been randomly assigned to a delayed treatment series which had been necessitated by the large number of program applicants. Their $35 deposit insured their place in the latter. After subjects in the three experimental groups had completed their 2-wk baseline and 6-wk treatment phases, Control subjects returned for an 8-wk weigh-in. They then began a self-control program which combined the strategies employed in the two Self-reward groups. That is, after receiving stimulus control information and self-monitoring their weight and eating habits for 2 wk, they were instructed to reward themselves on those weeks when they attained both their weight loss and habit improvement goals. During this second phase, subjects in the previous Self-reward and Self-monitoring groups entered a follow-up interval in which no treatment was received. Nine weeks after the termination of their treatment phase, a final weight-in was conducted.

Results

The "reduction quotient," obtained by dividing number of pounds lost by number of pounds overweight, served as the principle dependent measure. This index controls for variations in height, bodyweight, and degree of obesity (Feinstein, 1959).

Congruent with the findings of several other behavioral weight control programs (e.g., Penick *et al.*, 1971; Horan & Johnson, 1971), marked individual variability was encountered. Because group variances on measures of weight reduction, eating habits, and motivation differed significantly, nonparametric techniques were employed.

BASELINE SELF-MONITORING

Kruskal-Wallis analyses of reduction quotients, number of pounds lost, and percentage of bodyweight lost disclosed no significant differences between the three experimental groups on any of these measures during baseline. However, Wilcoxon analyses of within-subject reductions revealed highly significant losses on all three measures across groups ($p < .001$). As Fig. 1 shows, all three groups achieved substantial weight loss during the 2-wk self-monitored baseline.

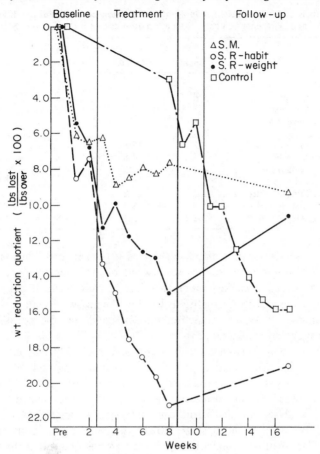

FIG. 1. Median weight changes displayed by subjects during baseline,
treatment, and follow-up phases.

TREATMENT EFFECTS

Kruskal-Wallis analyses revealed that the three groups differed significantly in weight reduction during the 6 treatment weeks. Mann-Whitney comparisons showed that subjects in the SR-Habit group lost significantly more weight than subjects in either the SR-Weight ($p < .05$) or Self-monitoring group ($p < .025$). The latter groups did not differ from each other (cf. Table 1). Wilcoxon analyses showed that, of the three groups, only SR-Habit subjects lost a significant amount of weight during the treatment period according to all three reduction measures ($p < .005$). Subjects who rewarded themselves for weight loss achieved significant reductions on two of the three measures, while those who only monitored their progress did not change during the treatment phase.

TABLE 1. Median weight reduction as a function of treatment condition and experimental phase. Reduction quotient = (lb lost/lb over) X 100

	SR-Weight	SR-Habit	Self-monitoring	Control
Baseline				
Reduction quotient	6.8	7.4	6.5	NA
Weight lost (lb)	3.5	3.5	2.0	NA
% Bodyweight lost	1.8	2.4	2.1	
Treatment				
Reduction quotient	8.2	13.8	1.2	NA
Weight lost (lb)	1.5	4.8	1.0	NA
% Bodyweight lost	1.3	2.7	0.7	NA
Total (week 8)				
Reduction quotient	15.0	21.2	7.7	3.1
Weight lost (lb)	5.0	8.3	3.0	2.5
% Bodyweight lost	3.1	5.1	2.8	1.3

The relative superiority of habit self-reward is further shown in comparisons between the groups at each successive week of treatment. Subjects in this condition displayed a marked progressive loss in weight and began to depart significantly from the other conditions beyond the mid-way point in treatment. By contrast, the SR-Weight and Self-monitoring conditions did not differ from each other at any stage of treatment.

Changes in the nontreated control group provide an additional index against which to evaluate the relative power of self-monitoring and self-rewarding influences in weight reduction. For this comparison, changes in weight were computed between the initial measurement and the one conducted 8 wk later. An overall analysis revealed significant inter-group variations in reduction quotients ($p < .005$), pounds lost ($p < .025$), and percentage of bodyweight lost ($p < .01$). Mann-Whitney comparisons between groups found that the SR-Habit group lost significantly more weight than control subjects on all three reduction measures ($p < .005$). SR-weight subjects were likewise superior to Controls in reduction quotients ($p < .01$), pounds lost ($p < .05$), and percentage of bodyweight lost ($p < .025$). Self-monitoring subjects, however, did not differ from Controls. The median weight reductions for each of the four groups between the initial and 8-wk assessment were 5.0 for SR-Weight, 8.3 for SR-Habit, 3.0 for Self-monitoring, and 2.5 for nontreated Controls.

MAINTENANCE OF WEIGHT LOSS

Subjects in all three treatment groups were highly successful in maintaining the weight losses they attained at the end of treatment and did not differ in this respect (cf. Fig. 1). However, significant weight reductions from pre-treatment to follow-up were displayed only by subjects who self-rewarded their performance. A one-year follow-up indicated marked superiority in maintenance on the part of SR-Habit subjects. In this group, 70% of the subjects maintained or improved their program losses as compared with 40%, 37.5%, and 40% on the part of the SR-Weight, Self-monitoring, and Treated Control subjects. Total losses after one year ranged from +4.0 to −74.0 pounds.

TREATED CONTROLS

Control subjects failed to lose any additional weight during their 2-wk self-monitored baseline compared to their weight at the end of the 8-wk delay period. Inter-group comparisons disclosed greater baseline reductions in the SR-Weight and Self-monitoring conditions, ($p < .025$) but no differences between Controls and SR-Habit subjects. However, after Control subjects rewarded themselves for attainment of both weight loss and habit improvement goals, their weight dropped progressively (Fig. 1) and differed significantly from their pre-treatment level ($p < .05$). Treated Controls fell intermediate between the Self-reward groups and did not differ significantly from them.

CHANGES IN EATING HABITS DURING TREATMENT

Subjects in all groups tended to report very high rates of appropriate eating habits throughout the period of treatment and did not differ in this respect. Although they displayed a comparable amount of inappropriate eating habits in the baseline period, highly significant inter-group variations were reported during the 6 wk of treatment. Specifically, SR-Habit subjects exhibited fewer inappropriate eating habits than either SR-Weight or Self-monitoring subjects. This difference was most pronounced in the category measuring situational restrictions of eating habits ($p < .001$). Wilcoxon tests indicated that only SR-Habit and Treated Control subjects significantly reduced their frequency of negative eating habits ($p < .01$).

The significant relationship between degree of habit change and magnitude of weight reduction was further demonstrated in correlational analyses. An overall Spearman rank correlation of −.60 ($p < .0005$) revealed that subjects' weight losses were inversely related to their success in eliminating inappropriate eating habits.

FREQUENCY OF SELF-REWARD

Mann-Whitney comparisons showed that Treated Control subjects rewarded themselves significantly less frequently than SR-Weight ($p < .05$) and SR-Habit subjects ($p < .001$). The latter two groups did not differ significantly from each other. Inter-group differences in the attainment of weekly weight loss and habit improvement goals were significant only for the habit category. Subjects who rewarded themselves for habit change attained their habit goals more frequently than SR-Weight and Self-monitoring subjects (43% versus 37 and 35%, respectively, $p < .05$). The infrequent attainment of both goals by Treated Control subjects reduced their frequency of self-reward. In all, nine subjects (5 Controls and 2 each in the Self-reward groups) went through the entire program without ever having rewarded themselves.

Consistency analyses were performed to assess adherence to suggested self-reward standards. Transgressions were defined as *unmerited self-reward* (when a goal was not met) and *self-denial* of a reward even though the appropriate goal had been attained. The rate of merited self-reward for the three groups was high (96.9, 92.7, and 90.4%, respectively). Of the eleven transgressions that did occur, eight were of the self-denial variety.

SUPPLEMENTARY MEASURES

Self-rated motivation to lose weight was relatively high in all groups during the baseline assessment. However, during the course of treatment subjects in the SR-Habit and Treated Control conditions reported substantially higher motivation than either SR-Weight or Self-monitoring subjects. At follow-up, the latter two groups had significantly dropped below their pre-treatment levels of motivation. Interpretation of changes in the Self-monitoring condition was complicated, however, because of a motivation decline in his group during the second baseline week.

In marked contrast to the attendance and attrition problems reported by the other researchers, near-perfect attendance was obtained in all four groups (98, 97, 99, and 97%, respectively). Only one subject was absent from the final follow-up assessment.

Analyses were performed to determine the relationship between possible predictor variables and degree of weight loss. Spearman rank correlations revealed no significant relationship between weight reduction and either chronicity ($r = .03$), pre-treatment eating patterns ($r = .02$), or perceived cause of obesity ($r = -.06$).

Discussion

Results of the present experiment clarify the short-term and enduring effects of self-monitoring and self-reinforcing influences in weight control. Daily recording of body weight and eating habits produced an initial loss in weight. However, even after the addition of weekly goal-setting, 8 wk of continuous self-monitoring failed to produce significant reductions. These findings are consistent with previous research reporting transient and variable results of self-monitoring operations (Mahoney, Moura, & Wade, 1973; Thoresen & Mahoney, 1974).

Generalizations regarding the effects of goal-setting and self-evaluation by weight reduction are complicated by the fact that the standardized goals in the present study were moderately high. Consequently, subjects attained their goals somewhat less frequently than may have been optimal to activate positive self-evaluative influences.

The addition of self-reward operations to self-monitoring and goal-setting resulted in significant improvements in weight reduction. Moreover, the magnitude of these improvements was substantially greater when subjects rewarded themselves for altering their daily eating habits rather than simply reducing their weight. The progressive weight losses of SR-Habit subjects convey the picture of a reliable influence method.

Results from the Treated Controls reveal potential problems that can arise from making self-reward contingent upon simultaneous attainment of multiple standards. Moreover, data from the present experiment suggest that therapists using self-reward operations in clinical cases should take care to encourage modest but realistic goal-setting. The ascetic self-denial of merited rewards further emphasizes the importance of initially monitoring and encouraging appropriate self-reward. These considerations may be particularly relevant in obesity programs. Most clients enter treatment with expectations of rapidly impressive weight loss. They may in fact have lost many pounds in the past through drastic dietary measures that have no lasting value. By conveying the set that ultimate goals are achieved through progressive rather than spectacular changes, moderate achievements may assume their proper significance.

Several lines of evidence indicate that the superior results accompanying the habit self-reinforcement group were mediated through alteration of eating styles. Subjects in the latter group were much more successful at modifying inappropriate eating patterns than subjects in the other treatment conditions. Moreover, correlation analyses showed that subjects' magnitude of weight reduction was significantly related to their eating habits. As the latter improved, weight losses increased.

Consistent with previous investigations of behavioral weight control strategies, there was marked individual variability in degree of weight loss. The exploration of this variability and isolation of effective predictor variables pose a contemporary challenge to obesity researchers (Mahoney, 1972c). In the present study, neither pre-treatment eating patterns, chronicity of weight problems, nor perceived cause of obesity accounted for the evident variance. However, the significant relationship between eating habit alteration and weight reduction during treatment suggests the need for more research on the pretreatment assessment of eating styles.

References

BANDURA, A. *Principles of behavior modification.* New York: Holt, Rinehart & Winston, 1969.

BANDURA, A. Vicarious and self-reinforcement processes. In R. Glaser (Ed.), *The nature of reinforcement.* New York: Academic Press, 1971. Pp. 228–278.

BRODEN, B., HALL, R. V., & MITTS, B. The effect of self-recording on the classroom behavior of two eighth grade students. *Journal of Applied Behavior Analysis*, 1971, **4**, 191–199.

FEINSTEIN, A. R. The measurement of success in weight reduction: An analysis of methods and a new index. *Journal of Chronic Diseases*, 1959, **10**, 439–456.

HIRSCH, J. Adipose cellularity in relation to human obesity. *Advances in Internal Medicine*, in press.

HORAN, J. J. & JOHNSON, R. G. Coverant conditioning through a self-management application of the Premack principle: Its effects of weight reduction. *Journal of Behavior Therapy and Experimental Psychiatry*, 1971, **2**, 243–249.

JOHNSON, S. M. & WHITE, G. Self-observation as an agent of behavioral change. *Behavior Therapy*, 1971, **2**, 488–497.

KANFER, F. H. The maintenance of behavior by self-generated stimuli and reinforcement. In A. Jacobs and L. B. Sachs (Eds.), *The psychology of private events: Perspectives on covert response systems*. New York: Academic Press, 1971. Pp. 39–59.

KAZDIN, A. E. Self-monitoring and behavior change. In M. J. Mahoney & C. E. Thoresen (Eds.), *Self-control: Power to the person*. Monterey: Brooks/Cole, 1974.

MAHONEY, M. J. Research issues in self-management. *Behavior Therapy*, 1972, **3**, 45–63. (a)

MAHONEY, M. J. Self-reward and self-monitoring techniques for weight control. Unpublished doctoral dissertation, Stanford University, 1972. (b)

MAHONEY, M. J. Self-control strategies in weight loss. Paper presented at the Sixth Annual Meeting of the Association for Advancement of Behavior Therapy, New York City, 1972. (c)

MAHONEY, M. J., MOURA, N. G. M., & WADE, T. C. The relative efficacy of self-reward, self-punishment, and self-monitoring techniques for weight loss. *Journal of Consulting and Clinical Psychology*, 1973, **40**, 404–407.

McFALL, R. M. The effects of self-monitoring on normal smoking behavior. *Journal of Consulting and Clinical Psychology*, 1970, **35**, 135–142.

McFALL, R. M. & HAMMEN, C. L. Motivation, structure, and self-monitoring: The role of nonspecific factors in smoking reduction. *Journal of Consulting and Clinical Psychology*, 1971, **37**, 80–86.

PENICK, S. B., FILION, R., FOX, S., & STUNKARD, A. J. Behavior modification in the treatment of obesity. *Psychosomatic Medicine*, 1971, **33**, 49–55.

STUART, R. B. & DAVIS, B. *Slim chance in a fat world: Behavioral control of obesity*. Champaign: Research Press, 1972.

THORESEN, C. E. & MAHONEY, M. J. *J. Behavioral self-control*. New York: Holt, Winston, in press.

CHAPTER 44

A Comparison of the Effects of External
Control and Self-control on the Modification
and Maintenance of Weight[1]

D. BALFOUR JEFFREY[2]

Emory University

Summary— In an experimental study of weight reduction, 62 obese men and women were administered a pretreatment questionnaire and randomly assigned to three experimental treatment groups: (a) an external control group with a non-refundable contingency; (b) a self-control group with a refundable contingency; and (c) a self-control group with a nonrefundable contingency. The results indicated that the self-control and external-control treatments were equally effective in producing reduction in weight. However, both self-control interventions were more effective than the external-control intervention in promoting maintenance of weight loss.

Current work in reinforcement and attribution theory suggests promising leads for treating even the most refractory behavioral problems. In view of the ineffectiveness of most weight loss programs (Stunkard & McLaren-Hume, 1959) these theories may have useful applications to the treatment of obesity. Reinforcement research has shown that much social behavior is operant and hence under the control of its consequences. Kanfer (1971) theorized that these stimuli, when self-dispensed, have the capacity to control behavior in the absence of externally dispensed consequences. This proposition has been supported by laboratory and field studies which have reported equal behavioral effects for external reinforcement and self-reinforcement (e.g., Bandura, 1971; Bolstad & Johnson, 1972).

Reprinted with permission from the *Journal of Abnormal Psychology*, 1974, **83**, 404–410.

[1] This study is based upon a dissertation submitted in partial fulfillment of the requirements for the PhD at the University of Utah. The author expresses his deep appreciation to Donald P. Hartmann, dissertation chairman, for his valuable support and suggestions. Gratitude is extended to the other committee members Donna M. Gelfand, Stewart Proctor, Howard N. Sloane, and David H. Dodd for their helpful feedback. The author also thanks Rashel Jeffrey, Roger C. Katz, and Michael J. Mahoney for their assistance and suggestions. This study was partially supported by a research fellowship to the author from the University of Utah Research Committee.

[2] Requests for reprints and additional information should be sent to D. Balfour Jeffery, Department of Psychology, Emory University, Atlanta, Georgia 30322.

449

An implicit aspect of training in self-reinforcement is that while the individual learns to dispense reinforcers to himself — reinforcers which in turn control his behavior — he also learns that he is the controller of his behavior. This perception of the locus of control and its subsequent influence on behavior has been the major focus of attribution theory (e.g., de Charms, 1968; Rotter, 1966). de Charms, for example, theorized that if a person believes that he is the cause of his own behavior, he is more likely to maintain his behavior in the absence of external rewards. In support of this proposition, Davison and Valins (1969) found that subjects who attributed to themselves the ability to withstand electric shock maintained their toleration of shock to a greater degree than did subjects who attributed their toleration of shock to a drug, which was actually a placebo.

In the treatment of obesity, recent clinical studies, employing various reinforcement procedures combined with other behavioral control techniques, have produced encouraging results.[3] For example, Mann (1972) has reported successful weight reduction using external-reinforcement procedures; Harris (1969) and Mahoney (1972) have reported successful weight reduction using self-control procedures which included self-reinforcement; other investigators have reported successful weight reduction using a combination of both external-control and self-control procedures (Jeffrey, Chistensen, & Pappas, 1972; Penick et al., 1971; Stuart, 1967). Unfortunately, none of these studies has compared the relative efficacy of external-control and self-control procedures on both the production and maintenance of weight loss.

Based on the speculations of Kanfer (1971) and de Charms (1968), it would be expected that self-control and external-control procedures would be equally effective in producing weight loss during therapy, but that self-control procedures would be more effective in promoting the maintenance of the weight loss in typical posttreatment environments where few reinforcers are available for the maintenance of weight loss. Thus the primary purpose of the present study was to compare the relative efficacy of external-control and self-control procedures on both the production and maintenance of weight loss.

---

[3]To avoid confusion in the use of self-hyphenated and external-hyphenated terms, definitions of these terms as used in the present study are provided. Self-reinforcement is the process of the individual dispensing reinforcers to himself, while external reinforcement is the process of somebody other than the individual (e.g., therapist) dispensing reinforcers to that individual. Self-control procedures are those procedures (e.g., self-reinforcement and self-attribution set) which require that the individual be primarily responsible for managing his own behavior. External-control procedures are those procedures (e.g., external reinforcement and external-attribution set) which require other people to be primarily responsible for managing an individual's behavior.

Method

DESIGN

Since previous behavior studies employing a variety of control groups — no treatment, waiting list, attention placebo, information only — have consistently reported insignificant changes in weight (see review by Stunkard & Mahoney, in press), it was reasoned that a control group in this study would be redundant and therefore was not included. In place of a standard control group, an additional self-control group was included in order to investigate a secondary hypothesis that a nonrefundable contingency self-control group would have a higher rate of inappropriate self-reinforcement (cheating) than a refundable self-control group.[4] In summary, obese adults were randomly assigned to (a) an external-control group which combined external reinforcement and an external-attribution set; (b) a self-control group which combined self-reinforcement with a refundable contingency and an internal-attribution set; and (c) a self-control group which combined self-reinforcement with a nonrefundable contingency and an internal-attribution set.

SUBJECTS

Adults from the community, who were solicited through newspaper and radio announcements, were told that the weight-control program would meet for seven weekly meetings in addition to a 6-week follow-up, that it would emphasize the alteration of eating habits, and that each person would need to deposit $35 at the first meeting, a portion of which he could earn back each week contingent on his performance. They were then questioned to determine whether they met the following eligibility criteria: (a) between 10% and 80% overweight by the national standard of obesity, (b) not pregnant, (c) not involved in any other current weight program, (d) not on any medication that might affect weight loss (e.g., "diet pills"), and (e) planning to be present in the area during treatment and follow-up. Out of an initial pool of 148 potential subjects, 57 females and 5 males met these criteria and were randomly assigned to the three treatment groups.

In general, these adults were typical of the "hard-core" overweight (Young, Berresford, & Moore, 1957). They were middle-aged (X = 39 years old, range 21–60); they were considerably overweight (42% on the average, range

---

[4] A fourth group, external control with a refundable contingency, was also considered; however, it was not included because (a) the refundable versus nonrefundable contingency condition was not the primary purpose of the study, and (b) the condition of external control with a refundable contingency does not approximate the usual experimental or naturally occuring use of external reinforcement.

12%–79%); and all had experienced previous unsuccessful attempts to regulate their weight either through medical means (88%) or through commercial weight programs (61%).

WEIGHT-CONTROL THERAPISTS

Three undergraduate students, one male and two females, were the principal weight-control therapists.[5] All three had taken psychology classes, but none had worked as a therapist. To insure a proper administration of the treatments, the therapists were rehearsed prior to the beginning of the study and monitored while administering the individual sessions. They were not informed of the hypotheses of the investigation until after its completion. In addition, their appointment schedules were balanced to insure an equivalent amount of contact between each therapist and subjects in all three treatment groups.

STANDARDIZED TREATMENT PROCEDURES

The general sequence of treatment meetings consisted of an initial group orientation meeting, seven individual weekly meetings, and finally a follow-up weigh-in 6 weeks after the end of treatment. As the subjects arrived for their group's orientation meeting, they were asked to fill out a questionnaire consisting of the internal–external control of reinforcement inventory (Rotter, 1966) and a brief weight-control questionnaire. A therapist then proceeded to explain the procedures that the subjects would use during the course.

Subjects were given a manual of weight-control procedures that provided (a) either an external-control or self-control orientation, depending on the subject's group assignment, and (b) brief instructions on how to record one's own weight and eating habits, basic facts of nutrition, and specific techniques of weight control.[6] These techniques consisted of a variety of stimulus control procedures – such as reducing the amount of food purchased, prepared, and consumed – suggested, for example, by Ferster, Nurnberger, and Levitt (1962), Stuart (1967, 1971), and Wollersheim (1970) in their research on obesity. The subjects were also given graphs and eating diaries with the instructions to record daily their weight and appropriate and inappropriate eating habits.

Two independent contingency systems, one for weight loss and one for eating habits, were applied to all subjects. The weight-loss contingency system required each subject to lose one or more pounds each week. The eating habits contingency system required each subject to make a 10-point improvement in appropriate eating habits and to make a 5-point decrement in inappropriate eating habits. Each subject deposited $35 at the end of the orientation meeting;

[5]Gratitude is extended to Scott Anderson, Vicky Harris, and Lesley Holloman, who served as therapists in this study.

[6]The weight manual and eating-habit recording system were modified version of the ones developed by Mahoney (1972).

each subsequent week, he could earn back $1.75 for achieving his weight goal and $2.50 for achieving his eating-habit goal. To minimize absences and dropouts, all subjects were told that they would be fined $5 for each absence and would forfeit their entire deposit if they should drop out of the program. Money not earned back or forfeited was given to a nonprofit agency.

After the procedures were explained, two copies of a behavioral contract were signed by the subject and the therapist. The contract simply summarized in writing the treatment procedures and subject's commitment to follow the procedures to the best of his ability.

The weekly treatment meetings consisted of seven individual 15-minute sessions with a therapist. The standard format of these meetings consisted of the therapist weighing the subject, checking his weight graph, counting the number of appropriate and inappropriate eating habits, setting the weight-loss and eating-habit goals for the following week, answering questions related to the program, and then writing checks (if appropriate) for weight improvement and for eating-habit improvement. Questions unrelated to the weight-control procedures were tactfully not answered.

Before the beginning of the last weekly meeting, the subjects were given a brief questionnaire similar to the pretreatment questionnaire. At the end of the meeting, the therapist scheduled an appointment six weeks later for a follow-up weigh-in and reminded the subjects that they would be paid $5.25, regardless of their weight at that time, for merely attending the final weigh-in.

TREATMENT GROUPS

External-control group. In addition to the standard procedures which were explained during the orientation meeting, the therapist told the external-control subjects that previous research has shown that weight loss is promoted if the therapist dispenses financial incentives (previously deposited by the subjects) for successful attainment of weight-control goals. The message emphasized the therapist's responsibility for weight loss by means of his control of rewards.

During the concluding portion of each weekly meeting, the therapist paid (with a check) the subjects $1.75 if he had met his weight-loss goals and $2.50 if he had met his eating-habit-improvement goal. If either or both goals were not met, the therapist deposited the corresponding check(s) through a slit into a locked cash box. The subjects understood that any money deposited into the security box would not be refunded.

Self-control refundable contingency group. In addition to the standard treatment instructions, self-control refundable contingency group subjects were told that each person was responsible for his own weight management. The therapist told them that previous research has shown that weight loss is promoted if they learn to appropriately reward themselves for successful attainment of weight-control goals. They were asked to deposit money with the weight program and then to reward themselves a proportion of their deposit each time they met their weekly goals.

The therapist explained that the subjects should reward themselves $1.75 when they made their weight-loss goal and $2.50 when they made their eating-habit-improvement goal. Conversely, they should not reward themselves when they did not make their weight-loss goal nor when they did not make their eating-habit goal. Although the therapist recommended the appropriate reward procedure, the subjects were reassured that they had complete control to pay or not to pay themselves, regardless of whether they had made their goals. To insure confidentiality and minimize any possible social pressure, each week the therapist wrote the checks to "cash" rather than to the person, placed them on the table at the end of the weekly meeting, and then left the interviewing room and closed the door. The subject was left completely alone to decide whether to reward himself by simply picking up the checks and leaving the room or not to reward himself by dropping the check or checks through the slit into the locked cash box. In addition, the subjects were told that any money they did not reward themselves during the weekly meetings would be refunded at the end of the program. To further minimize the possibilities of experimenter bias or social approval, the cash box was not opened until after the treatment was completed so the therapist literally did not know who had and who had not deposited their checks in the cash box.

Self-control nonrefundable contingency group. The procedures in this group were exactly the same as in the other self-control group except for one important clause in the contingency system. The self-control nonrefundable contingency group subjects were told that any money they deposited in the cash box would not be refunded. Thus, there was an externally imposed response cost penalty if they did not reward themselves during any given week.

Results

CHANGES IN WEIGHT WITHIN TREATMENTS

The unadjusted mean weights for the three groups across pretreatment, posttreatment, and follow-up are presented in Fig. 1.[7] The average weekly weight loss during treatment was .7 pound for the external-control group and .9 pound for the combined self-control groups.

Repeated-measures analyses of the unadjusted weights indicated significant weight changes across the three measurements periods for the external-control

[7] Three subjects in the external-control group and four subjects in the self-control noncontingency group dropped out during treatment. In addition, one subject from each group attended meetings regularly during treatment but did not come in for the follow-up weigh-in. Consequently, these subjects were excluded from all statistical analyses.

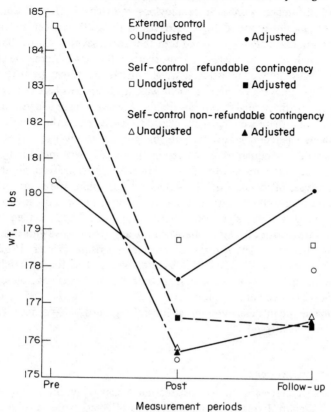

FIG. 1. Unadjusted mean weights and analysis of covariance adjusted
mean weights for the external-control, self-control refundable
contingency, and self-control nonrefundable contingency groups
across pretreatment, posttreatment, and follow-up.

group and the two self-control groups, with refundable and non-refundable
contingencies, respectively $(F = 10.20, df = 2/34, p < .001; F = 24.06, df = 2/36, p < .001; F = 14.77, df = 2/28, p < .001)$. The Newman-Keuls multiple-range
tests indicated that posttreatment and follow-up weights were significantly less
than the pretreatment weights for all three groups $(ps < .05)$. While there was no
significant change from posttreatment to follow-up for subjects in the two self-
control groups, subjects in the external-control group significantly increased in
weight from posttreatment to follow-up.

DIFFERENCES IN WEIGHT BETWEEN TREATMENTS

Feldt (1958), among others, has argued that based on considerations of
power, either blocking or covariance designs are preferred over designs

employing difference scores. Since previous research (Jeffrey & Christensen, 1972) has typically reported high correlations ($rs > .9$) between pretreatment and posttreatment weight — a condition that increases the relative power of a covariance analysis — the analysis of covariance rather than alternative statistical procedures was employed in assessing weight differences across groups.

Preliminary analyses of pretreatment weight differences between groups are not necessary with an analysis of covariance; however, these analyses indicated, as expected, that there were no significant differences across the three groups for actual weight, percentage overweight, or pounds overweight. The essential assumption of the equality of regression in all cells was met for both post-treatment and follow-up weight. The within-cell regressions were all above .98, and the analyses of variance of the within-cell regressions were correspondingly very significant. Based on the analyses of covariance, adjusted posttreatment and follow-up weights were calculated for each group (see Fig. 1, shaded symbols). The test of treatment differences between the adjusted postweights indicated no significant difference. The *a priori* planned comparisons (Winer, 1962) of the adjusted follow-up data indicated a greater weight loss for both self-control groups as compared with the external-control group (self-control refundable contingency/external-control groups, $F = 3.92$, $df = 1/48$, $p < .05$; self-control nonrefundable contingency/external-control groups, $F = 3.54$, $df = 1/48$, $p < .05$, one-tailed tests).

ADDITIONAL ANALYSES

Analyses of pretreatment to posttreatment changes within groups indicated that the self-control treatment manipulations affected scores on the internal—external control measures. In essence, these measures attempt to assess whether an individual believes he can control what happens to him (internal orientation) or whether he believes what happens to him is beyond personal control (external orientation). Correlated t tests performed on the subjects' Rotter internal—external scores showed (a) a significant increase in internal orientation for the self-control refundable contingency group ($t = -1.82$, $df = 18$, $p < .05$, one-tailed test); (b) a slight tendency toward a more internal orientation for the self-control nonrefundable contingency group ($t = -1.02$, $df = 14$); and (c) no change in internal—external orientation for the external-control group ($t = +.51$, $df = 17$). Similar trends were found on an item measuring internal—external orientation specifically related to weight; that is, both self-control groups reported a significant more internal orientation (Wilcoxon matched-pairs tests: self-control refundable contingency group $T = 6$, $p < .01$; self-control nonrefundable contingency group $T = 7$, $p < .01$) whereas the external-control group reported no change in orientation.

All cases of inappropriate reinforcement for weight loss among the self-control subjects (refundable contingency $= 4.4\%$; nonrefundable contingency = 15.1%) were a result of taking undeserved rewards. As expected, subjects in the self-control group with the non-refundable contingency cheated significantly more than subjects in the self-control group with the refundable contingency ($t = 1.98$, $df = 32$, $p < .05$, one-tailed test). In the external-control group, there was no cheating since the therapist controlled the dispensing of the monetary rewards.

Discussion

The findings of the present study demonstrated that the self-control and external-control treatment conditions were equally effective in producing weight reduction. The average weekly weight loss during the treatment of .9 pound for the combined self-control groups and .7 pound for the external-control group was consistent with the recommended goal of a gradual weight loss of approximately 1 pound per week (Stuart, 1967). Furthermore, this rate was comparable to the average weekly weight losses ranging from .7 to 1.1 pounds reported in previous behavioral studies (e.g., Hall, 1972; Harris, 1969; Mahoney, 1972; Stuart, 1967, 1971; Wollersheim, 1970).

An even more important finding was that both self-control treatments were more effective than the external-control treatment in promoting maintenance of weight loss. Subjects in the self-control conditions maintained their posttreatment weight loss, while subjects in the external-control condition gained back approximately 55% of their posttreatment weight loss.

Since the primary purpose of the present study was to contrast self-regulatory-enhancing procedures with external-control procedures and not to conduct a component analysis of all treatment ingredients, only speculative interferences can be drawn about the specific mechanisms involved in the superior maintenance displayed by subjects in the self-control groups. Perhaps this analysis would be facilitated by first examining the similarities among the treatments and results and then examining the differences.

Using Kanfer's (1971) three-phase model of self-regulation, all subjects were (a) given the same instructions for recording their weight and eating habits (self-monitoring), (b) given the same weekly performance goals and procedures for determining whether they had met their goals (standard setting and evaluation), and (c) provided the same monetary rewards (consequences). In addition, all subjects attended similar individual weigh-ins and were given copies of the same instruction booklet for improving their eating habits. In terms of the results during treatment, all three groups achieved similar weight losses. Consequently, it seems unlikely that these factors could have accounted for the superior maintenance of the self-control groups. Instead, it would seem that these differences in maintenance may best be accounted for by the specifically manipulated treatment components — locus of reinforcement control and attribution set.

Subjects in the self-control condition were trained to rely upon themselves for consequent control (self-reinforcement) and were implicitly as well as explicitly trained in self-attribution of control. In contrast, subjects in the external-control condition were trained to rely upon others for consequent control and were implicitly as well as explicitly trained in external-attribution of control.

According to the speculations of Kanfer (1971) and Thoresen and Mahoney (1974), training in the use of self-rewards increases the probability of continued incentives for the maintenance of a behavior in the virtual absence of external reinforcement. While there was no independent verification of the posttreatment use of self-reinforcement, previous research suggests that the superior maintenance of weight loss in the self-control groups was due in part to the self-dispensed incentives for appropriate weight control efforts.

In addition to the probable importance of the self-reinforcement manipulation, there also appears to be support for the importance of the attribution manipulation. Specifically, the self-control subjects made more self-attribution statements and reported a shift toward a more internal orientation at the end of treatment than the external-control subjects. According to de Charms (1968), an increase in internal orientation or personal causation for a set of behaviors should result in better maintenance of those behaviors in the absence of external reinforcement. It is not possible to determine within the context of the present study whether these changes in internal orientation were produced by the explicit attribution instructions or the training in self-reinforcement, or by both.

Subjects in the nonrefundable contingency self-control group cheated significantly more than subjects in the refundable contingency self-control group. Since subjects in the non-refundable contingency group were "punished" when they were honest and did not pay themselves undeserved rewards, it was not surprising that they cheated more than the refundable contingency subjects who were not "punished" for being honest. Because of the cheating problem, it would seem prudent to use self-control interventions with nonrefundable contingencies very carefully in clinical practice and experimental research.

While the effectiveness of self-control interventions offers promise for the treatment of obesity, additional information would be helpful to researchers and clinical practitioners. The following topics warrant investigation: One, replications of the self-control interventions which employ longer treatments and follow-ups are now needed before definitive conclusions can be made about the long-term efficacy of these procedures. Two, additional studies are needed to separate the relative contribution of self-reinforcement training procedures and attribution set manipulations. In the present study, these two components were intentionally combined; however, future studies should isolate these two components and assess their effects on weight loss and internal orientation. Three, investigations of the degree to which self-reinforcement is maintained over long periods of time and the variables controlling self-reinforcement are needed in order to more fully understand the mechanisms involved in the regulation of weight. Four, the possible effects of therapist approval need further examination. In the present study, the therapists did not know whether the subjects in the self-control groups appropriately rewarded themselves; consequently, it seems highly unlikely that their approval could systematically effect the rate of appropriate reinforcement. However, the issue of therapist expectancies is important, and future studies might test whether there are differences among self-reinforcement interventions when the therapist is and is not aware of how the subjects reinforce themselves.

In summary, the findings of the present study demonstrated that the self-control treatments were as effective as the external-control treatment in producing weight loss during therapy and were more effective in promoting maintenance during follow-up. These findings suggest that behavioral self-control procedures offer a promising approach to the treatment of obesity.

References

Bandura, A. Vicarious and self-reinforcement processes. In R. Glaser (Ed.), *The nature of reinforcement*. Columbus, Ohio: Merrill, 1971.

Bolstad, O. D. & Johnson, S. M. Self-regulation in the modification of disruptive behavior. *Journal of Applied Behavior Analysis*, 1972, 5, 443–454.

Davison, G. C. & Valins, S. Maintenance of self-attributed and drug-attributed behavior change. *Journal of Personality and Social Psychology*, 1969, 11, 25–33.

de Charms, R. *Personal causation*. New York: Academic Press, 1968.

Feldt, L. S. A comparison of the precision of three experimental designs employing a concomitant variable. *Psychometrika*, 1958, 23, 335–353.

Ferster, C. B., Nurnberger, J. E., & Levitt, E. E. The control of eating. *Journal of Mathetics*, 1962, 1, 87–109.

Hall, S. M. Self-control and therapist control in the behavioral treatment of overweight women. *Behaviour Research and Therapy*, 1972, 10, 59–68.

Harris, M. B. Self-directed program for weight control—a pilot study. *Journal of Abnormal Psychology*, 1969, 74, 263–270.

Jeffrey, D. B. & Christensen, E. R. The relative efficacy of behavior therapy, will power and no-treatment control procedures on the modification of obesity. Paper presented at the meeting of the Association for Advancement of Behavior Therapy, New York City, October 1972.

Jeffrey, D. B., Christensen, E. R., & Pappas, J. P. Developing a behavioral program and therapist manual for the treatment of obesity. *Journal of the American College Health Association*, 1973, 21, 455–459.

Kanfer, F. D. The maintenance of behavior by self-generated stimuli and reinforcement. In A. Jacobs and L. B. Sachs (Eds.), *Psychology of private events*. New York: Academic Press, 1971.

Mahoney, M. J. Self-reward and self-monitoring techniques for weight control. Unpublished doctoral dissertation, Stanford University, 1972.

Mann, R. A. The behavior-therapeutic use of contingency contracting to control an adult behavior problem: Weight control. *Journal of Applied Behavior Analysis*, 1972, 5, 99–109.

Penick, S. B., Filion, R., Fox, S., & Stankard, A. J. Behavior modification in the treatment of obesity. *Psychosomatic Medicine*, 1971, 33, 49–55.

Rotter, J. B. Generalized expectancies for internal vs. external control of reinforcement. *Psychological Monographs*, 1966, **80** (1, Whole No. 609).

Stuart, R. B. Behavioral control of overeating. *Behaviour Research and Therapy*, 1967, **5**, 357–365.

Stuart, R. B. A three-dimensional program for the treatment of obesity. *Behaviour Research and Therapy*, 1971, **9**, 177–186.

Stunkard, A. & Mahoney, M. J. Behavioral treatment of eating disorders. In H. Leitenberg (Ed.), *Handbook of behavior modification*. New York: Appleton-Century-Crofts, in press.

Stunkard, A. & McLaren-Home, M. The results of treatment for obesity. *Archives of Internal Medicine*, 1959, **103**, 79–85.

Thoresen, C. E., & Mahoney, M. J. *Behavioral self-control*. New York: Holt, Rinehart & Winston, 1974.

Winer, B. J. *Statistical principles in experimental design*. New York: McGraw-Hill, 1962.

Wollersheim, J. P. Effectiveness of group therapy based upon learning principles in the treatment of overweight women. *Journal of Abnormal Psychology*, 1970, **76**, 462–474.

Young, C. M., Berresford, K., & Moore, N. S. Psychological factors in weight control. *American Journal of Clinical Nutrition*, 1957, **5**, 186–191.

CHAPTER 45

Behavioral Techniques in the Treatment of Obesity: a comparative analysis[1]

RAYMOND G. ROMANCZYK, DOROTHY A. TRACEY, G. TERENCE WILSON and GEOFFREY L. THORPE

Psychological Clinic, Rutgers University, New Brunswick, New Jersey 08903, U.S.A.

Summary— The relative efficacy of the major techniques typically used in behavioral treatment programs for weight reduction was investigated using obese adult volunteers. Study 1 compared the effects of self-monitoring, self-control procedures, monetary rewards, aversive imagery and relaxation training. These procedures resulted in significantly greater weight reduction than either a no treatment group or subjects who graphed and recorded daily weight. Self-monitoring of daily caloric intake was as effective as the other methods, both singly and combined, over a 4 week treatment period. Study 2 compared the long-term effects of self-monitoring vs the full complement of behavioral techniques used in Study 1. The full behavior management program was significantly more effective, both during the treatment period and at 3 and 12 week follow-ups, although self-monitoring again produced substantial weight loss.

Stunkard (1972) recently concluded that behavior modification techniques constitute the only effective treatment of obesity, a clinical problem which has remained depressingly resistant to a variety of medical and psychotherapeutic interventions. Most of the behavioral methods employed are derived from Ferster, Nurnberger and Levitt's (1962) well-known detailed analysis of eating behavior and its control. Following Stuart's (1967) uncontrolled clinical investigation in which eight individually treated obese patients evidenced dramatic weight losses ranging from 29–47 lb over a 12-month period, several studies demonstrated that behavior modification is more successful than no treatment, diet planning and even supportive psychotherapy (Harris, 1969; Penick *et al.*, 1971; Stuart, 1971). Wollersheim (1970) showed that a comprehensive behavioral treatment program resulted in significantly greater weight reduction at an 8-week follow-up than both a social pressure group based upon the procedures of TOPS (Take Off Pounds Sensibly — Stunkard, Fox and Levine, 1970) and a non-specific therapy group designed to control for factors such as placebo, expectancy of therapeutic gain and therapist contact. Similarly, Hagen (1970)

Reprinted with permission from *Behaviour Research and Therapy*, 1973, **11**, 629–640.

[1] This research was supported in part by a Biomedical Science Support Grant to G. T. Wilson, to whom reprint requests should be sent at the following address: The Psychological Clinic, Rutgers University, New Brunswick, New Jersey, 08903, U.S.A.

found that behavioral treatment with a written manual describing the relevant principles was as effective as the same program applied by a therapist, and that both procedures were more effective than a delayed-treatment control group.

All of the above studies used a multifaceted treatment package including a variety of self-control techniques. A comparative analysis of the efficacy and limitations of the different components of the treatment package is important from both a theoretical and therapeutic cost-effectiveness standpoint. In general, the major components of behavior modification programs for the treatment of obesity can be subsumed under the following categories: self-monitoring, stimulus control strategies, behavior management methods, imagery techniques, relaxation training and contingency contracting or self- or experimenter-administered reinforcement for weight loss (cf. Stuart and Davis, 1972). Any or all of these procedures might account for successful therapeutic outcome since each technique has either independently been shown to be an effective behavior change agent or has been part of a successful broad-spectrum treatment program.

Experiment 1

Study 1 followed a "sequential dismantling" strategy (Lang, 1969) in which the techniques of a typical, full therapy package were identified and systematically removed one at a time.

Method

SUBJECTS

Of 150 people responding to an advertisement in a local newspaper, 102 subjects were selected according to the following criteria: age 18–55 yr; a minimum of 15 lb overweight based upon the 1959 Metropolitan Life Insurance Company norms (United States Department of Health, Education and Welfare 1967); not currently involved in any other weight control program or form of psychotherapy; the absence of obesity-related problems such as diabetes, thyroid condition, colitus or ulcers; and an expressed willingness to attend 5 weekly group treatment sessions and deposit $10 which was refundable contingent upon subjects attending sessions.

THERAPISTS

The authors acted as therapists. GTW had had extensive pre- and post-doctoral experience in the application of behavioral treatment programs; RGR, DAT and GLT were advanced clinical graduate students with strong backgrounds in the theory and practice of behavior modification. All three students had specialized training in the procedures administered in this study, and were rated by the clinical faculty as having outstanding therapeutic abilities.

PROCEDURE

Subjects were randomly assigned to seven treatment groups on the basis of within-sample matching with an *n* of 14 and 15 in each groups 1—3 and 4—7 respectively. The groups were constituted as follows:

Group 1: (*no-treatment control*). Subjects were weighed at the onset of the study and informed that there would be a 4-week delay before the program commenced. They were asked to wait and told that they would be contacted at the appropriate time.

Group 2: (*daily weight self-recording*). Subjects were told that the program would begin in 4 weeks and that they must weigh themselves daily and plot their daily weight on graph paper provided by the experimenter. Subjects were provided with written instructions explaining how to construct the graph together with weight-control pamphlets[2] which contained facts about obesity, suggested diets and nutritional information. Calorie counting booklets[3] were also given to each subject. Subjects were instructed that these materials were to be kept for use when the program started and that the graphs would provide useful information concerning normal weight fluctuations and that this procedure would be continued during the treatment program. Subjects were *not* told, however, to expect a loss. All subjects were given two sheets of graph paper and were told to mail in their first graph when it was completed in addressed envelopes provided. Each graph was adequate for approximately 20 calendar days. Subjects were also instructed to bring the second graph with them when the program started. This procedure of mailing completed graphs was used as a check on compliance with the instructions without necessitating a group meeting prior to treatment commencement.

Group 3: (*daily weight and caloric intake self-recording*). This group was identical to group 2 except that in addition they were given small pocket notebooks and were told to keep a *running cumulative* total of daily caloric intake of all foods and beverages ingested. They were also told that this would provide useful information on normal eating patterns and would be continued when the program started. Again, however, subjects were *not* told to expect a weight loss, *nor* where they told to restrict their caloric intake in any way. Subjects were informed that they need not mail their calorie records with their graphs due to the bulk of the notebooks, but that the notebooks would be collected before the program began.

Group 4: (*self-monitoring, symbolic aversion*). Subjects in this group, as well as in groups 5—7, participated in weekly 60-min group sessions for a period of 4 weeks. Subjects were instructed to self-monitor their behavior in the same manner as group three subjects, and to restrict caloric intake to approximately

[2] The authors are indebted to Smith, Kline, and French Laboratories for providing these materials.
[3] Dell Books, 1968.

1200 for women and 1500 for men. These self-observational data were collected by the therapist at each session, at which time all subjects were also weighed using a commercial bathroom scale. In addition, three trials of a symbolically generated aversive procedure similar to that described by Cautela (1967) were administered. Subjects were asked to close their eyes and imagine a favorite high calorie food which they had difficulty resisting. The therapist provided specific verbal cueing in order to help clarify and intensify the imagery by prompting subjects to concentrate on the color, texture, size, smell, taste and location of the food. Subjects were then instructed to imagine biting into the food, and experiencing a variety of individualized nausea-producing aversive consequences. The entire imagery sequence lasted approximately 3 min following which subjects were told to relax and clear their thoughts before the next trial began 60 sec later. Subjects were given the homework assignment of rehearsing this aversive imagery method three times a day at home, and to use the technique in specific food-tempting situations.

Group 5: (*self-monitoring, symbolic aversion, relaxation*). This group was the same as group 4 except that subjects were given abbreviated muscle relaxation training (Paul, 1966) for 10–15 min session. Subjects were informed that acquiring the skill to relax would assist them in coping with stressful situations which often triggered off unnecessary eating patterns in many overweight individuals. Homework assignments included practicing relaxation exercises on a daily basis. All sessions for groups ended with a general discussion of how well the group was progressing in controlling weight, with the therapist moderating the discussion in a nondirective fashion without making any specific behavioral suggestions or providing contingent social reinforcement for weight loss.

Group 6: (*self-monitoring, symbolic aversion, relaxation, behavioral management and stimulus control instructions*). In addition to the procedures used in group 5, subjects in this group received training in the modification and control of the eliciting, discriminatory and reinforcing stimuli governing eating, and the development of techniques to control the act of eating. This program[4] was modeled after Stuart's (1967, 1971) procedures. The emphasis during the sessions was on discussing the theoretical rationale and most effective ways of implementing these self-control principles.

Group 7: (*self-monitoring, symbolic aversion, relaxation, behavioral management and stimulus control instructions, and contingency contracting*). This group was identical to the former except that subjects' deposits were returned each week contingent upon weight loss at the rate of 50c per lb. Subjects were told that the deposit would be refunded in full at the end of the program irrespective of weight loss, but that this procedure would ensure a more rapid and more meaningful refund. In an attempt to still further increase the

---

[4] A copy of the expanded program may be obtained upon request from any of the authors.

reinforcing value of the weight loss, deposit money was refunded in the form of half dollars for 1 lb losses and silver dollars for multiple lb losses. All subjects in groups 4–7 were asked not to adhere to any fixed diet but to eat a variety of healthy and nutritious foods. All four therapists conducted treatment sessions for all four groups.

Following the 4-week treatment period groups 1–3 all received the therapeutic procedures described for group 6 above in a 6-week therapy program. Groups 4–7 were reassessed for weight loss at 2- and 8-week follow-up sessions. At the end of the first treatment session subjects in groups 4–7 were asked to rate on a 7-point scale the degree to which they felt the program described would help them to lose weight. At the final session groups 4–7 were asked to evaluate their satisfaction with the treatment program, and to indicate if they expected to gain, maintain or continue to lose weight.

Results

A number of people who had applied to the program failed to attend the initial therapy session resulting in unevenly sized groups. The number of subjects in groups 1–7 as of the first session was 14; 13; 14; 15; 12; 7 and 12. Subject attrition over the 4-week treatment period was as follows for groups 1–7; 1; 2; 1; 3; 1; 1 and 0. This attrition rate was fairly uniform across all groups, with the extreme difference in group size being mostly accounted for by subject attrition *before* the start of the therapy program. The composition of the groups at the end of the treatment was as follows: sixteen males, with at least one but not more than three in each of the groups: a mean age of 41.5 yrs (range 18–55); and mean pre-treatment body weight of 178.8 lb (range 131–263).

In order to compensate for individual differences in sex and height, each subject's weight was converted to percentage overweight in the following manner. First each subject's ideal weight was computed using the Metropolitan Life Co. tables; this was then subtracted from subject's pretreatment weight to yield an estimate of percentage overweight (cf. Mahoney, 1973).

The mean number of pounds overweight of all subjects in the study was 56.5 lb indicating that this population had a clinically significant problem with regard to obesity. The mean percentage overweight of all subjects in the study was 46 per cent. These data are presented in Table 1. A one-way analysis of variance revealed no significant differences between the seven groups prior to treatment on number of pounds overweight ($F < 1$; $df = 6/70$) or percentage overweight ($F < 1$; $df = 6/70$).

POST-TREATMENT

Table 1 summarizes the mean number of pounds overweight and percentage overweight for the different groups at the post-treatment evaluation and at the 2 week and 8 week follow-up. A one-way analysis of variance of percentage lb.

TABLE 1. Number of subjects, actual pounds lost and percentage of overweight lost for all groups

Group	Pre-treatment		Post-treatment			Follow-up 1			Follow-up 2		
	N	lb Overweight	N	lb Lost	Overweight lost (%)	N	lb Lost	Overweight lost (%)	N	lb Lost	Overweight lost (%)
1	14	52.7	12	+0.42	+2.07	—	—	—	—	—	—
2	13	55.3	11	+0.09	+1.36	—	—	—	—	—	—
3	14	55.6	13	5.30	9.10	—	—	—	—	—	—
4	12	60.7	12	8.50	13.95	11	5.32	8.50	5	7.10	13.27
5	11	61.2	11	5.50	9.22	7	5.00	8.47	4	6.38	10.30
6	7	74.9	6	8.17	11.86	3	10.67	17.93	5	8.83	16.56
7	12	51.3	12	6.42	18.11	12	5.63	15.37	7	2.64	9.09

overweight lost revealed that there was a significant difference between the groups ($F = 6.65$; $df = 6/70$; $p < 0.001$). Individual comparisons between pairs of means using Duncan's New Multiple Range test corrected for unequal Ns (Winer, 1971) indicated no differences between groups 1 and 2, or between groups 3, 4, 5, 6 and 7. Groups 3 and 6 differed from groups 1 and 2 at the $p < 0.05$ level, and groups 4, 5 and 7 differed from groups 1 and 2 at the $p < 0.01$ level.

FOLLOW-UP

Several subjects failed to return for follow-up evaluations as shown in Table 1. No significant differences between groups 4–7 emerged either at the 2 week ($F = 1.13$; $df = 3/29$; $P < 0.1$) or at the 8 week follow-up ($F < 1$; $df = 3/17$). These findings indicate that simply graphing daily weight is not significantly different from a no treatment condition, and that both are ineffective in producing weight loss. The other five treatment conditions were all equally effective in promoting significantly greater weight reduction than the daily graphing of weight and no treatment at all.

Table 2 presents the cumulative percentages of subjects in groups 4–7 who lost more than 10, 20, 30 and 40 per cent of pounds overweight at post-treatment and follow-up evaluations. There were no statistically significant differences between groups. Results from the expectancy questionnaires showed that the different groups did not differ from each other in terms of reported expectation of weight loss or in expressed satisfaction with the different treatment conditions.

TABLE 2. Cumulative percentage of subjects in each group losing given percentages of pounds overweight

Group	Evaluation	N	10%	20%	30%	40%
4	Post-treatment	12	83	17	0	0
	Follow-up 1	11	36	0	0	0
	Follow-up 2	5	60	20	0	0
5	Post-treatment	11	36	0	0	0
	Follow-up 1	7	43	14	0	0
	Follow-up 2	4	50	0	0	0
6	Post-treatment	6	50	0	0	0
	Follow-up 1	3	100	33	0	0
	Follow-up 2	5	60	40	0	0
7	Post-treatment	12	58	33	17	17
	Follow-up 1	12	58	17	8	8
	Follow-up 2	7	29	14	14	14

Discussion

The major finding of this study is that self-monitoring of daily caloric intake in the absence of therapist contact can be an effective method of producing weight loss in obese individuals. This is consistent with the evidence demonstrating the efficacy of self-monitoring as a behavior change procedure for obesity (cf. Romanczyk, 1973) and with different types of problem behavior (e.g. Gottman and McFall, 1972; Johnson and White, 1971). These results do, however, conflict with those reported by Mahoney (1973), Mahoney *et al.* (1973), and Stuart (1971), which show little effect of self-monitoring procedures on weight reduction.

The inconsistent findings on the reactive effects of self-monitoring might be attributable to the nature of the particular behavior being monitored. Subjects in group 2 of the present study monitored daily weight while subjects in the Stuart (1971) and Mahoney studies recorded eating habits and body weight. These strategies all failed to result in significant weight reduction. The reason for this failure, as well as the explanation for the success of group 3 — caloric intake monitoring — may lie in the specificity of the information yielded. Monitoring of caloric intake provides a definite criterion against which performance might be judged, and has a more specific and immediate functional relationship to the act of overeating than daily weighing. It may be that a specific, directly relevant criterion such as caloric intake facilitates the natural tendency for subjects to self-evaluate their progress, even if not explicitly instructed to do so, which then results in self-reinforcing and/or self-punishment for appropriate and inappropriate eating behaviors (Kanfer, 1971).

Although the results were in the predicted direction, the failure of the stimulus control, behavior management, aversive imagery and relaxation training methods to significantly improve upon the efficacy of the self-monitoring procedure, either singly or in combination, is surprising. One possible explanation is that a floor effect was reached such that subjects could not reduce weight faster without a drastic change in food consumption. Another possibility is that the program was too short for subject's maladaptive eating habits to be effectively modified and permanently incorporated into their behavioral repertoires. Unfortunately, the design of the study precluded any longterm comparison between the self-monitoring procedure and the effects of the additional techniques so that no conclusion with respect to the maintenance of weight loss is possible. It might be predicted that the full complement of self-control strategies would result in superior maintenance of weight loss which is considerably more difficult to accomplish than an initial treatment effect. Finally, group application of techniques precluded individual tailoring of self-control treatment strategies which is crucially important in the clinical application of behavioral principles (cf. Stuart, 1967).

Given the present results indicating that a single procedure, i.e. self-monitoring, can be as effective as a full treatment program in producing weight loss, comparative outcome studies on the different components of these multifaceted behavioral programs are essential.

It is noteworthy that every subject who completed treatment achieved some measure of weight reduction. Weight losses were substantial, and compared favorably with those reported in the clinical treatment literature. Finally, it is interesting that the group in which subjects were provided with contingent tangible reinforcement for weight loss at each session was the only group in which no attrition occurred. Subject attrition during treatment is a perennial problem with all obesity treatment programs, and the systematic use of similar reinforcement procedures might well be used to maintain participation in therapy programs as well as to accomplish actual weight loss (Mahoney, 1973).

Experiment 2

The results of study 1 indicated that self-monitoring of caloric intake plus daily graphing of weight has an initial treatment effect on weight reduction which is not noticeably enhanced by the addition of other self-control techniques. While it might be that the single self-monitoring procedure produces as significant an immediate treatment effect as the complete therapeutic package, the possibility remains that the latter would be superior to self-monitoring alone with respect to the *maintenance* of weight loss. Accordingly, the second study compared the successful self-monitoring procedure to a group employing the full range of behavioral techniques over an extended follow-up period. In order to create a stringent control group against which to test the efficacy of the full therapy package, relaxation training and relevant information concerning the nature of obesity were provided subjects in the self-monitoring condition so as to enhance the face validity and increase the expectancy of favorable therapeutic outcome in this group. Moreover, unlike Study 1, therapist contact was equated across both groups.

Method

SUBJECTS

Sixty subjects were selected from 75 people responding to an advertisement in a local newspaper. Selection criteria were the same as for Study 1.

THERAPISTS

The authors served as therapists, alternating across the groups they conducted to insure equal exposure of each group to each of the therapists.

PROCEDURE

Subjects were assigned to two treatment groups in the manner described in Study 1. Each of the treatment groups was subdivided into two groups of 15 subjects each and seen separately.

Group 1: (*Information, self-monitoring, relaxation*). Subjects in both groups participated in weekly 60 min group sessions for a period of 4 weeks. They were instructed to self-monitor daily weight and daily caloric intake in the same manner described in study 1. These data were collected at each session, at which time all subjects were weighed using a commerical bathroom scale. Subjects were given information concerning obesity based on recent research findings, e.g. Schachter (1971). No specific instruction was given on how to apply the results of the experimental studies presented. Relaxation training (Paul, 1966) was provided and subjects were encouraged to relax daily at home and to engage in relaxation when they felt urges to eat at inappropriate times. Any remaining time in the session was taken up by general non-directive discussion of problems related to eating with the therapist acting as group moderator. Subjects were told that obesity is caused by an imbalance between caloric intake and energy expenditure and that the only way to achieve enduring weight loss is to correct this imbalance.

Group 2: (*Information, self-monitoring, relaxation, behavioral management and stimulus control instructions, symbolic aversion*). In addition to the procedures used in group 1, subjects in this group were given the behavioral management program described in study 1 and received three trials of symbolic aversion in each session. They were told that obesity is due to faulty learning and that more adaptive eating patterns could be learned through application of behavior management and stimulus control procedures. All subjects were asked to eat a variety of healthy foods and not to adhere to any specific diet. They were advised that their $10 deposit would be refunded contingent on attendance at the sessions. At the conclusion of the program, subjects were informed that there would be 3- and 12-week follow-up meetings. Questionnaire measures of subjects' expectations of treatment were as in study 1.

Results

As in Study 1, a large number of subjects failed to keep the initial appointment resulting in unequal group sizes. Groups 1 and 2 contained 18 and 28 subjects respectively at the beginning of treatment. Subject attrition over the 4-week treatment period was 7 and 10 for the respective groups. The mean age was 42.1 yr (range 21–55), with a mean pre-treatment body weight of 173 lb (range 141–246). All subjects were females.

Percentage overweight was computed in the manner described in Study 1. The mean number of pounds overweight of all subjects was 51.1, while the mean percentage of pounds overweight was 42 per cent, again indicating a population with a clinically significant obesity problem. These data are presented in Table 3. A one-way analysis of variance revealed no significant differences between the two groups prior to treatment on number of pounds overweight ($F < 1$; $df = 1/27$) or percentage pounds overweight ($F < 1; df = 1.27$).

TABLE 3. Number of subjects, actual pounds lost and percentage of overweight lost for all groups

Group	Pre-treatment		Post-treatment			Follow-up 1			Follow-up 2		
	N	lb Overweight	N	lb Lost	Overweight lost (%)	N	lb Lost	Overweight lost (%)	N	lb Lost	Overweight lost (%)
1	18	54.9	11	5.54	10.3	9	4.89	8.3	9	6.11	12.0
2	28	48.8	18	8.05	19.2	17	9.81	23.8	11	8.82	25.6

POST-TREATMENT

Table 3 summarizes the mean number of pounds overweight and percentage pounds overweight for each group at the post-treatment evaluation and at the 3- and 12-week follow-ups. A one-way analysis of variance of percentage of pounds overweight lost revealed a significant difference between the two groups at the conclusion of the 4-week treatment period ($F = 4.8; df = 1/27; p < 0.05$).

FOLLOW-UP

Differences between the two groups were maintained at the 3-week follow-up ($F = 7.6; df = 1.25; p < 0.025$) and at the 12-week follow-up ($F = 4.9; df = 1/18; p < 0.05$). Table 4 presents the cumulative percentages of subjects in both groups who lost more than 10, 20, 30 and 50 per cent of pounds overweight at post-treatment and follow-up. Noteworthy too, is the tendency for these differences to increase over time, suggesting therapeutic gains subsequent to the treatment program.

TABLE 4. Cumulative percentage of subjects losing 10, 20, 30, and 40 per cent of overweight

Group		N	10%+	20%+	30%+	40%+
1	Post-treatment	11	63	0	0	0
	Follow-up 1	9	43	11	0	0
	Follow-up 2	9	55	11	11	0
2	Post-treatment	18	72	44	22	06
	Follow-up 1	17	88	53	24	17
	Follow-up 2	11	91	46	36	18

Discussion

The results achieved by the self-monitoring and information procedure closely replicate the findings from Study 1 and further support the efficacy of self-monitoring as a behavior change technique. In contrast to the previous study, however, the addition of other self-control methods resulted in a statistically significant greater treatment effect than that obtained with self-monitoring. Furthermore, this difference was maintained at both the 3- and 12-week follow-up evaluations, indicating the overall superiority of the full therapy package as compared to self-monitoring combined with information and relaxation instructions. While treatment effects of weight loss were maintained at follow-up for both groups, subjects receiving the full therapy package tended to show increasingly greater weight reduction from post-treatment to the second follow-up, suggesting that they had learned behavioral skills which they were able to implement on a continuing basis. These findings are especially encouraging in view of the difficulties with respect to achieving enduring weight losses in the treatment of obesity.

As in study 1, the magnitude of weight lost in the second study is impressive given the brevity of the treatment program and considering the nature of the subject population treated. Subjects were recruited on a largely unselected basis from the community and had a relatively advanced average age which does not make for a favorable prognosis (Stuart and Davis, 1972). Nonetheless, the percent of overweight lost by the full treatment subjects was greater at all evaluation periods than the results reported by Mahoney (1973) using the same dependent measure with college students.

References

CAUTELA, J. R. (1967) Covert sensitization. *Psychol. Rep.* **20,** 459–468.

FERSTER, C. B., NURNBERGER, J. I., and LEVITT, E. E. (1962) The control of eating. *J. Math.* **1,** 87–109.

GOTTMAN, J. M. and McFALL, R. M. (1972) Self-monitoring effects in a program for potential high school dropouts: a time series analysis. *J. consult. Clin. Psychol.* **39,** 273–381.

HAGEN, R. L. (1970) Group therapy vs bibliotherapy in weight reduction. Unpublished Doctoral Dissertation, University of Illinois.

HARRIS, M. B. (1969) Self-directed program for weight control: a pilot study. *J. abnorm. Psychol.* **74,** 263–270.

JOHNSON, S. M. and WHITE, G. (1971) Self-observation as an agent of behavior change. *Behav. Therapy* **2,** 488–497.

KANFER, F. H. (1970) Self-regulation: research, issues and speculations. In *Behavior modification in clinical psychology* (Eds. C. NEURINGER and J. L. MICHAEL), Appleton–Century–Crofts, New York.

LANG, P. J. (1969) The mechanics of desensitization and the laboratory study of fear. In *Behavior therapy: Appraisal and Status* (Ed. C. M. FRANKS), pp. 160–191. McGraw-Hill, New York.

MAHONEY, M. J., MOURA, N., and WADE, T. (1973) Self-reward and self-monitoring techniques for weight control. *J. consult. Clin. Psychol.* (in press).

MAHONEY, M. J. (1973) The relative efficacy of self-reward, self-punishment and self-monitoring techniques for weight loss. *Behav. Therapy* (in press).

PAUL, G. L. (1966) Outcome of systematic desensitization. II—Controlled investigations of individual treatment, technique variations, and current status. In *Behavior therapy: Appraisal and status* (Ed. C. M. FRANKS), pp. 105–159. McGraw-Hill, New York.

PENICK, S. B., ROSS, F., FOX, S., and STUNKARD, A. J. (1971) Behavior modification in the treatment of obesity. *Psychosomatic Med.* **33,** 49–55.

ROMANCZYK, R. G. (1973) Self-monitoring in the treatment of obesity: parameters of reactivity. *Behav. Therapy* (in press).

SCHACHTER, S. (1971) Some extraordinary facts about obese humans and rats. *Am. Psychol.* **26,** 129–144.

STUART, R. B. (1967) Behavioral control of overeating. *Behav. Res. & Therapy* **5,** 357–365.

STUART, R. B. (1971) A three-dimensional program for the treatment of obesity. *Behav. Res. & Therapy* **9,** 177–186.

STUART, R. B. and DAVIS, B. (1972) *Slim chance in a fat world: Behavioral control of overeating.* Champaign, Illinois: Research Press.

STUNKARD, A. (1972) New therapies for the eating disorders. *Archs gen. Psychiat.* **26,** 391–398.

STUNKARD, A., FOX, S., and LEVINE, H. (1970) The management of obesity: Patient self-help and medical treatment. *Archs of intern. Med.* **125,** 1067–1072.

WINER, B. J. (1971) *Statistical principles in experimental design*. McGraw-Hill, New York.
WOLLERSHEIM, J. P. (1970) Effectiveness of group therapy based upon learning principles in the treatment of overweight women. *J. abnorm. Psychol.* **76**, 462–474.

CHAPTER 46

A Therapeutic Coalition for Obesity:
behavior modification and patient self-help[1]

LEONARD S. LEVITZ and ALBERT J. STUNKARD[2]

Summary— The effectiveness of a self-help organization for the obese was significantly increased by behavior modification techniques. Sixteen chapters of TOPS (Take Off Pounds Sensibly), with a total of 234 members, received one of four treatments: behavior modification conducted by a professional therapist, behavior modification conducted by the TOPS leader, nutrition education conducted by the TOPS leader, and continuation of the usual TOPS program. During the 3-month treatment period, behavior modification produced significantly lower attrition rates and significantly greater weight losses than did the alternate treatment methods. At 9-month follow-up, the differences among treatments were even greater.

Self-help organizations for weight control are a large and growing vehicle for the control of obesity. Unfortunately, their effectiveness is limited; most members lose very little weight[1]. Behavior modification seems to be more effective in treating obesity than any traditional method, but it has not been widely applied. We designed this study to see if self-help and behavior modification could be combined. Behavior modification, we reasoned, might provide self-help organizations with a more effective treatment. At the same time, the self-help organizations could provide a means for the widespread application of behavior modification.

We asked ourselves four questions:

1. Can behavior modification be used in self-help groups for the obese?
2. If so, can it produce greater weight loss and/or lower attrition rates than other treatment approaches?

Reprinted with permission from the *American Journal of Psychiatry*, 1974, **131**, 423–427.

[1] A preliminary version of this paper was read at the 126th annual meeting of the American Psychiatric Association, Honolulu, Hawaii, May 7–11, 1973. This work was supported in part by Public Health Service grant MH–15383 from the National Institute of Mental Health.

[2] Dr. Levitz is Associate in Psychology, Department of Psychiatry, University of Pennsylvania, Philadelphia, Pa. 19174. Dr. Stunkard is Professor and Chairman, Department of Psychiatry, Stanford University School of Medicine, Stanford, Calif. 94305.

3. Can self-help group leaders who are given special training carry out a behavior modification program as successfully as professional therapists?
4. Are there any predictors of treatment success?

Method

TOPS (Take Off Pounds Sensibly) is a 25-year-old self-help organization for the obese. It has 320,000 members in more than 12,000 chapters nationwide; most are women. The 16 chapters in our study were selected from 21 chapters in the Philadelphia area whose weight reduction records we had monitored for the previous four years. Two of the other five chapters had disbanded, two had fewer than six members, and one chapter declined to participate.

At the beginning of the study the 16 chapters had 318 members. We deleted from data analysis the records of 20 members who were less than 10 percent above their ideal weight; they had already reached their ideal weight or had joined TOPS in order to lose only a small amount of weight. Sixty-four members joined TOPS between the time the study was announced and its start. Interviews revealed that knowledge of the impending study influenced at least some of these persons to join TOPS. Accordingly, we analyzed the data from this group separately. The main sample thus consisted of 234 subjects.

Each of the 16 chapters was assigned to one of four treatment conditions, with four chapters in each condition. Active treatment lasted 12 weeks.

BEHAVIOR MODIFICATION CONDUCTED BY A PROFESSIONAL THERAPIST

Three psychiatric residents and one graduate student in clinical psychology, all men, conducted these groups. At each weekly chapter meeting the therapist introduced two or three behavior modification techniques. Group members were asked to keep detailed records of their food intake. Each time a subject ate, she was asked to record the time, place, and duration of eating; the type, amount, and caloric value of the food consumed; and any associated emotions. At each meeting the therapist taught techniques designed to change any problem habits identified from the food intake records. Among the techniques, which are described more fully elsewhere,[2] were: (1) introducing changes in the act of eating, including slowing down the pace and leaving food at the end of a meal; (2) developing control over the stimuli signaling eating, including learning to eat at specific times and in a very limited number of places and removing excess food from the environment; (3) planning food intake well in advance of eating; (4) responding to boredom, fatigue, and emotional states with activities that do not involve eating; and (5) instituting group and individual rewards for behavior change and weight loss. In addition, a special effort was made to help subjects increase physical activity in their daily lives.

BEHAVIOR MODIFICATION BY THE TOPS CHAPTER LEADERS

After two preliminary training sessions, each leader and coleader attended 12 weekly training sessions conducted by the investigators. Concurrently, the leaders introduced the previously described behavior modification program to their members at the weekly chapter meetings.

NUTRITION TRAINING

TOPS leaders also attended a training program scheduled precisely as above. They were taught general principles of nutrition and in turn taught these principles to their members. The program was designed to control for nonspecific training and therapeutic effects. Attendance and weight records in each of these experimental conditions were given to the investigators each week.

CONTROL GROUP

In the fourth condition the usual TOPS program was continued. This program, which has been described extensively elsewhere,[3] includes a weigh-in, an announcement of weight gains and losses, rewards and sometimes punishments, group singing, and a general discussion of weight-related topics. Each week the chapters' attendance and weight records were mailed to the investigators. Aside from this data collection, the four chapters in this condition had no contact with the investigators and received no information from them.

Following the 12-week active treatment period, the therapist visits and training sessions were discontinued. For the 9-month follow-up period, leaders mailed weekly records of attendance and weights to the investigators.

The homogeneity of TOPS membership made it possible to match the subjects in the different experimental conditions very closely. Table 1 shows the remarkable match in age, current weight, percent overweight, length of membership in TOPS, and previous weight loss in TOPS. The average subject was a 45-year-old woman who had been a member of TOPS for 3 years and who had lost 5.0 kg. (11 lb.) during her membership. She currently weighed 81.6 kg. (180 lb.), 42 percent above her ideal weight.

Results

ATTRITION RATE

The first major therapeutic problem in obesity is the number of patients who drop out of treatment; attrition rates ranging from 20 percent to as high as 80 percent are reported.[4,5] Figure 1 presents the attrition rates of each experimental condition during the active-treatment and follow-up periods.

During the 3 months of active treatment fewer TOPS members dropped out

TABLE 1. Subjects' characteristics at the start of treatment

Condition	Number of subjects	Current weight (lb.) mean ± S.D.	Percent overweight mean ± S.D.	Previous weight loss (lb.) mean ± S.D.	Age (years) Mean ± S.D.	Length of membership (months) Mean ± S.D.
Professional behavior modification	73	180.80 ± 15.03	40.4 ± 23.8	10.80 ± 8.76	45.6 ± 10.6	38.2 ± 27.6
Chapter leaders						
Behavior modification	54	181.31 ± 11.27	44.5 ± 19.0	11.00 ± 9.95	48.7 ± 8.7	37.9 ± 20.5
Nutrition education	55	180.40 ± 14.42	42.5 ± 25.1	11.79 ± 11.95	43.3 ± 14.8	35.3 ± 27.4
TOPS control	52	177.50 ± 15.71	42.0 ± 22.1	11.31 ± 9.50	45.1 ± 11.6	33.6 ± 24.9

of the two behavior modification groups than out of the nutrition education and control groups. At 12 months this difference had become striking. Only 38 and 41 percent had dropped out of the behavior modification groups, compared with 55 and 67 percent for the nutrition education and control groups respectively $(\chi^2 = 12.35, p < .01)$.

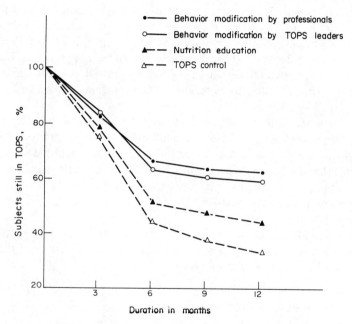

FIG. 1. Rates of attrition in the four treatment groups.

TABLE 2. Mean weight change during 12-week treatment period

Condition	Loss or gain	
	Pounds (mean ± S.D.)	Kilograms (mean)
Professional behavior modification	−4.24 ± 2.47	−1.92
Chapter leaders		
Behavior modification	−1.90 ± 1.88	−0.06
Nutrition education	−0.25 ± 1.83	−0.11
TOPS control	+0.71 ± 1.89	+0.32

WEIGHT LOSS DURING TREATMENT

What happened to the subjects who remained in treatment? It must be remembered that their lower dropout rates seriously bias the results against the behavior modification groups. Previous work has shown that poor weight-losers drop out at a more rapid rate than do those who lose greater amounts.[1] Decreasing the attrition rates thus means retaining the less successful members.

Despite this bias, groups using behavior modification lost significantly more weight than those in the control conditions ($F = 10.7, p < .001$). The chapters in which behavior modification was introduced by a professional therapist lost a mean of 1.92 kg. (4.2 lb.), significantly more ($p < .001$) than the weight loss in both the nutrition education condition (−0.11 kg. or 0.2 lb.) and the TOPS control condition, in which subjects actually gained 0.32 kg. (0.7 lb.). Chapters in which behavior modification was introduced by professionals lost significantly more weight ($p < .05$) than those taught the same program by the TOPS chapter leaders (−0.86 kg. [1.9 lb.]).

Consider now the three conditions in which leadership was provided by the TOPS chapter leaders. The behavior modification program produced significantly greater weight loss ($p < .05$) than did the continuation of the usual TOPS program. The difference between the behavior modification and nutrition education programs was not statistically significant, although the results favored the behavior modification program. The two control conditions did not differ significantly from each other.

Behavior modification thus kept more persons in TOPS during and after treatment. It also produced greater weight losses, despite the bias against weight loss produced by the lower attrition rates.

WEIGHT LOSS DURING FOLLOW-UP

Figure 2 shows the mean weight changes of subjects who stayed in each experimental condition for 12 months. Subjects in the behavior modification groups led by professionals not only maintained their higher weight loss for one year but even increased it slightly. This final mean weight loss of 2.63 kg. (5.8 lb.) was significantly higher ($p < .001$) than that of any of the other conditions. It also represented half the weight lost by these subjects in their three previous years in TOPS.

The initial weight loss of subjects in the behavior modification program conducted by TOPS group leaders was not maintained during follow-up, and the subjects' weights returned to their pretreatment levels. However, these subjects did better than the control and nutrition education groups. Subjects in these two conditions actually gained 1.27 kg. (2.8 lb.) and 1.81 kg. (4.0 lb.) during the follow-up period.

In addition to the mean weight changes, we also examined the percentage of subjects gaining and losing certain amounts of weight. Table 3 shows the

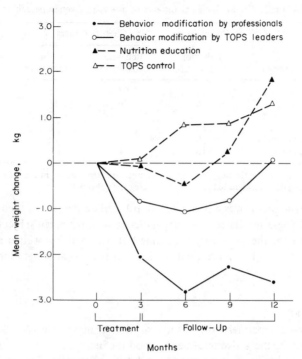

FIG. 2. Mean weight change during treatment and follow-up.

percentage of subjects in each experimental condition who attained three levels of weight change at the end of 12 months. The two behavior modification programs produced significantly greater rates of weight loss, and significantly lower rates of weight gain, at three criterion levels: 2.3 kg. (5 lb.) (χ^2 = 39.69, $p < .001$), 4.5 kg. (10 lb.) (χ^2 = 12.85, $p < .05$), and 9.1 kg. (20 lb.) (χ^2 = 18.38, $p < .01$). In the professional-led behavior modification program, over 50 percent of the subjects lost more than 5 pounds, while only 15 percent gained that much weight. By contrast, in the TOPS control condition, 37 percent *gained* more than 5 pounds while only 17 percent of the subjects lost that amount of weight. Behavior modification by TOPS leaders was similar to the nutrition education condition in its rate of weight loss, but resulted in a far lower rate of weight gain.

A 9.1 kg. (20 lb.) criterion has often been used as a single measure of effectiveness. Only subjects in the professional-led behavior modification program achieved this degree of weight loss. The subjects who lost more than 9.1 kg. shared a striking similarity: all eight had been members of TOPS for more than 2 years and during that time, all had gained weight! This criterion seemed an effective predictor of success in treatment. The mean weight loss of

TABLE 3. Weight change at the end of one year, given in percents*

Weight change	Professional Behavior modification	Chapter leaders Behavior modification	Nutrition education	TOPS control
Gained 5 pounds	15	21	46	37
Lost 5 pounds	54	24	15	17
Gained 10 pounds	5	6	23	21
Lost 10 pounds	24	9	8	10
Gained 20 pounds	0	0	8	0
Lost 20 pounds	15	0	0	0

*The percents given here for weight changes are cumulative, in that the greater losses and gains are included in the lesser categories above them.

all subjects who met it was 8.35 kg. (18.4 lb.), and 88 percent of them lost more than 9.1 kg. These results contrast dramatically with the seven subjects who had been in TOPS for the same length of time but who had *lost* weight during that time. None of these lost more than 9.1 kg. and their mean weight loss was only 0.54 kg. (1.2 lb.).

NEW MEMBERS

We analyzed separately the results of the small sample (*N* = 64) of new members. During the active treatment period the behavior modification program again produced lower attrition rates than did the control conditions: 11 percent for each of the behavioral conditions, 32 percent for nutrition education, and 20 percent for the TOPS control.

Mean weight losses during treatment followed the same pattern as that of longer-term members. The two behavior modification conditions achieved mean weight losses of 4.54 kg. (10 lb.) and 3.46 kg. (7.6 lb.) respectively. Subjects receiving nutrition education lost an average of 3.23 kg. (7.1 lb.), and those in the TOPS control condition 1.36 kg. (3.0 lb.). Because of the small sample size, differences among the groups did not reach statistical significance.

During the follow-up period, the dropout rates showed a different pattern from those of old members. Subjects in the three active treatment conditions dropped out at a *higher* rate than those in the TOPS control condition. Three months after termination of treatment, the attrition rates in the behavior modification conditions were 57 and 58 percent; in the nutrition education condition it was 52 percent. By contrast, the TOPS control showed a dropout rate of only 27 percent. At one year, 78 and 89 percent dropped out of the behavior modification groups, 73 percent out of the nutrition education condition, but only 53 percent from the TOPS control groups. Because of the small initial sample and the extremely high dropout rates in the active treatment conditions, not enough subjects remained in the treatment groups at one year to permit a comparison of final mean weight loss.

Comments

The introduction of behavior modification techniques substantially improved the effectiveness of patient self-help groups on two interacting and critical measures of success. The program resulted in far lower dropout rates and in greater weight losses for those who remained in treatment, both during the treatment period and at follow-up.

The overall ineffectiveness of self-help groups for the obese was recently demonstrated in a 2-year study of 485 TOPS members.[1] Attrition rates were 47 percent in one year and 70 percent in two. Furthermore, attrition was not a result of successful weight reduction; members who dropped out were those who had lost less weight: "Although a small percentage of persons joining TOPS are able to lose substantial amounts of weight and to maintain the weight loss, for the vast majority of members, TOPS is a relatively ineffective method of weight control." The present investigation reaffirmed this conclusion; the four TOPS chapters that served as controls *gained* weight during the year of study.

The behavior modification program helped TOPS members to lose weight. But the amount of weight lost was less than in other studies using similar treatment techniques.[6-8] At least four factors may account for this difference.

1. TOPS members are older, less well-educated, and of lower socioeconomic status than were the subjects of previous behavior modification programs. Each of these factors may unfavorably influence the effectiveness of behavior modification.

2. The TOPS subjects had already lost weight (mean = 5.0 kg.), whereas other behavior modification studies used subjects new to treatment. A high percentage of obese persons lose weight at the outset of *any* weight reduction program.

3. Members who had reached or approximated their ideal weight before intervention were excluded from the data analysis. We thus started with a sample selected for their inability to lose weight.

4. Probably most important, each TOPS group was considerably larger than those in earlier studies, which had rarely exceeded eight members. By contrast, our chapters averaged 19 members. This larger size made it impossible to individualize treatment for each member.

In addition to these theoretical reasons, a recent study provides further empirical evidence that the performance of TOPS members is poorer than that of the subjects in earlier behavior modification research. A behavior modification program of individualized treatment for a small selected sample of TOPS members produced dropout rates and weight losses quite similar to ours.[9]

Professional therapists achieved significantly greater weight losses in their subjects than TOPS chapter leaders, even though both used the same behavioral program. Equally important, subjects in the professional-led (but not TOPS leader-led) groups maintained their weight loss after the end of treatment. In one year, these subjects increased by one-half the weight loss they had attained in three previous years of TOPS membership. Moreover, only in the professional-led groups were there members who lost as much as 20 pounds.

We believe this is the clearest demonstration to date of the greater effectiveness of professional over nonprofessional therapeutic intervention. We have earlier shown that it is possible for a nonprofessional, carefully selected for successful weight reduction and leadership qualities, to promote substantial weight losses in a behavior modification group.[10] But within the context of TOPS, a professional therapist was able to produce greater weight losses than were the TOPS group leaders using any of a variety of treatment approaches.

Neither investigators of obesity nor investigators of behavior modification have been able to predict an individual's response to treatment. The identification of even a small group who can predictably lose weight is thus of considerable theoretical importance. Further, the favorable response of persons whose motivation, unreinforced by weight loss, was high enough to stay in TOPS for 2 years is of practical importance. TOPS may be particularly useful in screening large numbers of obese persons to identify those with a good prognosis for weight loss. This would permit the more effective deployment of limited professional treatment resources.

References

1.   Garb, J. and Stunkard, A. A further assessment of the effectiveness of TOPS in the control of obesity. In *Proceedings of the Fogarty International Center Conference on Obesity*, Bray, G. (Ed.) Washington, D.C., U.S. Government Printing Office (in press).
2.   Stuart, R. B. and Davis, B. *Slim Chance in a Fat World: Behavioral Control of Obesity*. Champaign, Ill., Research Press, 1972.
3.   Stunkard, A., Levine, H. and Fox, S. The management of obesity: patient self-help and medical treatment. *Arch. Intern. Med.* **125**, 1067–1072, 1970.
4.   Stunkard, A. and McLaren-Hume, M. The results of treatment of obesity. *Arch. Intern. Med.* **103**, 79–85, 1959.
5.   Seaton, D. A. and Rose, K. Defaulters from a weight reduction clinic. *J. Chronic Dis.* **18**, 1007–1011, 1965.
6.   Stuart, R. B. Behavioral control of overeating. *Behav. Res. Ther.* **5**, 357–365, 1967.
7.   Penick, S. B., Filion, R. and Fox, S. *et al.*, Behavior modification in the treatment of obesity. *Psychosom. Med.* **33**, 49–55, 1971.
8.   Stunkard, A. J. New therapies for the eating disorders: behavior modification of obesity and anorexia nervosa. *Arch. Gen. Psychiatry* **26**, 391–398, 1972.
9.   Hall, S. M. Self-control and therapist control in the behavior treatment of overweight women. *Behav. Res. Ther.* **10**, 59–68, 1972.
10.   Jordan, H. A. and Levitz, L. S. Behavior modification in a self-help group. *J. Am. Diet. Assoc.* **62**, 27–29, 1973.

CHAPTER 47

Behavioral Treatment of Obesity:
a two-year follow-up

SHARON M. HALL

University of Wisconsin, Milwaukee

Summary— Data obtained from a 2-year follow-up of ten obese women treated via behavioral methods is presented. Failure to obtain lasting results was noted, and reasons for this failure suggested. Implications of these data for investigators in the area of obesity were discussed.

A review of the recent literature indicates a number of studies with encouraging results obtained via the behavioral treatment of obesity (Hall and Hall, unpublished). However, long-term follow-up data are generally lacking. This lack of long-term data is especially troublesome in the area of obesity. With regard to traditional treatment methods, such as drugs, psychotherapy, and nutritional counseling, it has generally been noted that those overweight individuals who complete a course of treatment, and who lose weight, regain the weight lost (Stunkard and McClaren-Hume, 1958). Within the literature on the behavioral treatment of obesity, only one study (Stuart, 1967) has provided weight data for as long as 1 year after initiation of treatment. Stuart's data indicated a gradual loss of weight over the year. However, these data did not reflect S's ability to control weight following termination of treatment, for during the year, follow-up sessions were scheduled monthly, and thus, therapist contact was available.

The present paper, in an attempt to fill the need for long-term follow-up data, presents data obtained 2 years after the termination of a behavioral treatment program. None of the Ss had been in contact with the therapist since the termination of the study 2 years earlier.

Method

SUBJECTS

The Ss were ten females who had participated in a behavioral weight reduction program which was held June–September 1970. At that time, all Ss were members of Take Off Pounds Sensibly (TOPS), a self-help reducing organization. During treatment, all Ss had received two forms of behavioral treatment over a 10-week period. One treatment was instruction in self-management techniques; the second treatment was an experimenter administered program wherein Ss earned tangible reinforcers through weight loss. Both programs were described in detail elsewhere (Hall, 1972).

Reprinted with permission from *Behaviour Research and Therapy*, 1973, 11, 647–648.

PROCEDURES

In the month of August 1972, all Ss who participated in the 1970 study were sent a questionnaire requesting information concerning present weight, recent weight history, and participation in supervised weight programs since the termination of the 1970 study. Of the original ten Ss, four returned the questionnaire. Five of the remaining six Ss were contacted by telephone and data necessary to complete the questionnaire solicited. One S had moved from the area and could not be located.

Results

Pretreatment and post-treatment weight, weight at 1-month follow-up and 2-year follow-up, and ideal weight are shown in Table 1 for each S.

Binomial tests performed on differences between pretreatment weight and post-treatment weight, and pretreatment weight and 2-year follow-up weight revealed direction of changes were distributed differently than would be expected by chance at post-treatment ($N = 10$, $p < 0.01$), but not at 2-year follow-up ($N = 9$, $p < 0.25$). Tests were not computed for 1-month follow-up because data for 30% of the Ss were lacking.

TABLE 1. Post-treatment, follow-up and ideal weights for subjects treated via two behavioral methods

Subject	Pretreatment weight (lb)	Post-treatment weight (lb)	1-month follow-up weight (lb)	2-year follow-up weight (lb)	Ideal weight (lb)
1	207.00	184.00	184.00	176.00	165.00
2	227.75	215.00	217.00	183.00	150.00
3	177.50	174.00	171.00	167.00	140.00
4	190.50	171.00	–	200.00	140.00
5	168.00	166.75	169.00	170.00	154.00
6	143.00	137.00	–	150.00	131.00
7	130.00	120.75	120.00	–	115.00
8	197.75	191.00	190.00	178.00	160.00
9	200.00	202.50	203.00	196.00	160.00
10	141.25	138.00	–	139.00	125.00

In order to determine those variables important in continuing weight loss, directions of weight changes for those Ss who indicated they had participated in additional supervised programs (S3, S9, S10) were compared with those obtained from the remaining six Ss. A Fisher's Exact Probability Test did not reach significance ($p < 0.17$). Similarly, differences in direction of weight change for those Ss continuing in TOPS (S6 and S8) as compared to those who did not continue were not significantly different ($p < 0.41$). Finally, it should be noted that, as inspection of Table 1 indicates, no S reached her ideal weight during the 2-year follow-up period.

Discussion

The results do not indicate a long-lasting effect resulting from behavioral treatment of obesity. The present data would appear to warn against complacency concerning the efficacy of these techniques in the treatment of a disorder as refractory as obesity. They indicate the need for larger, better controlled investigations over long time periods, to determine if, in fact, the encouraging results reported over shorter time periods do last, and if so, under what circumstances. The failure of even one *S* to reach her ideal weight would appear to indicate the great need for increased emphasis upon efficient techniques which truly do equip *S*s with the tools for self-regulation after treatment is terminated.

Lest these results appear too discouraging, the failure to find long-term effects may be at least partially due to the relative inefficiency of the particular self-management techniques employed in this study, at least as compared with the *E* administered treatment, which was noted even during the actual treatment period. Since one would expect success during follow-up to be highly dependent upon the extent to which *S*s had learned *self*-management, the failure to obtain lasting results may reflect an earlier deficiency in the particular program used, and might not be present in other programs.

References

HALL, S. M. (1972) Self-control and therapist control in the behavioral treatment of overweight women. *Behav. Res. & Therapy* **10**, 59–68.

STUNKARD, A. J. and McCLAREN-HUME (1958) The results of treatment for obesity. *Arch. Int. Med.* **103**, 79–85.

CHAPTER 48

Permanence of Two Self-managed Treatments of Overweight in University and Community Populations[1]

SHARON M. HALL[2]

University of Wisconsin, Milwaukee

and

ROBERT G. HALL,[3] RICHARD W. HANSON, and BETTY L. BORDEN[4]

Wood Veterans Administration Center, Milwaukee

      Summary– Males and females from community and university samples were assigned to two self-management treatments, nonspecific, or no-treatment controls. At post-treatment, self-management conditions differed from controls in percentage of body weight and percentage of overweight lost. At 3-month follow-up, the simpler self-management procedure differed from the nonspecific control on both dependent variables. The more complex self-management treatment differed only on percentage of body weight lost. At 6-month follow-up, differences were not significant. Treatments X Time of Assessment analysis on body weight indicated a significant interaction and significant losses during treatment and gains during posttreatment for both self-management conditions. Results are discussed in terms of conceptualizations of self-management and the utility of treatments employed.

      Behavioral treatment of obesity has attracted the attention of the popular press (e.g., Gross, 1973; Lake, 1973a, 1973b), the medical profession (Stunkard, 1972), and that of researchers. It would appear that psychology has devised a treatment useful in ameliorating a serious, widespread health problem (U.S. Public Health Service, undated). Training programs in "self-management" have received the most attention (Ferster, Nurnberger, & Levitt, 1962; Stuart, 1967; Stuart & Davis, 1972). Evaluations have generally indicated the superiority of such training over nontreated or other controls (Hagen, 1970; Harris, 1969;

      Reprinted with permission from *Journal of Consulting and Clinical Psychology*, 1974, **42**, 781–786.

    [1] The authors wish to thank Carla Garnham, Fred Ostapik, and Stephen Maisto for their generous assistance with data presentation and analysis.
    [2] Requests for reprints should be sent to Sharon M. Hall, who is now at the Langley-Porter Neuropsychiatric Institute, University of California, San Francisco, California 94143.
    [3] Also at the Medical College of Wisconsin.
    [4] Now at the University of Wisconsin–Milwaukee.

Wollersheim, 1970). However, two methodological difficulties obscure the clinical usefulness of results obtained. Subjects have been young, mildly overweight college students; thus, samples were not representative of the obese population, since obesity is more prevalent in middle and later life (U.S. Public Health Service, 1965). Also, follow-up periods have not been sufficiently long to determine permanence of weight losses, and they have failed to demonstrate that losses continue or are maintained.

In the treatment of obesity through self-management training, maintenance of change is of primary importance. Many methods provide temporary losses, but weight lost is usually regained (Stunkard & McClaren-Hume, 1959). An effective treatment must produce improvement over this pattern. Also, repeated weight gains and losses may be associated with accretion of serum cholesterol in the circulatory system (U.S. Public Health Service, undated). Finally, the purported goal of self-management training is to enable the client to modify his behavior during and following therapy (Cautela, 1969). Since most subjects participating in weight loss studies cannot reach ideal weight within the typical 10–12-week treatment period, an effective treatment should produce continuing losses to ideal weight. Available data indicate that continuing losses do not generally occur. While differences between treated and nontreated groups generally remain significant at follow-up, treated groups usually show weight increases after termination (Hagen, 1970; Wollersheim, 1970). Follow-up periods in these studies have been short (1–2 months); when these periods are increased (Harris & Bruner, 1971), differences are no longer significant.

The first purpose of the present study was to determine the long-term effectiveness of self-management procedures and to examine weight changes after treatment. The second purpose was to compare performance of a university sample and a more representative community sample.

A final purpose was to evaluate a treatment based on techniques reported by Fowler *et al*. (1972) and Shulman (1971). This method, referred to as simple self-management, consists of instructing the subject to monitor and record bites of food ingested per day and successively decrease the number of bites ingested until a satisfactory weight loss rate is achieved. The simplicity of the method, the lack of professional involvement, plus promising preliminary data reported by Shulman (1971) and Fowler *et al*. (1972) suggested it might prove at least equal to combined self-management, particularly during follow-up periods.

Method

SUBJECTS

Percentage over ideal weight was computed from the Metropolitan Height and Weight Tables (U.S. Public Health Service, undated) for individuals with medium bone structure. Only those individuals who were 10% or more above mean weight were considered. Individuals with metabolic disorders were excluded, as were those whose status with respect to populations was unclear. Ninety-four subjects were randomly selected from the 150 suitable individuals who answered advertisements in newspapers and who returned questionnaires. Subjects were designated members of university or community samples by meeting both of two criteria: (a) location of the advertisement to which the subject had responded (campus versus community newspaper) and (b) student status at the University of Wisconsin, Milwaukee, or lack of such status. Thirty-three subjects (12 males, 21 females) were members of the university population. Fifty-one subjects (8 males, 43 females) were members of the community sample. Mean ages of university and community samples were 20.80 and 42.00 years, respectively. Overall mean was 43 years. Median percentage overweight was 32% and 52% for university and community subjects, respectively; overall median was 43%. Subjects from both samples separately were randomly assigned to combined self-management ($n = 25$), simple self-management ($n = 24$), nonspecific treatment ($n = 23$), or no treatment ($n = 22$).

APPARATUS AND PROCEDURE

Subjects were weighed at pretreatment, posttreatment, and follow-up on a balance-beam scale. In group meetings, two spring-balance bathroom scales were used to provide feedback to subjects.

All subjects attended one of two preliminary meetings. Written commitment to complete the study was obtained, and importance of completing treatment and attendance was emphasized. Subjects were given permission forms to be signed by their physicians, completed data sheets and release forms, were weighed, and were given the time and place of their first group meetings. Subjects in the no-treatment control were asked to refrain from joining any supervised weight loss effort and were promised treatment following the post-treatment assessment. For the other three groups, meetings began the next week.

Three of the therapists (two males, one female) had Ph.D. degrees in clinical psychology. The fourth (female) had completed all degree requirements and was on a clinical internship. All considered social learning as their primary orientation; expectations as to the outcome of the study differed. Each therapist met with one group from each treatment condition.

All treatment groups received booklets containing caloric and nutritional information at the first treatment meeting and discussed the need to limit calories. Subjects were encouraged to think of themselves as permanently changing their lives, rather than as being on a temporary "diet". At the last three meetings, subjects were instructed to practice techniques exactly as they had during treatment after termination. Subjects in each of these three conditions met weekly for 10 weeks in groups of 5–7 individuals.

Combined self-management techniques. Groups met for 75 minutes each week. Subjects were taught weight and food monitoring, stimulus control over eating, applications of deprivation and satiation, self-reinforcement and self-punishment, techniques leading to breaking the chain leading to eating, and the development of a prepotent repertory (Wollersheim, 1970).

At each meeting subjects were weighed and reported weight changes to the group. Losses were met with approval from the therapist; failures were met with encouragement to do better. The initial portion of the meetings following weight reports was used to discuss techniques introduced at previous meetings. New material was presented verbally by the therapist, and subjects were provided with written material reiterating the information given. With the presentation of each new technique, the therapist attempted to evoke from each subject specific instances of planned application. The sixth, ninth, and tenth meeting served as review meetings. Group participation and interaction were encouraged and reinforced throughout the meetings. Missed meetings were handled by scheduling individual meetings.

Simple self-management. All meetings except the first lasted approximately 10–15 minutes; the first meeting lasted 30 minutes. At the meeting, the subjects were told that they were to monitor the number of bites of food ingested per day and to record this daily on data sheets. Subjects were given a Borm wrist response counter[5] to monitor bites of food. At the next meeting, subjects were instructed to take the average of bites per day for the previous week and to begin systematically decreasing bites per day by three from this average. At the end of 2 weeks, if the subject had lost 1–2 pounds per week for both weeks, he was instructed to keep bites per day at the average level for the previous week; if a loss of this magnitude had not occurred, the subject was instructed to decrease bites per day by three until he was losing 1–2 pounds per week. If, at any time, a subject lost more than 2 pounds per week for two successive weeks, he was to increase the number of bites per day by three until no more than 2 pounds per week were lost. Throughout the experiment, subjects decreased, held steady, or increased the number of bites of food per day in accord with weight changes.

The rationale and instructions were explained by the therapist, and written material reiterating the explanations was provided. During the fifth week, subjects recorded their daily food intake. These data were used to insure that no subject was endangering his health by unsound food consumption.

The subjects were weighed at group meetings. Weight changes were not announced to the group, although the therapist did respond to changes individually in the combined technique.

There was no attempt to develop group interaction. Subjects met in groups for efficiency. Missed sessions were handled as in combined self-management.

---

[5] Borm Golf Company, 708 E. Auer, Milwaukee, Wisconsin 53216.

Nonspecific treatment. Subjects met for 75 minutes each session. At the first meeting, the following rationale was presented:

A common complaint of the obese is that tension aggravates, and sometimes instigates overeating. Deep muscle relaxation has been demonstrated helpful in reducing tension. Thus, relaxation training should serve as a useful adjunct to weight reduction, particularly if individuals practice relaxation in conjunction with imaginal representations of tension producing situations.

For the remainder of the first meeting, and in Sessions 2–10, subjects practiced relaxation and developed hierarchies of stressful situations. Subjects were told that this training would aid in weight loss but that they must also limit their caloric intake.

The therapists attempted to avoid discussion of situations directly related to eating. If asked about use of relaxation as a self-control device to decrease eating directly, the therapist remarked that this might be helpful but that other situations should also be considered. Subjects were given homework assignments and were asked to complete data sheets concerning home practice. Weighing and therapist reactions to weight changes were identical to those in the behavioral treatment groups, and absences were handled in the same manner as in those groups. Weight changes were reported to the group as in combined self-management, and group interaction and discussion of problem situations were encouraged.

No-treatment control. The no-treatment control was weighed at the pretreatment meeting and at another meeting taking place during the tenth week of treatment for the three treated groups.

For the treatment groups, weights were obtained at 3 and 6 months after the termination of treatment. At both follow-ups, subjects were weighed by a research assistant, and questioned about their use of techniques.

Results

The criterion for exclusion at posttreatment was failure of the subject to attend two group meetings and two scheduled make-up meetings. Premature termination rates were 16% for combined self-management, 20% for simple self-management, and 21% for nonspecific treatment. In addition, 13% of the no-treatment control subjects refused to return for posttreatment assessment. The frequency of premature terminators did not differ significantly among treatments $(\chi^2 = .826, df = 3, p > .95)$ or populations $(\chi^2 = .001, df = 1, p > .95)$. At posttreatment, $n = 21$ for combined self-management, 19 for simple self-management, 18 for nonspecific treatment, and 20 for the no-treatment control group.

At posttreatment, groups differed significantly in percentage of body weight lost $(F = 14.52, df = 3/73, p < .001)$. The two behavioral treatments differed significantly from both control conditions $(p < .01)$ but did not differ from one another.[6] Differences between the control conditions were not significant. Mean percentage body weight lost was -6.60, -5.67, $-.47$, and $+.92$ for complex self-management, simple self-management, nonspecific, and no-treatment conditions, respectively. Therapist and Therapist $\times$ Treatment effects were not significant ($F < 1$ for all comparisons).[7]

At 3-month follow-up, data were obtained for 19 subjects in the combined techniques conditions, 15 in the simple self-management, and 15 subjects in the nonspecific treatment. Excluded subjects were not predominantly from either population. Analyses of variance indicated significant differences in percentage of body weight lost ($F = 4.40$, $df = 2/45$, $p < .05$), Comparisons of means indicated that the behavioral treatments both differed from nonspecific treatment ($p < .05$) but not from each other. Mean percentage of body weight changed from pretreatment was -4.86, -4.78, and $+1.58$ for complex self-management, simple self-management, and nonspecific treatment, respectively.

At 6-month follow-up, $n = 19$ for complex self-management, 15 for simple self-management, and 14 for nonspecific treatment. Groups no longer differed from each other on percentage of body weight lost ($F = 2.11$, $df = 2/44$, $p > .25$). Mean percentage of body weight changed from pretreatment was -2.98, -3.30, and $+1.24$ for combined self-management, simple self-management, and nonspecific treatment, respectively. Weight losses at each assessment period for all groups in percentage of body weight are shown in Fig. 1.

A Treatment $\times$ Time of Assessment analysis of variance was performed on body weight of those subjects available at all assessment periods ($n = 19, 13$, and 14 for combined self-management, simple self-management, and nonspecific treatments, respectively). The results were significant for both time of assessment ($F = 9.66$, $df = 3/129$, $p < .01$) and the Treatments $\times$ Time of Assessment interaction ($F = 6.01$, $df 6/129$, $p < .01$). Analysis of simple effects indicated that differences between treatments were not significant at any assessment period, although they approach significance in the predicted direction at posttreatment and at 3 months. Differences between assessment periods were significant for combined self-management ($F = 8.56, df = 3/129$, $p < .001$) and simple self-management ($F = 4.58, df = 3/120, p < .001$) but not for nonspecific treatment ($F = 1.28$).

Comparisons of differences between means of the two-self-management conditions indicated significant decreases in pounds from pretreatment to posttreatment (-11.89 for combined self-management and -10.34 for simple self-

---

[6] All comparisons between means were via Tukey's honestly significant difference test (Tukey, 1953, as cited in Kirk, 1968).

[7] Subjects assigned to the experimental conditions were not found to differ on pretreatment body weight, pounds over ideal weight, or percentage over ideal weight, at posttreatment or at either follow-up. Differences on these three dependent variables also failed to reach significance when only those subjects completing treatment were included.

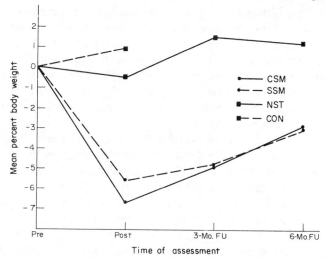

FIG. 1. Mean change in percentage of body weight from pretreatment
to posttreatment and at the 3- and 6-month follow-up.

-management) and at the 3-month follow-up (−6.44 and −8.58, respectively).
However, both groups showed significant gains from posttreatment to the
6-month follow-up (+9.61 and +4.83, respectively), and, in the case of combined
self-management, the 3-month follow-up (+5.52).

A Treatment × Population analysis of variance was performed for percentage
of body weight lost. All F ratios failed to reach significance at either posttreatment or the 6-month follow-up, but at the 3-month follow-up university
and community populations differed significantly ($F = 4.43, df = 1/37, p < .05$;
university $M = -6.63$; community $M = 5.74$). However, when initial percentage
of overweight was held constant via analysis of covariance, differences between
samples were no longer significant at any assessment period.

Treatment × Sex analyses indicates marginally significant differences at the
3-month follow-up ($F = 3.98$, $df = 1/37$, $p < .10$; male $M = -8.51$, female
$M = -3.32$) but not at posttreatment or the 6-month follow-up.

Discussion

The most important finding was the failure of self-management treatments to
produce maintenance or continued weight loss. Supposedly the most important
benefit of self-management training is continued therapy without the therapist
(Cautela, 1969); clearly this was not evident in the present study.

In almost every respect, results obtained replicated those of earlier
demonstration studies for posttreatment and short-term follow-up. It should be
noted that although differences between groups were statistically significant, the

magnitude of the differences may be of limited practical importance. For the longer term, the treatments studied are lacking. Data obtained by Stuart (1967) suggest that occasional follow-up contact with the therapist may be of value for continued weight loss. Manipulation of the demands made upon the subject to apply techniques and continued peer support might also be helpful as well as instructions to deal with each subject's "weak spots" after treatment.

Both self-management treatments produced similar results. Pattern of weight changes observed may be related to the demands of the experimental situation. Demands of participation in an experiment compel the subject to follow the experimenter's suggestions since the subject has volunteered for the study and is working toward a goal he reputedly desires. Termination of treatment removes the subject from this situation and from the demand to perform the techniques. It might be expected that group pressure would enhance this effect. The somewhat more marked treatment loss—posttreatment gain by subjects in the combined training program supports this formulation, as did informal questioning of the subjects at the 3-month follow-up. Virtually all of the subjects trained in combined self-management reported that they no longer used any of the techniques taught them; approximately three-fourths of the subjects in the simple self-management condition reported abandoning the method. The implicit assumption of this formulation is that behavioral methods are effective if applied. The determination of those conditions of which application is a function is crucial and has received little attention.

Differences between samples and the relation of these differences to initial percentage of overweight suggest that caution is warranted in generalizing from university samples to more severely afflicted populations.

Premature termination rates in both self-managed and nonspecific groups approached the lower limit for traditional treatments of obesity (20%; Stunkard & McClaren-Hume, 1959). These rates may have been higher had subjects not felt an obligation to remain in treatment because of initial commitment. Therefore, the premature termination rates may not approximate those to be expected in clinical situations but are probably as close as can be obtained within an experimental situation (as opposed to deposit procedures).

The sheer number of articles on obesity in the popular press indicate that it is a problem of great national concern. Caution must be used when presenting the results and limitations of treatment procedures to the public interested in this problem.

References

Cautela, J. R. Behavior therapy and self-control: Techniques and implications. In C. W. Franks (Ed.), *Behavior therapy: Appraisal and status*. New York: McGraw-Hill, 1969.

Ferster, C. B., Nurnberger, J. E. & Levitt, E. E. The control of eating. *Journal of Mathetics*, 1962, 1, 87–109.

Fowler, R. S., Fordyce, W. E., Boyd, V. D., & Masock, A. J. A mouthful diet: A behavioral approach to overeating. *Rehabilitation Psychology*, 1972, **10**, 98–106.

Gross, A. Fat control. *Mademoiselle*, August 1973, 318–319, 402–405.

Hagen, R. G. Group therapy versus bibliotherapy in weight reduction. Unpublished doctoral dissertation. University of Illinois, 1970.

Hall, S. M. Self-control and therapy control in the behavioral treatment of overweight women. *Behaviour Research and Therapy*, 1972, **10**, 59–68.

Harris, M. G. Self-directed program for weight control: A pilot study. *Journal of Abnormal Psychology*, 1969, **74**, 263–270.

Harris, M. G. & Bruner, C. G. A comparison of self-control and a contract procedure for weight control. *Behaviour Research and Therapy*, 1971, **9**, 347–354.

Lake, A. Get thin, stay thin; New way to lose weight. *McCall's* , January 1973, 90–91, 135–138 (a).

Lake, A. Take pounds off and keep them off with behavior therapy. *Reader's Digest*, July 1973, 131–134 (b).

Shulman, J. The behavioral control of overeating. Unpublished master's thesis, University of Montana, 1971.

Stuart, R. G. Behavioral control of overeating. *Behaviour Research and Therapy*, 1967, **5**, 357–365.

Stuart, R. B. & Davis, B. *Slim chance in a fat world: Behavioral control of overeating.* Champaign, Ill.: Research Press, 1972.

Stunkard, A. New therapies for the eating disorders: Behavior modification of obesity and anorexia nervosa. *Archives of General Psychiatry*, 1972. **26**, 391–398.

Stunkard, A. & McClaren-Hume, M. The results of treatment for obesity. *Archives of Internal Medicine*, 1959, **103**, 79–85.

Tukey, J. W. The problem of multiple comparisons. Unpublished manuscript, Princeton University, 1953. Cited by R. G. Kirk, *Experimental design: Procedures for the behavioral sciences.* Belmont, Calif.: Brooks-Cole, 1968.

U.S. Public Health Service. *Weight, height and selected body dimensions of adults.* Washington, D.C.: U.S. Government Printing Office, 1965.

U.S. Public Health Service. *Obesity and health.* Washington, D.C.: U.S. Government Printing Office, undated.

Wollersheim, J. P. Effectiveness of group therapy based on learning principles in the treatment of overweight women. *Journal of Abnormal Psychology*, 1970, **76**, 462–474.

Author Index

Subject Index

PERGAMON GENERAL PSYCHOLOGY SERIES

Editors: Arnold P. Goldstein, *Syracuse University*
Leonard Krasner, *SUNY, Stony Brook*

The terms of our inspection copy service apply to all the
above books. A complete catalogue of all books in the
Pergamon International Library is available on request.
The Publisher will be pleased to receive suggestions for
revised editions and new titles.